Technical Advances in AIDS Research in the Human Nervous System

Technical Advances in AIDS Research in the Human Nervous System

Edited by

Eugene O. Major

National Institute of Neurological Disorders and Stroke
Bethesda, Maryland

and

Jay A. Levy

University of California, San Francisco
San Francisco, California

Technical Editor

Devera Schoenberg

National Institute of Neurological Disorders and Stroke
Bethesda, Maryland

Plenum Press • New York and London

Library of Congress Cataloging in Publication Data

Technical advances in AIDS research in the human nervous system / edited by Eugene
O. Major and Jay A. Levy.
    p.   cm.
    Proceedings of an NIH Symposium on Technical Advances in AIDS Research in
the Human Nervous System, held October 4–5, 1993 in Washington, D.C.—T.p. verso.
    Includes bibliographical references and index.
    ISBN 0-306-45000-3
    1. Nervous system—Infections—Congresses. 2. AIDS (Disease)—Complications—
Congresses. I. Major, Eugene O. II. Levy, Jay A. III. NIH Symposium on Technical
Advances in AIDS Research in the Human Nervous System (1993: Washington, D.C.)
    [DNLM: 1. Central Nervous System Diseases—etiology—congresses. 2. Central Ner-
vous System Diseases—virology—congresses. 3. Acquired Immunodeficiency Syndrome—complications—congresses. 4. HIV-1—congresses. 5. Polymerase Chain Reaction—methods—congresses. WL 300 T255 1995]
RC385.T43   1995
616.8′047—dc20
DNLM/DLC
for Library of Congress
    95-17558
    CIP

Proceedings of an NIH symposium on Technical Advances in AIDS Research in the Human Nervous
System, held October 4–5, 1993, in Washington, D.C.

ISBN 0-306-45000-3

© 1995 Plenum Press, New York
A Division of Plenum Publishing Corporation
233 Spring Street, New York, N. Y. 10013

10 9 8 7 6 5 4 3 2 1

PREFACE

It is remarkable that each month the quantity of articles published on AIDS still numbers in the thousands. The basic, clinical and sociological aspects that address this epidemic have been vigorously investigated, and equally as extensively reported in traditional as well as new journals. Therefore, what can the reader of this volume expect to find that is different from the information already found in the literature? The authors of this text met in October 1993 to discuss not only AIDS and its effects on the nervous system but also to address the problem from the point of view of the diverse technologies that are used in understanding the disease. Just as the recognition of oncogenic viruses gave us insights into cellular genes that govern growth, the study of HIV-1 in the nervous system has opened new areas of investigation in the nervous system. Use of human fetal and glioma-derived cell cultures, discovery of toxins in the nervous system, release and damage of cytokines in the brain, the neuropathic effects of HIV proteins, the investigation of new treatment for neuro-AIDS, and virus detection strategies to identify latent HIV-1 infection are described in this volume. Basic and clinical investigators from more than thirty laboratories around the world contributed to the ideas discussed at the meeting, "Technical Advances in AIDS Research in the Human Nervous System." By applying various technologies, the study of AIDS has taught us much that is new about the nervous system. Moreover, HIV-induced disease in the brain has been a driving force for seeking new methods to answer important questions of pathogenesis and therapies for this complex disease process. It was the intention of the organizers and participants of this meeting to blend together much of their knowledge so that a multidisciplinary appreciation of the challenges ahead can be achieved. The solution of neurologic AIDS can have widespread application to other other diseases in the human nervous system.

Jay A. Levy, M.D.
San Francisco, California

Eugene O. Major, Ph.D.
Bethesda, Maryland

SPEAKERS

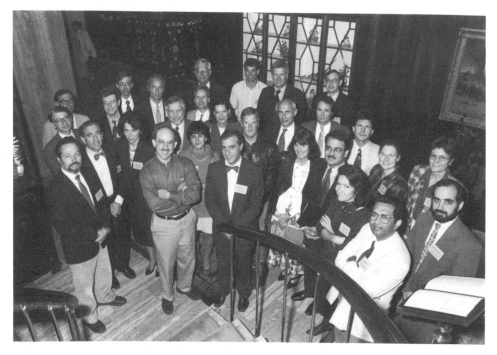

(all are left-to-right)

Front row:	F. Gonzalez Scarano, J. Levy, P. Grady, R. Pomerantz, F. Chiodi, J. Berger, J. Clements, O. Bagasra
2nd row:	L. Epstein, D. Volsky, E. Major, L. Pulliam, M. Heyes, M. Dubois-Dalcq, K. Khalili, H. Gendelman
3rd row:	A. Haas, D. Clifford, P. Schmid, H. Gelbard, P. Lantos, A. Rees, D. Benos, V. Dawson, R. Brack-Werner
Back row:	R. Johnson, S. Wesselingh, J. Nelson, J. Griffin

Not shown in photograph: G. Nuovo, S. Wolinsky, V. Erfle, G. Pavlakis

CONTENTS

NEW CONCEPTS IN THE PATHOGENESIS OF HIV-1 ENCEPHALOPATHY

Chapter 1. HIV Encephalopathy: Clinical and Diagnostic Considerations 3

J.R. Berger and R. Kaderman

Chapter 2. Cellular and Molecular Pathology of Novel Cerebral Diseases in AIDS 27

P.L. Lantos

Chapter 3. Peripheral Neuropathy in AIDS: New Investigative Approaches 41

J.W. Griffin, S.L. Wesselingh, and J.C. McArthur

MODELS OF HIV-1 INFECTION AND NEUROTOXICITY IN THE HUMAN FETAL NERVOUS SYSTEM

Chapter 4. Overview: Models of HIV-1 Infection and Neurotoxicity in the Human Fetal Nervous System 57

L.G. Epstein

Chapter 5. HIV-1-Derived Neurotoxic Factors: Effects on Human Neuronal Cultures 61

H.A. Gelbard, K.A. Dzenko, L. Wang, A. Talley, H. James, and L. Epstein

Chapter 6. Experimental Model Systems for Studies of HIV Encephalitis 73

H.E. Gendelman, P. Genis, M. Jett, and H.S.L.M. Nottet

Chapter 7. Cell Cultures from Human Fetal Brain Provide a Model for HIV-1 Persistence and Reactivation in the Central Nervous System 89

E.O. Major, W.A. Atwood, K. Conant, K. Amemiya, J. Boston, and R.G. Traub

Chapter 8. Use of Human Brain Cell Aggregates for AIDS Research in the Nervous System 105

L. Pulliam

Chapter 9. Infection of Human Fetal Astrocytes with HIV 117
A. Nath and M. Na

MODEL CELL CULTURES FROM ADULT BRAIN AND GLIOMA CELL LINES

Chapter 10. Molecular Interaction of HIV-1 in Glioma Cells 125

V. Erfle, A.Kleinschmidt, M. Neumann, A. Ludvigsen, B.K. Felber, G.N.
Pavlakis, B. Kohleisen, and R. Brack-Werner

Chapter 11. Transcription of Human Immunodeficiency Virus Promoter
in CNS-Derived Cells: Effect of TAT on Expression on Viral and
Cellular Genes 135

K. Khalili, J.P. Taylor, C. Cupp, M. Zeira, and S. Amini

Chapter 12. Tumor Necrosis Factor Alpha Derived from Human Microglia Enhances HIV-1 Replication and Is Toxic for Rat Oligodendrocytes in Vitro 151

S.G. Wilt, J.M. Zhou, S. Wesselingh, C.V. Kufta, and M. Dubois-Dalcq

Chapter 13. Nitric Oxide Mediates a Component of gp120 Neurotoxicity
in Primary Cortical Cultures 163

V.L. Dawson and T.M. Dawson

NEUROTROPISM OF HIV-1 STRAINS

Chapter 14. Contribution of V3 and Reverse Transcriptase Sequence
Analysis to Understanding the Concept of HIV-1 Neurotropism 177

F. Chiodi, M. Di Stefano, and F. Sabri

Chapter 15. Sequence Analysis of Neuroinvasive and Blood-Derived
HIV-1 nef Genes 189

R. Brack-Werner, T. Görblich, T. Werner, F. Chiodi, L. Gürtler,
J. Eberle, A. Schön, and V. Erfle

Chapter 16. An Organ Model for HIV Infection of the Blood-Brain
Barrier 205

A.V. Moses and J.A. Nelson

Chapter 17. The Role of the Astrocyte in the Pathogenesis of the AIDS
Dementia Complex 223

D.J. Benos, J.K. Bubien, B.H. Hahn, B.M. Shaw, and E.N. Beneviste

Chapter 18. Alternative Receptors for HIV-1 in Nervous System
Tissues 235

F. Gonzalez-Scarano, J. Fantini, D.G. Cook, and N. Nathanson

MOLECULAR TECHNOLOGY FOR THE DETECTION AND ANALYSIS OF HIV-1 IN NERVOUS SYSTEM TISSUE

Chapter 19. Detection of HIV-1 Gene Sequences in Brain Tissue by
in Situ Polymerase Chain Reaction 251

O. Bagasra, T. Seshamma, J.P. Pestaner, and R.J. Pomerantz

Chapter 20. The Utility of PCR *in Situ* Hybridization for the Detection
of HIV-1 DNA and RNA 267

G.J. Nuovo

Chapter 21. Electrochemiluminescence-Based Detection System for the
Quantitative Measurement of Antigens and Nucleic Acids: Application to HIV-1 and JC Viruses 281

J.J. Oprandy, K.Amemiya, J.H. Kentren, R.G. Green, E.O. Major, and
R. Massey

DEVELOPMENT OF NEW TECHNIQUES AND METHODS APPLIED TO AIDS

Chapter 22. Techniques in PCR and PCR Evaluation Technology
and Its Application to the Study of Cerebrospinal Fluid in HIV
Disease 301

P. Schmid, A. Conrad, K. Syndulko, E.J. Singer, X. Li, G. Tao,
D. Handley, B. Fahy-Chandon, and W.W. Tourtellotte

Chapter 23. Quantification of Quinolinic Acid Metabolism of Macrophages and Astrocytes 317

M.P. Heyes, E.O. Major, K. Sato, and S. M. Markey

Chapter 24. Targeted Defective Interfering HIV-1 Particles as
Renewable Antivirals? 327

M. Schubert, A.C. Banerjea, S-Y. Paik, G.G. Harmison, and C-J. Chen

FOCUS ON AIDS AND THE NERVOUS SYSTEM: CHALLENGES DURING THE DECADE OF THE BRAIN

Chapter 25. Treatment of Neurological Complications in AIDS: The
AIDS Clinical Trials Group in the 1990s 355

D.B. Clifford

Chapter 26. Technical Advances and the Challenge of HIV-1 Related
Neurological Diseases 363

R.T. Johnson

Contributors 367

Index 371

NEW CONCEPTS IN THE PATHOGENESIS OF HIV-1 ENCEPHALOPATHY

HIV ENCEPHALOPATHY: CLINICAL AND DIAGNOSTIC CONSIDERATIONS

Joseph R. Berger,[1] and Richard Kaderman[2]

[1]Department of Neurology
University of Miami School of Medicine
Miami, Florida 33136

[2]Departments of Neurology and Psychology
University of Miami
Miami, Florida 33136

INTRODUCTION

Clinically apparent and frequently debilitating neurological disease is common with human immunodeficiency virus type 1 (HIV-1, hereafter "HIV") infection. More than 50% of HIV-infected persons will eventually develop symptomatic neurological disease. Early retrospective studies,[1,2] performed at a time in the course of this pandemic when life expectancies were considerably shorter and many of the neurological illnesses associated with the infection unrecognized, proffered rates of neurological complications of approximately 40% in patients with AIDS. Other studies have demonstrated significantly higher rates of neurological disease.[3] Although neurological disease typically occurs with advanced disease and profound immunosuppression, it is not infrequently the harbinger of AIDS. Neurological disease heralds AIDS in 10%[4] to 20%[3] of HIV-infected persons. As many as 100,000 HIV-infected individuals develop neurological disease annually in the United States. The frequency with which neuropathological abnormalities are observed at the time of autopsy is substantially higher than the frequency of clinically recognized neurological disease. In some series, more than 90% of patients dying with AIDS display some form of neuropathology at postmortem examination.[5,6] It is not surprising that careful neurological examination, even in the absence of specific complaints by the HIV-infected patient, frequently reveals evidence of central or peripheral nervous system dysfunction.

Not only is the spectrum of neurological disorders that complicates HIV-1 extremely broad, but any part of the neuraxis may be affected. In general, the illnesses affecting the nervous system can be classified into those that are believed to be the direct result of HIV-1, although the precise mechanism by which HIV results in the pathogenesis of these neurological disorders remains uncertain, and those that result from other identifiable etiologies. Among the disorders in the former category are encephalopathy, myelopathy, peripheral neuropathy and inflammatory myopathy. The illnesses in the latter category are chiefly a consequence of the severe abnormalities of cellular immunity accompanying AIDS with opportunistic infections leading the list. As a rule, these

Technical Advances in AIDS Research in the Human Nervous System
Edited by E.O. Major and J.A. Levy, Plenum Press, New York, 1995

opportunistic neurological infections are the consequence of a dissemination or recrudescence of a latent or persistent infection rather than a recently acquired infection. Often these infections relapse after initially successful therapy. Therefore, secondary antibiotic prophylaxis is warranted in certain infections, such as toxoplasma encephalitis and cryptococcal meningitis. Other causes of neurological disease seen in association with the immunosuppression of HIV infection include primary and metastatic neoplasms, metabolic-nutritional disorders, drug neurotoxicity, and cerebrovascular complications. This chapter deals exclusively with the clinical manifestations of HIV infection of the brain.

ACUTE HIV MENINGITIS AND MENINGOENCEPHALITIS

HIV enters the nervous system shortly after infection.[7-11] In an anecdotal instance of acute infection, the virus was demonstrated within the brain two weeks following primary infection.[12] Typically, this brain infection is clinically silent or unrecognized. In a minority of acutely infected persons, an acute meningitis or meningoencephalitis may supervene within 3-6 weeks of primary infection. The latter is characterized by systemic disease similar to many other acute viral infections. The symptoms of this illness include arthralgias, myalgias, nausea and vomiting, sore throat, abdominal cramps and diarrhea. Examination reveals fever, generalized lymphadenopathy, pharyngeal injection, splenomegaly and splenic tenderness, and rash.[13,14] The illness precedes seroconversion to HIV which generally requires 8-12 weeks from the time of infection to develop.

The meningitis[13,15] or meningoencephalitis[16] is characterized by headache, meningismus, photophobia, generalized seizures and altered mental state. On rare occasions, other neurological complications may accompany acute HIV infections including ataxia,[17,18] cranial neuropathies,[19] acute meningoradiculitis,[20] acute myelopathy,[21] cauda equina,[22] and brachial plexus.[17,23] In the face of acute HIV meningitis or meningoencephalitis, CSF examination usually reveals an increased protein (<100 mg%), mononuclear pleocytosis (≤ 200 cells/mm^3) and normal glucose.[15] CSF viral cultures or viral antigen studies may establish the diagnosis before the development of either a systemic or local antibody response. However, neither the presence of HIV in the CSF by culture or antigen assay[24] nor the demonstration of intrathecal antibody synthesis specific for HIV indicate the coexistence of clinically symptomatic neurological disease. Viral recovery from the CSF[25] may be as common in the absence of neurological disease as in its presence. Similarly, intrathecal HIV-specific IgG synthesis during early infection occurs commonly in asymptomatic HIV-seropositive individuals.[11,26]

A small percentage of individuals with HIV meningitis will present in subacute fashion and have features of the illness persisting for months. Hollander and Stringari[15] proposed that two forms of meningitis may accompany HIV infection. In a study of 14 patients with relatively preserved immune function, an unexplained CSF lymphocytic pleocytosis was associated with an acute, self-limited, meningitis in seven, and chronic headaches with or without meningeal signs in the other seven.[15] In four of five CSF specimens studied,[15] HIV was recovered. The authors concluded that in addition to the acute HIV meningitis associated with recent seroconversion, sporadic episodes of acute and chronic meningitis may complicate HIV infection.[15] Even in the absence of any symptoms, abnormal CSF findings are extraordinarily common in HIV-infected individuals.[26-30] Marshall et al. found some CSF abnormalities in 63% of 424 HIV-infected United States Air Force personnel, 80% of whom were entirely asymptomatic.[28] These CSF abnormalities are diverse in nature and include mononuclear pleocytosis, elevated protein increased IgG, and the presence of oligoclonal bands. As with CSF viral recovery, these abnormalities and the demonstration of CSF p24 antigen[24] do not appear to be predictive of the subsequent development of clinically manifest neurological disease.[28]

HIV ENCEPHALOPATHY (HIV-1 ASSOCIATED COGNITIVE/MOTOR COMPLEX)

Prevalence and Incidence

Shortly after the initial description of AIDS, an unusual, slowly progressive, dementing illness was recognized in association with this disorder.[1,31] This disorder was at first referred to as a "subacute viral encephalitis" and cytomegalovirus was considered the likely etiology.[1,31,32] Subsequently, compelling evidence accumulated directly linking HIV to this encephalopathy. This illness has been referred to by several appellations, including "AIDS dementia complex," "AIDS dementia," AIDS encephalopathy," and "HIV encephalopathy." Because of the spectrum of abnormalities observed in association with this disorder, a Working Group of the American Academy of Neurology (AAN) chose the somewhat cumbersome name "HIV-1-associated cognitive/motor complex" which includes a group with severe manifestations as well as individuals with milder illness.[33] The distinction between the mild cognitive deficits associated with HIV infection and clinically evident dementing illness is hardly semantic (*vide infra*). Whether these disorders exist on the same continuum remains uncertain. Criteria established by the AAN Working Group for the diagnosis of HIV-1-associated cognitive/motor complex are listed in Table 1.

The exact incidence of this disorder in HIV-infected individuals remains uncertain. Of 144,184 persons with AIDS reported to the Centers for Disease Control (CDC) between September 1, 1987 and August 31, 1991, 10,553 (7.3%) were reported to have HIV encephalopathy, and in 2.8% of the adult patients with AIDS and 5.3% of the pediatric patients with AIDS,[34] HIV encephalopathy was the initial manifestation of AIDS. In other studies, the frequency with which HIV encephalopathy was the initial AIDS-defining illness has ranged from 0.8%[3] to 2.2%[35] of adult AIDS patients. It has been reported as the initial manifestation of AIDS in as many as 17.9% of children.[36] In their admittedly "selected clinical experience," Price and colleagues have estimated that at the time of AIDS diagnosis, approximately one-third of patients exhibit overt and one-quarter subclinical AIDS dementia complex.[37] These investigators[38,39] correlated the clinical manifestations of dementia in 70 AIDS patients tracked for three years with neuropathological findings obtained postmortem. Forty-one patients with evidence of focal nervous system disease were excluded from analysis, and of the 70 remaining patients, 46 (66%) suffered from a progressive dementia according to DSM-III-R criteria. The unexplained cognitive and motor changes were presumed to be attributable to HIV and were characterized as moderate to severe in terms of functional impairment Indeed, no patient was capable of fully independent living.

Deriving the prevalence of HIV encephalopathy from the published literature is difficult due to the prior lack of a standardized definition, differences in the study populations, and disparities in study designs, Price and colleagues have estimated, extrapolating from their experience, that approximately one-third of patients with AIDS-related complex or Kaposi sarcoma-defined AIDS have unequivocal evidence of HIV encephalopathy, and another one-fourth have subclinical affliction.[40] These same investigators have estimated that the preterminal prevalence of the overt AIDS dementia complex is approximately 66%, and that an additional 25% of preterminal AIDS patients have a subclinical form of the disorder.[37] Other studies have suggested a prevalence of HIV encephalopathy of 50% in patients with AIDS.[41] However, McArthur found only 30 cases in a series of 186 HIV-seropositive patients.[10] Our own experience suggests a lower prevalence, particularly with respect to cognitive disorders rendering the patient dependent. In part, the development of effective antiretroviral therapy, such as zidovudine (AZT), may have altered the natural history of this disorder and changed the frequency with which it is observed.[42,43] Dementia as the presenting, manifestation of HIV infection is rare in adults. Data from the Multicenter AIDS Cohort Study indicates that there is a 4% incidence of dementia coincident with the diagnosis of AIDS and that the annual incidence of dementia

Table 1. Criteria for clinical diagnosis of central nervous system disorders in adults and adolescents.

HIV-1-Associated Cognitive/Motor Complex

All of the following diagnoses require laboratory evidence for systemic HIV-1 infection (ELISA test confirmed by Western blot, polymerase chain reaction, or culture).

I. Sufficient for diagnosis of AIDS
    A. HIV-1-associated dementia complex*
    Probable (must have each of the following):

1. Acquired abnormality in at least 2 of the following cognitive abilities (present for at least 1 month): attention/concentration, speed of information processing, abstraction/reasoning, visuospatial skills, memory/learning, and speech/language. This decline should be verified by reliable history and mental status examination. In all cases, when possible, history should be obtained from an informant, and examination should be supplemented by neuropsychological testing.

Cognitive dysfunction causing impairment of work or abilities of daily living§ (objectively verifiable or by report of a key informant). This impairment should not be attributable solely to severe systemic illness.

2. At least one of the following:
    a. Acquired abnormality in motor function or performance verified by clinical examination (e.g., slowed rapid movements, abnormal gait, limb incoordination, hyperreflexia, hypertonia, or weakness), neuropsychological tests (e.g., fine motor speed, manual dexterity, perceptual motor skills), or both.
    b. Decline in motivation or emotional control or change in social behavior. This may be characterized by any of the following changes in personality with apathy, inertia, irritability, emotional lability, or new onset of impaired judgment characterized by socially inappropriate behavior or disinhibition.

3. Absence of clouding of consciousness during a period long enough to establish the presence of #1.

4. Evidence of another etiology, including active CNS opportunistic infection or malignancy, psychiatric disorders (e.g., depressive disorder), active alcohol or substance use, or acute or chronic substance withdrawal, must be sought from history, physical and psychiatric examination, and appropriate laboratory and radiologic investigation (e.g., lumbar puncture, neuroimaging). If another potential etiology (e.g., major depression) is present, it is not the cause of the above cognitive, motor, or behavior symptoms and signs.

Possible (must have one of the following):
1. Other potential etiology present (must have each of the following):
    a. As above (see Probable) #1, 2, 3.
    b. Other potential etiology is present but the cause of #1 above is uncertain.
2. Incomplete clinical evaluation (must have each of the following):
    a. As above (see Probable) #1, 2, 3.
    b. Etiology cannot be determined (appropriate laboratory or radiologic investigations not performed).

*For research purposes, HIV-1-associated dementia complex can be coded to describe the major features:

    HIV-1-associated dementia complex requires criteria 1, 2a, 2b, 3, 4.

    HIV-1-associated dementia complex (motor) requires criteria 1, 2a, 3, 4.

    HIV-1-associated dementia complex (behavior) requires criteria 1, 2b, 3, 4.

§ The level of impairment due to cognitive dysfunction should be assessed as follows:

    Mild: Decline in performance at work, including work in the home, that is conspicuous to others. Unable to work at usual job, although may be able to work at a much less demanding job. Activities of daily living or social activities are impaired but not to a degree making the person completely dependent on others. More complicated daily tasks or recreational activities cannot be undertaken. Capable of basic self-care such as feeding, dressing, and maintaining personal hygiene, but activities such as handling money, shopping, using public transportation, driving a car, or keeping track of appointments or mediations is impaired.

    Moderate: Unable to work, including work in the home. Unable to function without some assistance of another in daily living, including dressing, maintaining personal hygiene, eating, shopping, handling money, and walking, but able to communicate basic needs.

    Severe: Unable to perform any activities of daily living without assistance. Requires continual supervision. Unable to maintain personal hygiene, nearly or absolutely mute.

---

is 7% thereafter.[44] Anemia, low weight, and constitutional symptoms seem to be associated with an increased risk of dementia.[44] A phase II placebo-controlled study of the AZT in patients with AIDS and ARC suggests that the annual rate of clinical dementia in patients with CDC stage IV disease is approximately 14%.[43] In children, HIV-associated dementia is more common. Belman and colleagues[45] estimate that as many as 62% of HIV-infected children will develop dementia. Current estimates based on the number of HIV-infected persons in the United States and clinical data indicating that at least one-third of adults with AIDS will exhibit dementia before death suggest that the annual incidence of AIDS dementia in the U.S. approximates 40,000.

The incidence of HIV encephalopathy determined at autopsy has varied among different series. In a Swiss study of the findings of 345 consecutively performed autopsies of patients dying with AIDS, 68 (19%) had morphological features of HIV encephalopathy.[46] In a large series incorporating seven separate neuropathological studies,[6] that included a total of 926 patients, the estimates for HIV encephalopathy ranged from 13.3-62.9% with a composite total of 30.9% Navia and colleagues have suggested that as many as two-thirds of autopsied AIDS patients have this encephalopathy,[39] whereas other investigators have found a higher incidence, ranging between 70% and 93%.[5,32,47-51] A study from San Diego, California of 107 brains of AIDS autopsies collected during a three-year period revealed that while only 16% had the characteristic hallmarks of "HIV encephalitis," more than 50% exhibited evidence of HIV infection.[52]

Cognitive Deficits in Otherwise Healthy HIV-Infected Persons

In 1987 Grant and colleagues[53] reported cognitive impairment in 7 of 16 (44%) asymptomatic HIV-infected individuals raising concerns of incipient CNS deterioration in early HIV infection. Subsequently, considerable effort has been invested in attempts to clarify the nature of cognitive decline among otherwise healthy HIV-infected individuals. To date, no empirical consensus has emerged. Complaints of mental slowing and difficulties in concentration, forgetfulness, mood disturbances, and motor and coordination symptoms have been observed before the onset of AIDS defining illness.[54] These self-perceived cognitive declines should not be dismissed as solely an artifact of psychological distress,[55] but their relationship to depression and anxiety may be complex.[54]

The detection of subtle cognitive-motor deficit may be difficult as a consequence of the adopted definitions of impairment, comparison of group means, small sample sizes, assumption of homogeneity among asymptomatic individuals studied, differential sensitivity of tests utilized and potential confounding factors, such as, age, education, substance abuse, language, and antiretroviral and other therapies. Each of the preceding issues has prevented unequivocal conclusions to be reached with regard to neurological dysfunction during the early course of HIV infection. Reviews of the literature describing the neuropsychology of HIV exhibit divergent opinions with regard to early neurobehavioral effects of HIV, suggesting that the results are inconclusive,[56] do not support the existence of increased neuropsychological abnormalities among asymptomatic HIV-seropositive individuals relative to HIV-seronegative controls,[55] or are indicative of only small to moderate levels of impairment in certain areas.[57,58] A meta-analysis[58] of 8 studies published between 1986 and 1988 concluded that small to moderate decrements [effect size: + 1.0 = performance worse than 82% of controls] occurred in visuomotor/attention (0.43), motor speed (0.39), auditory discrimination/ attention (0.31), and abstraction/novel problem solving abilities (0.33). Perry[57] reviewed studies of early neuropsychological impairment with predominantly homosexual or bisexual risk groups from diverse sites and noted impairment in 10 of the 20 investigations, particularly those which utilized more extensive neuropsychological batteries.

A brief review of methodologically more sophisticated studies conducted between 1989-1991 indicates that all controlled for multiple potential confounds, including: age, education, ethnicity, substance abuse, experimental antiretroviral therapy, psychotropic medication, learning disability, preexisting neurological or psychiatric condition and depression/anxiety. While considerable variability remains with regard to the manner in which impairment is defined, criteria typically include performance deficits 1-2 standard deviations below either uninfected control or extant normative mean values in either multiple domains or on multiple independent tests. The predominant finding across several well-controlled studies utilizing multiple neuropsychological domains and various definitions of impairment is that no discernible group differences exist between HIV-seropositive asymptomatic and HIV-seronegative controls[58-63] and the cognitive deficits seen among a minority of otherwise healthy HIV-seropositive asymptomatic individuals may be attributable in some cases to causes other than HIV such as anxiety/depression, alcohol/drug abuse, or education/dyslexia.[60] Although not universally observed,[54,64] some studies found no relationship between neuropsychological performance, and duration of infection[58,59,63] or immunological parameters or CSF profiles,[60] CD4 lymphocyte counts or CD4:CD8 ratio.[58-60,63] Strong practice effects may also obscure any subtle declines in some studies.

Many of the preceding investigations employed only 5-6 tests per battery which provided equivocal assessment of the major domains of cognitive functioning and lack of sensitivity to subtle deficits. Some studies[54,65] using multiple tests per domain that had been selected on the basis of their sensitivity to subtle deficits and to subcortical functioning, detected significant differences between HIV-seropositive asymptomatic and uninfected controls. However, these differences were not clinically relevant. A review of the literature published to date on early cognitive impairment in otherwise healthy, HIV-infected patients is presented in Table 2.

Cognitive Deficits with ARC and AIDS

Considerable variability for the rate of neuropsychologic abnormalities observed in ARC and AIDS have been reported, ranging from 12-87%.[41,53,70,72,73] Factors which contribute to these discrepant findings include: (1) stage of disease progression; (2) various aspects of the study sample, including, random selection of patients, selection on the basis of suspected cognitive dysfunction, and the use or absence of antiretroviral therapy; and (3) lack of established criteria for the definition of abnormality.

Neuropsychological abnormalities among ARC patients have ranged from 5.6-54%.[53,71,73] Conservative estimates utilizing a 2 standard deviation cut-off

Table 2. Neuropsychology literature examining early cognitive impairment in otherwise healthy, asymptomatic HIV-1-infected patients.

Study	Number	Impairment	Result: Asymptomatic Group
Skoraszewski, 1991[72]	8	Effect size	Visual-motor attention (0.43); auditory attention (0.31); abstraction-novel problem solving (0.33).
Lunn et al.1991[66]	20 AIDS 20 Asympt. 20 HIV-	Mann-Whitney U	Psychomotor speed; verbal memory; 35% asymptomatics impaired
van Gorp et al., 1991[55]	233 Asympt. 256 HIV-	MANOVA	No differences; depressed mood, independent of serostatus or neuropsychologic impairment, associated with increased cognitive complaints.
Sinforiani et al.,1991[67]	41 Asympt. 41 HIV-	1-way ANOVA	No differences
Stern et al., 1991[54]	75 Sympt. 49 Asympt. 84 HIV-	>1 SD/2SD clinical impression; MANOVA	Borderline deficits (>1 SD) for memory, executive functioning, attention, and abstract reasoning; statistically but not clinically significant.
Miller et al. 1990[63]	84 AIDS 727 Asympt. 769 HIV-	MANOVA MANOVA	No differences.
Selnes et al., 1990 (MACS)[68]	238 Asympt. 170 HIV-	Multivariate auto-regressive analysis	No differences over 2 yrs.
Wilkie et al., 1990[65]	46 Asympt. 13 HIV-	>1-2 SD	Verbal memory; speed of processing & visual inform.
Gibbs et al. 1990[61]	20 ARC 20 Asympt. 20 HIV-	1-way ANOVA	No differences.
Koralnik et al., 1990[62]	29 Asympt. 33 HIV-	1 of 6 >2 SD, and 1 of 6 >1 SD, or 3 of 6 >1 SD	No differences.
Levin et al., 1990[69]	99 Asympt. 36 HIV-	MANOVA	Verbal fluency; arithmetic design fluency; set shifting; delayed recall of logical discourse material.

Table 2. (continued)

Study	Number	Impairment	Result: Asymptomatic Group
van Gorp, et al., 1989[55]	Review		As a group, asymptomatics don't exhibit increased prevalence of neuropsychologic abnormalities compared with HIV-; do not appear to demonstrate clinical neurobehavioral effects of CNS involvement as a result of HIV; greater incidence occurs with advancing infection in context of immunosuppression.
Goethe et al., 1989[58]	176 RE 1-2 18 HIV-	ANOVA	No differences.
Janssen et al., 1989[59]	26 ARC 31 G. Lymphad. 43 Asympt. 157 HIV-	1.5 SD on tests in >2 functional domains,	No differences between asymptomatics and HIV.
McArthur et al., 1989 (MACS)[60]	270 Asympt. 193 HIV-	Mann-Whitney rank sum test 2 SD on 2 or 3 SD on 1.	No difference in prevalence rate of neuropsychological abnormalities relative to HIV-.
Grant et al., 1987[53]	15 AIDS 13 ARC 16 Asympt.	Mann-Whitney U definite impairment on 1; probable impairment on 2.	Asympt. abnormalities on verbal delayed recall and abstraction.

on $\geq$3 tests[73] to $\geq$9 tests[71] indicated that approximately 24% of ARC patients experienced severe neuropsychological impairment. Dunbar and colleagues[73] compared ARC patients who did and did not progress to AIDS after 1 year, and noted that 27% of those patients progressing to AIDS were impaired at follow-up. Neuropsychological performance at baseline did not differentially predict the development of AIDS in the two groups, and lack of significant differences at 1-year follow-up may have been due to the relatively short duration between onset of AIDS and testing. Tross and colleagues[70] examined 44 newly diagnosed (mean of 4.2 months since diagnosed with AIDS) and 40 late (mean 13 months since diagnosed with AIDS) AIDS patients with suspected cognitive dysfunction and reported a 32% and 71% rate of impairment, respectively, utilizing a 1 SD cut-off score on 2 or more tests. In a sample of 20 newly diagnosed AIDS patients, none of whom were taking antiretroviral medication, 50% were impaired according to a 2 SD cut-off on >2 tests.[41] Perdices and Cooper[71] reported similar findings for 17 AIDS patients who were selected from a cohort of 531 patients for evaluation based upon suspected cognitive dysfunction. Approximately 54% of their sample $\geq$2 SD below HIV-seronegative means on 3 or more tests. Grant and colleagues[53] provided the most liberal estimate for rates of neuropsychological abnormality among AIDS patients (87%) by using criteria for impairment of either 2 SD below normative means on 1 test or 1 SD on $\geq$2 tests. Taken together, conservative estimates indicate that approximately $\overline{24\%}$ of ARC patients suffer from clinically significant cognitive dysfunction. Rate of cognitive impairment appears to increase throughout the course of AIDS, affecting approximately 32%

of newly diagnosed AIDS patients and possibly accelerating with advanced infection to affect over 50% of those in later stages.

Any conclusions with regard to the cognitive integrity of asymptomatic HIV-seropositive individuals remain tentative. Well-controlled investigations which have utilized multiple tests to assess different functional domains have consistently identified deficits in memory, aspects of executive functioning, attention, abstract reasoning, motor speed, and timed psychomotor tasks relative to either HIV-seronegative controls[58,65-67] or extant normative values.[54] The degree of impairment has typically been characterized as clinically insignificant insofar as it affects social and work functioning. An incipient process of cognitive deterioration may affect 20-30% of HIV-infected asymptomatic individuals. More severe dysfunction is reportedly rare, with an estimated prevalence of approximately 3.7:1,000.[60] Conclusions regarding the lack of cognitive impairment among nonsymptomatic HIV-seropositive individuals should be tempered with reference to the potential operation of cohort effects. Many of the patients in large, long-term studies tend to be better educated and may be more able/motivated for medical and self-care. The low prevalence of cognitive deficits noted in these individuals may not be representative of all HIV-infected individuals, particularly intravenous drug users and the impoverished. In addition, the inability to detect impairment may be, in part, due to declines from superior to normal levels of functioning among better educated cohorts. It has been frequently asserted that among HIV-infected individuals, neurological deterioration typically occurs within the context of immunosuppression. However, no reliable relationship has been demonstrated between neuropsychological performance among aympytomatics and immunological parameters across studies. Finally, there are no data convincingly demonstrating that these minor cognitive deficits in HIV-seropositive patients or in patients with more advanced disease are necessarily predictors for the development of AIDS dementia.

Overt HIV Encephalopathy (AIDS Dementia Complex)

This disorder typically occurs in the setting of advanced immunosuppression and coexistent systemic disease,[37,40,54,55,58,61,67,68] but may be the presenting or even sole manifestation of HIV infection before the infected individual exhibits any other illnesses characteristic of impaired immunity.[74-76] It is characterized clinically by an insidious onset of a disturbance in intellect often accompanied by fatigue, malaise, headaches, increasing social isolation and loss of sexual drive. On rare occasion, the disorder may begin abruptly and progress rapidly. Salient complaints include increasing forgetfulness, difficulty concentrating and reading, and a slowness in thinking and in motor skills. Job performance declines and,ultimately, assistance in activities of daily living are required. Initially, a diagnosis of depression is often considered; however, dysphoria is typically absent.[37] Unlike cortical dementias, language skills are typically affected late in the course of the disease and are chiefly characterized by word-finding difficulties. Aphasia is typically not observed. Many patients complain of incoordination, imbalance, gait disturbances, or tremor. Painful peripheral dyesthesias are generally the consequence of superimposed HIV-related peripheral neuropathy. Sleep disturbances are reported with polysomnographic studies indicating a distortion of sleep architecture,[77,78] and both focal and generalized seizures have been described.[79-82] In a significant percentage of HIV-infected persons with seizures, no etiology other than HIV could be identified for the seizures.[79,80]

Physical Examination. These patients, although not invariably, appear debilitated and chronically ill as a consequence of advanced immunosuppression. Hallmarks of full-blown AIDS include temporal and general body wasting, alopecia, seborrheic dermatitis and generalized lymphadenopathy. Bedside mental status examination in advanced HIV encephalopathy reveals a slowing of mental processing. It is not unusual for a hiatus of several seconds to occur before the patient responds to a simple question or command posed by the examiner.

Ocular motility is disturbed. Abnormalities that may be observed include slowed saccadic eye movements,[83-85] hypometric saccades,[86] overshoot dysmetria,[87] fixational instability,[86] dissociative nystagmus,[88] and defective smooth pursuits.[86] Currie and colleagues[86] found these eye movement abnormalities useful predictive markers for the development of HIV encephalopathy. The face becomes less expressive and speech hypophonic, monotonous and slow. Stuttering has also been reported.[89] Coordination is impaired even in the early stages of the illness.[90] Fine movements are performed slowly and awkwardly. Tasks such as buttoning shirts, writing, cutting food and shaving, may prove difficult.[91] A fine, irregular tremor that is most evident during sustained postures of the upper limbs is frequently detected. Despite many features reminiscent of parkinsonism, a resting tremor is usually not observed. Generalized weakness is not uncommon. When weakness is confined to the lower extremities, particularly when accompanied by long tract signs and incontinence, the possibility of an associated myelopathy needs to be considered. In advanced stages of the illness, the patient is bed-bound and incontinent. Muscle tone is increased and dystonia may be observed in the absence of neuroleptic exposure.[92] Muscle stretch reflexes may be increased; however, the frequent superimposition of peripheral neuropathy may result in a loss of diminution of ankle jerks as well as diminished sensory perception in distal extremities. Evidence of corticospinal tract involvement may include Hoffman's and Babinski's signs and crossed adductor reflexes. In early stages of HIV encephalopathy, brisk walking, pivoting, and walking heel-to-toe may betray abnormalities,[91] and later in the disorder, the gait may be slow and clumsy with diminished arm swing and postural instability. There is an exquisite sensitivity to the administration of dopamine receptor blockers, including prochlorperazine and metoclopropamide,[93-96] and the patient may literally be "frozen" in bed as a consequence of their use. Frontal release signs including, snout, suck, involuntary grasps, palmomentals, nuchocephalic and glabellar, are typically elicitable.

Neuropsychological Function. The pattern of neuropsychological performance deficits and reported changes observed in cognition, motor function, and behavior are consistent with a subcortical dementia.[97] With respect to performance,the abnormalities most reliably observed in patients with AIDS have been on measures having a substantial motor and pscyhomotor speed component. However, the overall pattern of impairment among these patients includes such higher cortical functions as abstraction, memory, and verbal spontaneity.[58] Some investigators have suggested that HIV-induced cognitive dysfunction manifests with more variability, including dementia with cortical deficits, subcortical dementia, and subcortical cognitive deficits in the absence of global intellectual deterioration.[98]

Tross and colleagues[70] report that the following tests are particularly helpful in detecting cognitive disturbances in these patients: (1) fine motor control [grooved pegboard, finger tapping]; (2) rapid sequential problem solving [trail making, digit symbol]; (3) spontaneity [verbal fluency]; (4) visuospatial problem solving [block design]; and (5) visual memory [visual reproduction].

Psychiatric Disorders. A broad spectrum of psychiatric disorders may be seen with HIV encephalopathy.[99-104] These psychiatric manifestations occur in isolation and may actually herald the clinical recognition of HIV encephalopathy.[75,100] In one study,[105] delirium, characterized by a clouding of consciousness with reduced capacity to shift, focus and sustain attention to stimuli and accompanied by excessive psychomotor activity and hallucinations and delusions, was the most frequent diagnosis in patients with AIDS for which a psychiatric consultation had been requested. The abuse of alcohol and recreational drugs and prior brain damage were risk factors for its development.[106] Psychoses may also be observed.[104] In perhaps up to 10% of affected individuals, the disorder may present as a frank psychosis. A triad of mood disturbance, thought disorder with grandiose delusions, and severe memory deficits has been noted.[103] Organic affective disorders, mania and depression, may also accompany HIV encephalopathy.[104] Severe depression often poorly responsive to antidepressant therapy may be a consequence of organic disease.[107] An improvement in refractory depressive symptoms following the administration of AZT has been anecdotally reported.[108] The possible contribution of drugs to the genesis of the psychiatric disorder should always be considered; mania has been reported as a consequence of AZT use,[109] and aggressive psychosis occurs following corticosteroid administration.[110] As previously mentioned, an exquisite sensitivity to anticholinergic drugs with resultant confusion,[111-113] and to dopamine receptor blockers, such as metoclopropamide and a variety of widely used neuroleptics, may result in severe parkinsonism.[15]

HIV Encephalopathy in Children

Children infected with HIV also develop a progressive encephalopathy.[114,115] The neurologic manifestations may precede features suggesting immunodeficiency.[116] Generally, the neurologic disease progresses in tandem with worsening immunological function.[117] In one study of 36 infected children,[117] the incubation period from initial infection in the perinatal period to the development of the encephalopathy varied from 2 months to 5 years. The encephalopathy is characterized by a developmental delay or the loss of motor milestones and intellectual abilities that had been previously acquired.[117,118] Examination may reveal weakness with pyramidal tract and extrapyramidal signs, pseudobulbar palsy, ataxia, and secondary microcephaly. Myoclonus and seizures may also be observed.

Diagnostic Studies for HIV Encephalopathy

Cerebrospinal Fluid. A mononuclear pleocytosis of the cerebrospinal fluid (CSF) is observed in one-fifth of individuals with HIV encephalopathy.[119] The mononuclear pleocytosis observed is generally low,[38] usually with counts less than 50 cells/mm³. Cytological analysis may reveal reactive lymphocytes, plasma cells, and, in rare instances, multinucleated giant cells.[120] The CSF glucose is normal or borderline. Values that are one-third to one-half of serum glucose levels are not uncommon. Two-thirds have an increased CSF protein.[113] Typically, the protein levels are below 200 mg/dl.[38] Intrathecal synthesis of HIV-specific antibody and oligoclonal bands can be frequently demonstrated,[121] but do not appear to be predictive of the CNS disease.[122] Controversy surrounds the issue of whether the presence of CSF HIV p24 antigen is a useful predictor of HIV encephalopathy. Some studies report that its presence is associated with a progressive encephalopathy in children[123,124] and adults,[125] whereas other studies have failed to confirm these findings.[24,126] Not unexpectedly, the isolation of HIV from CSF is not a useful marker for HIV encephalopathy.[126] Although serological conversion to HIV has occurred in almost all patients with HIV encephalopathy, in rare instances both adults[119] and children[127] may present with the encephalopathy before seroconversion.

Detection of a variety of cytokines in the CSF, particularly those hypothesized to play a role in the pathogenesis of the disorder, is under active investigation. Interleukin-1β (IL-1β) was found in the CSF of 58% of patients with HIV infection, and interleukin-6 (IL-6) was found in 42% in one study.[128] Although both could be detected in the absence of clinical neurological disease, they appeared to be more frequently detected in the presence of HIV encephalopathy.[128] Other cytokines that are detected in elevated levels in the CSF of some patients with AIDS include the macrophage products, tumor necrosis factor-α (TNF-α), neopterin, and β2-microglobulin, and the T-cell products, soluble CD8 and γ-interferon (INF-γ).[129] CSF TNF-α may be correlated with the severity of the encephalopathy,[129] but this observation is not universally accepted.[130] Discrepancies in these studies may simply reflect the sensitivity of the assays used. Elevated β2-microglobulin, a low molecular weight protein that is bound to the major histocompatibility protein and expressed on the cell surface of almost all nucleated cells, has been detected in the CSF. Elevated CSF β2-microglobulin appears to be more common in the presence of neurological disease,[131-133] but its levels do not appear to be correlated with the degree of CSF pleocytosis or the alteration in the blood-brain barrier.[132] Brew and colleagues argue that its concentration is a useful surrogate marker for the severity of HIV encephalopathy.[132,133] Levels of CSF β2-microglobulin greater than 3.8 mg/l occurring in the absence of opportunistic infection appear to be a clinically useful marker for HIV encephalopathy.[134]

Quinolinic acid, a potent neuroexcitant in the CNS,[135] is induced in macrophages infected with HIV,[136] and may be detected in the CSF during HIV infection. A correlation between levels of CSF quinolinic acid and poorer neuropsychological performance across the spectrum of HIV has been reported.[137] Some investigators have found myelin basic protein in the CSF of patients with HIV encephalopathy and have related its presence to the associated demyelinating process.[138] Conversely, other studies have found it in only a small minority of patients with HIV encephalopathy.[139] It is generally not observed in asymptomatic HIV-infected individuals.[140]

Radiographic Studies. The chief value of radiographic imaging of the brain, computed tomography (CT scan) of the brain, and cranial magnetic resonance imaging (MRI), in patients with suspected HIV encephalopathy is to exclude from diagnostic consideration other neurological disorders that may also

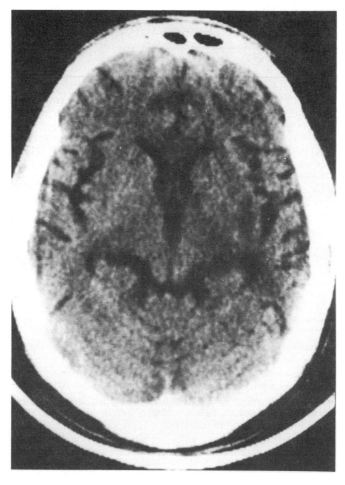

Figure 1. Computed tomographic scan of the brain. This CT scan shows both central atrophy characterized by ventricular dilatation and cortical atrophy.

result in a neuropathy.[141] The most commonly reported abnormality on brain CT is cerebral atrophy (Fig. 1). A correlation has been noted between neuro-psychological function, namely a slowing of response time, and severity of brainatrophy determined by cerebral ventricular enlargement on CT scan and on MRI.[69] Similarly, brain atrophy detected on MRI may be correlated with the presence of HIV in CSF and with elevated levels of β2-microglobulin has been demonstrated.[144] Olsen and colleagues[145] have described a number of white matter lesions commonly visualized on MRI in HIV encephalopathy. They cate-gorized these lesions into various patterns, including: (1) "diffuse," a widespread involvement of a large area, most commonly observed; (2) "patchy," localized involvement with ill-defined margins; and (3) "punctate," small loci[145] less than 1 cm in diameter (Fig. 2). Minimal brain abnormalities detected on cranial MRI, including slight brain atrophy, need not reflect the presence of underlying HIV encephalopathy[146] nor show progression over time.[147]

Preliminary studies with positron emission tomography (PET) using [18F]fluorodeoxygluose (FDG) assessing regional cerebral metabolic rates for

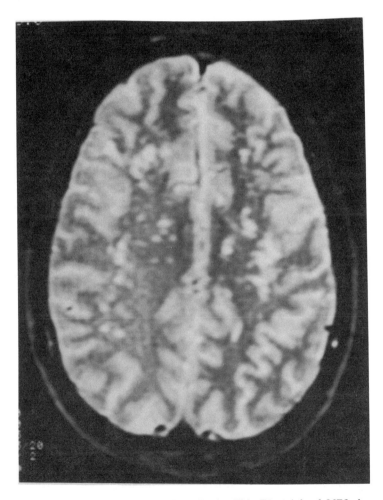

Figure 2. Magnetic resonance imaging of the brain. This T2 weighted MRI shows multiple punctate areas of high signal intensity in a patient with HIV encephalopathy. These lesions did not enhance following the administration of gadolinium and were unassociated with mass effect or focal findings on neurological examination.

glucose demonstrated relative subcortical (thalamus and basal ganglia) hypermetabolism in early HIV encephalopathy and cortical and subcortical gray matter hypometabolism in advanced stages of the disease.[148] The alterations in subcortical metabolism appear to correlated with impairment of fine motor control and that of cortical metabolism with impairments in verbal fluency and problem solving. Suggestions that FDG/PET may be an objective method of diagnosing the onset of HIV encephalopathy and providing data on response to antiviral therapy[148] requires further investigation. Single photon emission tomography (SPECT) employing $99mTc$-hexmethyl propyleneamineoxime (HMPAO) studying cerebral blood flow has revealed decreases in the temporal and parietal lobes.[149] Utilizing [123I]IMP SPECT, two other groups[150,151] have found analogous perfusion defects in comparable groups of patients.

As a correlate of the neuronal loss detected with quantitative morphometry, studies using proton magnetic resonance spectroscopy reveal significant reductions in levels of N-acetyl aspartate (NAA) relative to creatine (Cr) and elevations in choline-containing compounds relative to Cr in patients with moderate to severe HIV encephalopathy.[152] NAA is a metabolic marker for normal neuronal functions and its decrease relative to Cr suggests neuronal dropout in this disorder. The alteration of the choline/Cr ratio is possibly the result of changes in membrane metabolism.[152]

Electrophysiological Studies. Electroencephalography (EEG) has been suggested as a sensitive method to detect subclinical cerebral disease in HIV-infected individuals.[153] Some investigators claim that there is a correlation between EEG abnormalities and clinical illness.[154] A variety of EEG abnormalities have been reported in the HIV-infected individual including increased amounts of generalized episodic or persistent, predominantly anterior slow wave activity,[153,155] lower maximal amplitudes of dominant background activity and more marked generalized and anterior disturbances when compared to uninfected controls.[153] However, other studies found no definitely abnormal EEG tracings that could be attributed to HIV infection in otherwise asymptomatic individuals.[156,157] The application of computerized spectral analysis of the EEG, a technique that may be more sensitive than routine EEG,[158] has been used to evaluate HIV-infected persons.[158-160] Whether it will be meaningful in this disorder remains uncertain.

Brainstem auditory evoked potential studies (BAERs) have detected significant delays in waveforms I-V and II-V in HIV-infected individuals compared to controls, indicating abnormalities in the upper brainstem.[85,161,162] Multiple regression analysis in studies of BAERs fail to reveal a significant influence of other factors, such as past medical history or drug use, in these waveforms.[162,163] A delayed response time has also been seen in studies employing cognitive event-related potentials.[90,164] All electrophysiological studies still remain unproven predictors of the presence or progression of HIV encephalopathy.

Survival

Adults with HIV encephalopathy have an average survival of approximately 6 months.[10,165] This survival is less than one-half of that observed in patients with AIDS without dementia.[10,165] In children, survival is generally between 6 and 24 months.[165] Effective therapy is likely to improve survival statistics.

Treatment

AZT penetrates the blood-brain barrier reasonably well. CSF levels may briefly exceed 1 μmol/L when AZT is administered as 5 mg/kg intravenously every 4 hours.[166] The CSF to plasma ratios vary between 135% following an oral administration of 15 mg/kg to 15% at an oral dose of 2 mg/kg.[166] Brain tissue levels may not reflect CSF levels of the drug. Portegies and others[43] reported a decline in the overall incidence of HIV encephalopathy after the introduction of AZT. The anecdotal clinical reports[167,168] demonstrated improvement in HIV encephalopathy in adults with AZT use were shortly confirmed by more comprehensive studies.[169,173] Both the smaller study by Price and colleagues[113] and the larger one of Schmitt et al.[169] showed only partial improvement in neuropsychological abnormalities associated with HIV. Parallel studies of the effect of AZT on brain metabolic abnormalities with HIV encephalopathy employing [18F]-FDG show reversal of large focal cortical,abnormalities of glucose utilization.[170] The optimal dose of AZT is uncertain, but higher doses (1000-1500 mg) than generally administered are used in the treatment of HIV encephalopathy and higher doses (2000 mg) may be required.[171] AZT-related side effects, such as anemia and leukopenia, may be controlled with erythropoietin (EPO) and granulocyte colony stimulating factor (Neupogen), respectively. If AZT is not helpful or not tolerated, dideoxyinosine (ddI) 600 mg daily is a rational choice, although this value in adults for dementia remains unproven.

In children, a similar and perhaps more dramatic improvement in encephalopathy was demonstrated by Pizzo et al. with the use of continuous infusion of AZT.[172] This improvement may be noted in the absence of an improvement in immunological parameters.[172] The optimal intravenous dose of AZT in children appeared to be between 0.9 and 1.4 mg/kg/hour.[172]

The value of other antiretroviral therapies for HIV encephalopathy is unanswered. Neither ddI nor dideoxycytosine (ddC) appear to cross the blood-brain barrier as well as AZT. Drugs that do not have a primary effect on HIV, such as CNS stimulants (methylphenidate and dexedrine) and corticosteroids have been used in a limited and nonrigorous fashion in attempts at symptomatic improvement of HIV encephalopathy. ddI has been shown to improve scores on standardized tests of intelligence in children with HIV-related cognitive disturbances.[173] Plasma ddI levels correlated with this cognitive improvement.[173] Anecdotally, prednisone has been reported to improve HIV encephalopathy in children.[174] No data are available regarding its value in adults with this disorder. Although there are legitimate concerns relative to the potential deleterious effect of corticosteroids on HIV-infected patients with an already compromised immune system, one study of HIV-infected children receiving prednisone showed no consistent or significant change in the number or percentage of CD3, CD4, CD8 or CD19 lymphocytes.[175] Other drugs under investigation for AIDS dementia include agents which block components of the viral envelope gp120, e.g., the pentapeptide, peptide T,[176] calcium channel antagonists, e.g., nimodipine and cytokine blockers, e.g., pentoxifylline which opposes the activity of TNF-α.[177]

REFERENCES

1. W.D. Snider, D.M. Simpson, S. Neilsen, et al. Neurological complications of the acquired immunodeficiency syndrome: analysis of 50 patients. *Ann. Neurol.* 14:403 (1981).
2. R.M. Levy, D.E. Bredesen, and M.L. Rosenblum. Neurological manifestations of the acquired immunodeficiency syndrome (AIDS): experience at UCSF and review of the literature. *J. Neurosurg.* 62:475 (1985).
3. J.R. Berger, L. Moskowitz, M. Fischl, and R.E. Kelley. Neurologic disease as the presenting manifestation of acquired immunodeficiency syndrome. *South. Med. J.* 80:683 (1987).
4. D.E. Bredesen, and R. Messing. Neurological syndromes heralding the acquired immunodeficiency syndrome. *Ann. Neurol.* 14:141 (1983).
5. F. Gray, R. Gherardi, F. Scaravilli. The neuropathology of the acquired immune deficiency syndrome (AIDS). *Brain* 111:245 (1988).
6. K. Kure, J.F. Llena, W.D. Lyman, et al. Human immunodeficiency virus 1 infection of the nervous system: an autopsy study of 268 adult, pediatric, and fetal brains. *Hum. Pathol.* 22:700 (1991).
7. D.H. Gabuzda, D.D. Ho, S.M. de la Monte, et al. Immunohistochemical identi-

fication of HTLV-III antigen in brains of patients with AIDS. *Ann. Neurol.* 20:289 (1986).

8. S. Gartner, P. Markovits, D.M. Markovits, et al. Virus isolation from and identification of HTLV-III/LAV-producing cells in brain tissue from patients with AIDS. *J.A.M.A.* 256:2365 (1986).

9. M.H. Stoler, T.A. Eskin, S. Benn, et al. Human T-cell lymphotropic virus type II infection of the central nervous system - a preliminary *in situ* analysis. *J.A.M.A.* 2546:2360 (1986).

10. J.C. McArthur. Neurological manifestations of AIDS. *Medicine* 66:407 (1987).

11. L. Resnick, J.R. Berger, P. Shapshak, and W.W. Tourtellotte. Early penetration of the blood-brain barrier by HIV. *Neurology* 38:9 (1988).

12. L.E. Davis, B.L. Hjelle, V.E. Miller, et al. Early viral brain invasion in iatrogenic human immunodeficiency virus infection. *Neurology* 42:1736 (1992).

13. D.D. Ho, M.G. Sarngadharan, L. Resnick, et al. Primary human T-lymphotropic virus type III infection. *Ann. Intern. Med.* 103:880 (1987).

14. D.A. Cooper, J. Gold, P. Maclean,e t al,. Acute AIDS retrovirus infection: definition of a clinical illness associated with seroconversion. *Lancet* 1:537 (1985).

15. H. Hollander, and S. Stringari. Human immunodeficiency virus-associated meningitis. Clinical course and correlations. *Am. J. Med.* 83:813 (1987).

16. C.A. Carne, R.S. Tedder, A. Smith, et al. Acute encephalopathy coincident with seroconversion for anti-HTLV-III. *Lancet* 2:1206 (1985).

17. B.J. Brew, M. Perdices, P. Darveniza, et al. The neurological features of early and 'latent' human immunodeficiency virus infection. *Aust. N.Z. J. Med* 198:700 (1989).

18. E. Scarpini, G. Sacilotto, A. Lazzarin, et al. Acute ataxia coincident with seroconversion for anti-HIV. *J. Neurol.* 238:356 (1991).

19. P.J. Hughes, K.A. McLean, and R.J.M. Lane. Cranial polyneuropathy and brainstem disorder at the time of seroconversion in HIV infection. *Int. J. Stud. AIDS* 3:60 (1992).

20. P. Paton, J. Poly, P.-M. Gonnaud, et al. Acute meningoradiculitis concomitant with seroconversion to human immunodeficiency virus type 1. *Res. Virol.* 141:427 (1990).

21. D.W. Denning, J. Anderson, P. Rudge, and H. Smith. Acute myelopathy associated with primary infection with human immunodeficiency virus. *Br. Med. J. [Clin. Res.]* 294:143 (1987).

22. A. Zeman, and M. Donaghy. Acute infection with human immunodeficiency virus presenting with neurogenic urinary retention. *Genitourin. Med.* 67:345 (1991).

23. L.H. Calabrese, M.R. Profitt, K.H. Levin, et al. Acute infection with human immunodeficiency virus (HIV) associated with acute brachial neuritis and exanthematous rash. *Ann. Intern. Med.* 197:849 (1987).

24. P. Portegies, L.G. Epstein, S.T.A. Hung, J. de Gans, and J. Goudsmit. Human immunodeficiency virus type 1 antigen in cerebrospinal fluid. *Arch. Neurol.* 46:261 (1989).

25. D.C. Gajdusek, H.L. Amyx, C.J. Gibbs, Jr., et al. Infection of chimpanzees by human T-lymphotropic retroviruses in brain and other tissues from AIDS patients. *Lancet* 1:55 (1985).

26. I. Elovaara, M. Iivanainen, S.-L. Valle, et al. CSF protein and cellular profiles in various stages of HIV infection related to neurological manifestations., *J. Neurol. Sci.* 78:331 (1987).

27. A.C. Chalmers, B.S. Aprill, and H. Shephard. Cerebrospinal fluid and human immunodeficiency virus: findings in healthy, asymptomatic, seropositive men. *Arch. Neurol.* 150:1538 (1990).

28. D.W. Marshall, R.L. Brey, W.T. Cahill, et al. Spectrum of cerebrospinal fluid findings in various stages of human immunodeficiency virus infection. *Arch. Neurol.* 35:954 (1988).

29. D.W. Marshall, R.L. Brey, C.A. Butzin, et al. CSF changes in a longitudinal

study of 124 neurologically normal HIV-1-infected U.S. Air Force personnel. *J. AIDS* 4:777 (1991).

30. M.E. Appleman, D.W. Marshall, R.L. Brey, et al. Cerebrospinal fluid abnormalities in patients without AIDS who are seropositive for the human immunodeficiency virus. *J. Infect. Dis.* 158:193 (1988).

31. C.B. Britton, and J.R. Miller. Neurologic complications in acquired immunodeficiency syndrome. *Neurol. Clin.* 2:315 (1984).

32. S.L. Nielsen, C.K. Petito, C.S. Urmacher and J.B. Posner. Subacute encephalitis in acquired immune deficiency syndrome: a postmortem study. *Am. J. Clin. Pathol.* 82:768 (1984).

33. R.J. Janssen, D. R. Cornblath, L.G. Epstein, et al. Nomenclature and research case definitions for neurologic manifestations of human immunodeficiency virus type 1 (HIV-1) infection. *Neurology* 41:778 (1991).

34. R.S. Janssen, O.C. Nwanyanwu, R.M. Selik, and J.K. Stehr-Green. Epidemiology of human immunodeficiency virus encephalopathy in the United States. *Neurology* 42:1472 (1992).

35. R.M. Levy, and D.E. Bredesen. Central nervous system dysfunction in acquired immunodeficiency syndrome. *J. AIDS* 1:41 (1988).

36. G.B. Scott, C. Hutto, R.W. Makuch, et al. Survival in children with perinatally acquired human immunodeficiency virus type 1 infection. *N. Engl. J. Med.* 321:1791 (1989).

37. R.W. Price, B. Brew, J. Sidtis, et al. The brain in AIDS: central nervous system HIV-1 infection and AIDS dementia complex. *Science* 239:586 (1988).

38. B.A. Navia, B.D. Jordan, and R.W. Price. The AIDS dementia complex: I. Clinical features. *Ann. Neurol.* 19:517 (1986).

39. B.A. Navia, B.D. Jordan, and R.W. Price. The AIDS dementia complex: II. Neuropathology. *Ann. Neurol.* 19:525 (1986).

40. R.W. Price, and B.J. Brew. The AIDS dementia complex. *J. Infect. Dis.* 158:1079 (1988).

41. I. Reinvang, S.S. Froland, and V. Skripeland. Prevalence of neuropsychological deficit in HIV infection. Incipient signs of AIDS dementia complex in patients with AIDS. *Acta Neurol. Scand.* 83:2389 (1991).

42. P. Portegies, J. de Gans, J.M.A. Lange, et al. Declining incidence of AIDS dementia complex after introduction of zidovudine treatment *Br. Med. J.* 299:819 (1989).

43. J.J. Day, I. Grant, J.H. Atkinson, et al. Incidence of AIDS dementia in a two-year follow-up of AIDS and ARC patients on initial phase II AZT placebo-controlled study: San Diego cohort. *J. Neuropsychiatry* 4:15 (1992).

44. J.C. McArthur, D.R. Hoover, H. Bacellar, et al. Dementia in AIDS patients: incidence and risk factors. (in press)

45. A.L. Belman, G.Diamond, D. Dickson, et al. Pediatric acquired immunodeficiency syndrome. Neurologic syndromes. *Am. J. Dis. Child.* 142:29 (1988).

46. P. Kleihues, S.L. Leib, C. Strittmatter, O.D. Wiestler, and W. Lang. HIV encephalopathy: incidence, definition and pathogenesis. *Acta Pathol. Jap.* 41:197 (1991).

47. S.M. de la Monte, D.D. Ho, R.T. Schooley, et al. Subacute encephalomyelitis of AIDS and its relation to HTLV-III infection. *Neurology* 37:562 (1987).

48. F. Gulotta, K. Kuchelmesiter, T. Masini, P. Ghidoni, and E. Cappricci. Zur morphologie der HIV-encephalopathies. *Zentralbl. allg. Pathol. pathol. Anat.* 135:5 (1989).

49. T. Kato, A. Hirano, J.F. Llena, and H.M. Dembitzer. Neuropathology of acquired immune deficiency syndrome (AIDS) in 53 autopsy cases with particular emphasis on microglial nodules and multinucleated cells. *Acta Neuropathol. (Berl.)* 77:287 (1987).

50. P. Kleinhues, W. Lang, P.C. Burger, et al. Progressive diffuse leukoencephalopathy in patients with acquired immune deficiency syndrome (AIDS). *Acta Neuropathol. (Berl.)* 68:333 (1985).

51. C. Petito. Review of central nervous system pathology in human immunodeficiency virus infection. *Ann. Neurol.* 23 (suppl.):S54 (1988).

52. E. Masliah, C.L. Achim, N. Ge, et al. Spectrum of human immunodeficiency virus-associated neocortical damage. *Ann. Neurol.* 32:321 (1992).
53. I. Grant, J.H. Atkinson, J.R. Hesselink, et al. Evidence of early central nervous system involvement in the acquired immunodeficiency syndrome (AIDS) and other human immunodeficiency virus (HIV) infections. Studies with neuropsychologic testing and magnetic resonance imaging. *Ann. Intern. Med.* 107:828 (1987).
54. Y. Stern, K. Marder, K. Bell, et al. Multidisciplinary baseline assessment of homosexual men with and without human immunodeficiency virus infection. III: Neurologic and neuropsychologic findings. *Arch. Gen. Psychiatry* 48:131 (1991).
55. W.G. van Gorp, E.N. Miller, P. Satz, and B. Visscher. Neuropsychological performance in HIV-1 immunocompromised patients: A preliminary report. *J. Clin. Exp. Neuropsychol.* 11:763 (1989).
56. K.L. Kaemingk, and A.W. Kazniak. Neuropsychological aspects of human immunodeficiency virus infection. *Clin. Neuropsychol.* 3:309 (1989).
57. S.W. Perry. Organic mental disorders caused by HIV: Update on early diagnosis and treatment. *Am. J. Psychiatry* 147:696 (1990).
58. K.E. Goethe, J.E. Mitchell, D.W. Marshall, et al. Neuropsychological and neurological function of human immunodeficiency virus seropositive asymptomatic individuals. *Arch. Neurol.* 46:129 (1989).
59. R.S. Janssen, A.J. Saykin, L. Cannon, et al. Neurological and neuropsychological manifestations of HIV-1 infection: Association with AIDS-related complex but not asymptomatic HIV-1 infection. *Ann. Neurol.* 26:592 (1989).
60. J.C. McArthur, B.A. Cohen, O.A. Selnes, et al. Low prevalence of neurological and neuropsychological abnormalities in otherwise healthy HIV-1-infected individuals: Results from the Multicenter AIDS Cohort Study. *Ann. Neurol.* 26:601 (1989).
61. A. Gibbs, D.G. Andrewes, G. Szmukler, B. Mulhall, and S.C. Bowden. Early HIV-related neuropsychological impairment: Relationship to stage of viral infection. *J. Clin. Exp. Neuropsychol.* 12:766 (1990).
62. I.J. Koralnik, A. Beaumanoir, R. Hausler, et al. A controlled study of early neurologic abnormalities in men with asymptomatic human immunodeficiency virus infection. *N. Engl. J. Med.* 323:864 (1990).
63. E.M. Miller, O.A. Selnes, K.J.C. McArthur, et al. Neuropsychological performance in HIV-1-infected homosexual men. The Multicenter AIDS Cohort Study (MACS). *Neurology* 40:197 (1990).
64. R.A. Bornstein, H.A. Nasrallah, M.F. Para, et al. Rate of CD4 decline and neuropsychological performance in HIV infection. *Arch. Neurol.* 48:704 (1991).
65. F.L. Wilkie, C.Eisdorfer, R., Morgan, D.A. Lowenstein, and J. Szapocznik. Cognition in early HIV infection. *Arch. Neurol.* 47:433 (1990).
66. S. Lunn, M. Skydbjerg, H. Schulsinger, et al. A preliminary report on the neuropsychologic sequelae of human immunodeficiency virus. *Arch. Gen. Psychiatry* 48:139 (1991).
67. E. Sinforiani, M. Mauri, G. Bono, et al. Cognitive abnormalities and disease progression in a selected population of asymptomatic HIV-positive subjects. *AIDS* 5:1117 (1991).
68. O.A. Selnes, E. Miller, J. McArthur, et al. HIV-1 infection: No evidence of cognitive decline during the asymptomatic stages. *Neurology* 40:204 (1990).
69. H.S. Levin, D.J. Williams, M.J. Borucki, et al. Magnetic resonance imaging and neuropsychological findings in human immunodeficiency virus infection. *J. AIDS* 3:757 (1990).
70. S. Tross, R.W. Price, B. Navia, et al. Neuropsychological characterization of the AIDS dementia complex: a preliminary report. *AIDS* 2:81 (1988).
71. M. Perdices, and D.A. Cooper. Neuropsychological investigation of patients with AIDS and ARC. *J. AIDS* 3:555 (1990).
72. M.J. Skoraszewski, J.D. Ball, and P. Mikulka. Neuropsychological functioning of HIV-infected males. *J.Clin. Exp. Neuropsychol.* 13:278 (1991).

73. N. Dunbar, M. Perdices, A. Grunseit, and D.A. Cooper. Changes in neuro-psychological performance of AIDS-related complex patients who progress to AIDS. *AIDS* 6:691 (1992).
74. B.A. Navia, and R.W. Price. The acquired immunodeficiency syndrome dementia complex as the presenting or sole manifestation of human immunodeficiency virus infection. *Arch. Neurol.* 44:64 (1987).
75. A. Beckett, P. Summergrad, T. Manschreck, et al. Symptomatic HIV infection of the CNS in a patient without clinical evidence of immunosuppression. *Am. J. Psychiatry* 144:1342 (1987).
76. J.-C. Chermann. HIV-associated diseases: acute and regressive encephalopathy in a seropositive man. *Res. Virol.* 141:137 (1990).
77. S.E. Norman, A.D. Chediak, M. Kiel, and M.A. Cohn. Sleep disturbances in HIV-infected homosexual men. *AIDS* 4:775 (1990).
78. S.E. Norman, L. Resnick, M.A. Cohn, et al. Sleep disturbances in HIV-seropositive patients. (Letter) *J.A.M.A.* 260:922 (1988).
79. D.M. Holtzman, D.A. Kaku, Y.T. So. New-onset seizures associated with human immunodeficiency virus infection: causation and clinical features in 100 cases. *Am. J. Med.* 87:173 (1989).
80. F. Bartolomei, P. Pellegrino, C. Dhiver, et al. Crises d'épilepsie au cours de l'infection par le VIH: 52 observations. *La Presse Méd.* 20:2135 (1991).
81. A. Parisi, M. Strosselli, A. Pan, R. Maserati, and L. Minoli. HIV-related encephalitis presenting as convulsant disease. *Clin. Electroencephal.* 22:1 (1991).
82. M.C. Wong, N.D.A. Suite, and D.R. Labar. Seizures in human immunodeficiency virus infection. *Arch. Neurol.* 47:640 (1990).
83. N. Nguyen, S. Rimmer, B. Katz. Slowed saccades in the acquired immunodeficiency syndrome. *Am. J. Ophthalmol.* 107:356 (1989).
84. P.T. Merrill, G.D. Paige, R.A. Abrams, R.G. Jacoby, and D.B. Clifford. Ocular motor abnormalities in human immunodeficiency virus infection. *Ann. Neurol.* 30:130 (1991).
85. U. Rosenhall, C. Häkansson, G.-B. Löwhagen, P. Hanner, and B. Johnsson-Ehk. Otoneurological abnormalities in asymptomatic HIV-seropositive patients. *Acta Neurol. Scand.* 79:140 (1989).
86. J. Currie, E. Benson, B. Ramsden, M. Perdices, and D. Cooper. Eye movement abnormalities as a predictor of the acquired immunodeficiency syndrome dementia complex. *Arch. Neurol.* 45:949 (1988).
87. D.I. Friedman, and S.E. Feldon. Eye movements in acquired immunodeficiency syndrome. (Letter) *Arch. Neurol.* 46:841 (1989).
88. H.W. Pfister, K.M. Einhaupl, U. Buttner, et al. Dissociated nystagmus as a common sign of ocular motor disorders in HIV-infected patients. *Eur. Neurol.* 29:277 (1989).
89. L. Fantry. Stuttering and acquired immunodeficiency syndrome. (Letter) *J.A.M.A. 263:38 (1990)*.
90. G. Arendt, H. Hefter, V. Hoemberg, et al. Early abnormalities of cognitive event-related potentials in HIV-infected patients without clinically evident CNS deficits. *Clin. Neurophysiol.* 41:370 (1990).
91. K.R. Robertson, and C.D. Hall. Human immunodeficiency virus-related cognitive impairment and the acquired immunodeficiency syndrome dementia complex. *Sem. Neurol.* 12:18 (1992).
92. W.S. Metzer. Movement disorders with AIDS encephalopathy: case report. *Neurology* 37:1438 (1987).
93. H. Hollander, J. Golden, T. Mendelson, et al. Extrapyramidal symptoms in AIDS patients given low-dose metoclopropamide or chlorpromazine. (Letter) *Lancet* 2:1186 (1985).
94. E. Hriso, T. Kuhn, J.C. Masdeu, and M. Grundman. Extrapyramidal symptoms due to dopamine-blocking agents in patients with AIDS encephalopathy. *Am. J. Psychiatry* 11:1558 (1991).
95. J.R. Swenson, M. Erman, J. Labelle, and J.E. Dimsdale. Extrapyramidal reactions: neuropsychiatric mimics in patients with AIDS. *Gen. Hosp. Psychiatry* 11:248 (1989).

96. H. Edelstein, and R.T. Knight. Severe parkinsonism in two AIDS patients taking prochlorperazine. (Letter). *Lancet* 2:341 (1987).
97. P.R. McHugh, and M.F. Folstein. Psychiatric syndromes of Huntington's chorea: a clinical and phenomenologic study, *in*: "Psychiatric Aspects of Neurological Disease," F. Benson, and D. Blumer, eds., Grune and Stratton, New York (1975).
98. M.M.A. Derix, J. de Gans, J. Stam, and P. Portegies. Mental changes in patients with AIDS. *Clin. Neurol. Neurosurg.* 92:215 (1990).
99. M.R. Faulstich. Acquired immune deficiency syndrome: an overview of central nervous system complications and neuropsychological sequelae. *Int. J. Neurosci.*, 30:249 (1986).
100. M.A. Cummings, K.L. Cummings, M.H. Rapaport, et al. Acquired immunodeficiency syndrome presenting as schizophrenia. *West. J. Med.* 146:615 (1987).
101. H.G. Nurnberg, J. Prudic, M. Fiori, et al. Psychopathology complicating acquired immune deficiency syndrome (AIDS). *Am. J. Psychiatry* 141:95 (1985).
102. C.S. Thomas, B.K. Toone, A. El Komy, et al. HTLV-III and psychiatric disturbance (Letter). *Lancet* 1:395 (1985).
103. E.J. Kermani, J.C. Borod, P. Brown, et al. New psychopathologic findings in AIDS: case report. *J. Clin. Psychiatry* 46:240 (1985).
104. M. Maj. Organic mental disorders in HIV-1 infection. *AIDS* 4:831 (1990).
105. M.A. O'Dowd, and F.P. McKegne. Does AIDS reduce psychiatric illness: AIDS patients compared with other medically ill HIV+ patients seen in consultation [abstract 2006]. *VI International Conference on AIDS,* San Francisco, June, 1990.
106. H.N. Ochitill, and J.W. Dilley. Neuropsychiatric aspects of acquired immunodeficiency syndrome, *in*: "AIDS and the Nervous System," R.M. Levy, and D.E. Bredesen, eds., Raven Press, New York (1988).
107. S.W. Burton. The psychiatry of HIV infection. *Br. Med. J.* 295:228 (1987).
108. B.O. Perkins, and D.L. Evans. HIV-related major depression: response to zidovudine [abstract SB 392]. *VI International Conference on AIDS*, San Francisco, June 1990.
109. J.M. Wright, P.S. Sachdev, R.J. Perkins, and P. Rodriguez. Zidovudine-related mania. *Med. J. Austral.* 150:339 (1989).
110. I.A. Campbell. Aggressive psychosis in AIDS patient on high-dose steroids. *Lancet* 2:750 (1987).
111. R.J. Lowenstein, and S. S. Sharfstein. Neuropsychiatric aspects of acquired immune deficiency syndrome. *Int. J. Psychiatr. Med.* 13:255 (1984).
112. S. Perry, and P. Jacobsen. Neuropsychiatric manifestations of AIDS-spectrum disorder. *Hosp. Community Psychiatry* 37:135 (1986).
113. W.A. Price, and J. Forejt. Neuropsychiatric aspects of AIDS: a case report. *Gen. Hosp. Psychiatry* 68:7 (1986).
114. L.G. Epstein, L.R. Sharer, V.V. Joshi, et al. Progressive encephalopathy in children with acquired immune deficiency syndrome. *Ann. Neurol.* 17:488 (1985).
115. A.L. Belman, M.H. Ultmann, D. Horoupian, et al. Neurological complications in infants and children with acquired immune deficiency syndrome. *Ann. Neurol.* 18:560 (1985).
116. S.L. Davis, C.C. Halsted, N. Levy, and W. Ellis. Acquired immune deficiency syndrome presenting as progressive infantile encephalopathy. *J. Pediatr.* 110:884 (1987).
117. L.G. Epstein, L.R. Sharer, J.M. Oleske, et al. Neurologic manifestations of human immunodeficiency virus infection in children., *Pediatrics* 78:678 (1986).
118. M.H. Ultmann, A.L. Belman, H.A. Ruff, et al. Developmental abnormalities in infants and children with acquired immune deficiency syndrome (AIDS) and AIDS-related complex. *Dev. Med. Child. Neurol.* 27:563 (1985).
119. R.W. Price, and B.A. Navia. Infections in AIDS and in other immunosup-

pressed patients, in: "Infections of the Nervous System," P.G.E. Kennedy and R.,T. Johnson, eds. Butterworth, London (1987).

120. R.L. Katz, C. Alappattu, J.P. Glass, and J.M. Bruner. Cerebrospinal fluid manifestations of the neurologic complications of human immunodeficiency virus infection. *Acta Cytol.* 33:233 (1989).

121. L. Resnick, F. diMarzo-Veronese, J. Schupbach, et al. Intra-blood-brain barrier synthesis of HTLV-III-specific IgG in patients with neurologic symptoms associated with AIDS or AIDS-related complex. *N. Engl. J. Med.* 313:1498 (1985).

122. K.K. Gotswami, S. Kaye, R. Miller, R. McAllister, R. Tedder. Intrathecal IgG synthesis and specificity of oligoclonal IgG in patients infected with HIV-1 do not correlate with CNS disease. *J. Med. Virol.* 33:106 (1991).

123. L.G. Epstein, J. Goudsmit, D.A. Paul, et al. Expression of human immunodeficiency virus in cerebrospinal fluid of children with progressive encephalopathy. *Ann. Neurol.* 21:397 (1987).

124. J. Goudsmit, J.M. Lange, W.J. Krone, et al. Pathogenesis of HIV and its implications for serodiagnosis and monitoring of antiviral therapy. *J. Virol. Meth.* 17:19 (1987).

125. J. Goudsmit, F. de Wolf, D.A. Paul, et al. Expression of human immunodeficiency antigen (HIV-Ag) in serum and cerebrospinal fluid during acute and chronic infection. *Lancet* 2:177 (1986).

126. R. Buffet, H. Agut, F.Chieze, et al. Virological markers in the cerebrospinal fluid from HIV-1-infected individuals. *AIDS* 5:1419 (1991).

127. M.V. Ragni, A.H. Urbach, S. Taylor, et al. Isolation of human immunodeficiency virus and detection deficiency syndrome and progressive encephalopathy. *J. Pediatr.* 110:892 (1987).

128. P. Gallo, K. Frei, C. Rordorf, et al. Human immunodeficiency virus type 1 (HIV-1) infection of the central nervous system: an evaluation of cytokines in cerebrospinal fluid. *J. Neuroimmunol.* 23:109 (1989).

129. W.R. Tyor, J.D. Glass, J.W. Griffin, et al. Cytokine expression in the brain during the acquired immunodeficiency syndrome. *Ann. Neurol.* 31:349 (1992).

130. P. Gallo, M.G. Piccinno, L. Krzalic, and B. Tavolato. Tumor necrosis factor alpha (TNFα) and neurological diseases: failure in detecting TNFα in the cerebrospinal fluid from patients with multiple sclerosis, AIDS dementia complex, and brain tumors. *J. Neuroimmunol.* 23:41 (1989).

131. I. Elovaara, M. Iivanainen, E. Poutiainen, et al. CSF and serum β2-microglobulin in HIV infection related to neurological dysfunction. *Acta Neurol. Scand.* 79:81 (1989).

132. B.J. Brew, R.B. Bhalla, M. Fleischer, et al. Cerebrospinal fluid β2 microglobulin in patients with human immunodeficiency virus. *Neurology* 39:830 (1989).

133. B.J. Brew, R.B. Bhalla, M. Paul, et al. Cerebrospinal fluid β2 microglobulin in patients with AIDS dementia complex: an expanded series including response to zidovudine treatment. *AIDS* 6:461 (1992).

134. J.C. McArthur, T.E. Nance-Sproson, D.E. Griffin, et al. The diagnostic utility of elevation in cerebrospinal fluid β2 microglobulin in HIV-1 dementia. *Neurology* 42:1707 (1992).

135. T.W. Stone, and M.N. Perkins. Quinolinic acid: a potent endogenous excitant at amino acid receptors in CNS. *Eur. J. Pharmacol.* 72:411 (1981).

136. B.J. Brew, J.Corbeil, C.J. Pemberton, et al. Quinolinic acid and the pathogenesis of AIDS dementia. Presented at the Neuroscience of HIV Infection. *Basic and Clinical Frontiers*, Amsterdam, (July 14-17, 1992).

137. M.P. Heyes, B.J. Brew, A. Martin, et al. Quinolinic acid in cerebrospinal fluid and serum in HIV-1 infection: Relationship to clinical and neurological status. *Ann. Neurol.* 29:202 (1991).

138. C.M. Mastroianni, G.M. Liuzzi, and P. Ricco. AIDS dementia complex: on the relationship between HIV-1 infection, immune-mediated response and myelin damage in the brain. *Acta Neurol.* 13:184 (1991).

139. H.W. Pfister, K.M. Einhaupl, A. Fateh-Moghadam, et al. Myelin basic

protein in the cerebrospinal fluid of patients infected with HIV. *J. Neurol.* 236:288 (1989).

140. D.W. Marshall, R.L. Brey, C.A. Butzin. Lack of cerebrospinal fluid myelin basic protein in HIV-infected asymptomatic individuals with intrathecal synthesis of IgG. *Neurology* 39:1127 (1989).

141. M.J.D. Post, J.R. Berger, and G.T. Henley. The radiology of central nervous system disease in acquired immunodeficiency syndrome (Chapter 38A), *in*: "Radiology: Diagnosis-Imaging-Intervention," J.B. Lippincott Co., Philadelphia (1988).

142. E.M. Burstzyn, B.C.P. Lee, and J. Bauman. CT of acquired immunodeficiency syndrome. *A.J.N.R.* 5:711 (1984).

143. R.M. Levy, S. Rosenbloom, and L.V. Perrett. Neuroradiology findings in AIDS: a review of 200 cases. *A.J.N.R.* 7:833 (1985).

144. A. Sönnerborg, J. Sääf, B. Alexius, et al. Quantitative detection of brain aberrations in human immunodeficiency virus type 1-infected individuals by magnetic resonance imaging. *J. Infect.Dis.* 162:1245 (1990).

145. W.L. Olesen, F.M. Longo, C.M. Mills, and D. Norman. White matter disease in AIDS: findings at MR imaging. *Radiology* 169:445 (1988).

146. I. Elovaara, E. Poutianinen, R. Raininko, et al. Mild brain atrophy in early HIV infection: the lack of association with cognitive deficits and HIV-specific intrathecal immune response. *J. Neurol. Sci.* 99:121 (1990).

147. M.J.D. Post, B. Levin, J.R. Berger, et al. Sequential cranial MR findings of asymptomatic and neurologically symptomatic HIV+ subjects. *A.J.N.R.* 13:359 (1992).

148. D.A. Rottenberg, J.R. Moeller, S.C. Strother, et al. The metabolic pathology of the AIDS dementia complex. *Ann. Neurol.* 22:700 (1987).

149. P.J. Ell, D.C. Costa, and M. Harrison. Imaging cerebral damage in HIV infection. *Lancet* 2:569 (1987).

150. E. Schielke, K. Tatsch, W. Pfister, et al. Reduced cerebral blood flow in early stages of human immunodeficiency virus infection. *Arch. Neurol.* 47:1342 (1990).

151. J.C. Masdeu, A. Yudd, R.L. Van Heertum, et al. Single photon emission computed tomography in human immunodeficiency virus encephalopathy: a preliminary report. *J. Nucl. Med.* 32:1471 (1991).

152. D.K. Menon, J.G. Ainsworth, J. Cox, et al. Proton MR spectroscopy of the brain in AIDS dementia complex. *J. Comput. Assist. Tomogr.* 16:538 (1992).

153. I. Elovaara, P. Saar, S.-L. Valle, et al. EEG in early HIV-1 infection is characterized by anterior dysrhythmicity of low maximal amplitude. *Clin. Electroencephal.* 22:131 (1991).

154. A. Beaumanoir, P. Vurkhard, G. Gauthier, et al. EEG dans 19 cas de SIDA avec atteinte de l'encephale. *Neurophysiol. Clin.* 18:313 (1988).

155. D.H. Gabuzda, S.R. Levy, and K.H. Chiappa. Electroencephalography in AIDS and AIDS-related complex. *Clin. Electroencephal.* 19:1 (1988).

156. M.R. Nuwer, E.N. Miller, B.R. Visscher, et al. Asymptomatic HIV infection does not cause EEG abnormalities: results from the Multicenter AIDS Cohort Study (MACS). *Neurology* 42:1214 (1992).

157. P. Tinuper, P. de Carolis, M. Gaelotti, et al. Electroencephalogram and HIV infection: a prospective study in 100 patients. *Clin. Electroencephal.* 21:145 (1990).

158. A. Parisi, M. Strosselli, G. DiPerri, et al. Electroencephalography in the early diagnosis of HIV-related subacute encephalitis: analysis of 185 patients. *Clin. Electroencephal.* 20:1-5 (1989).

159. A. Parisi, G. DiPerri, M. Strosselli, et al. Usefulness of computerized electroencephalography in diagnosing, staging and monitoring AIDS-dementia complex. *AIDS* 3:209 (1989).

160. T.M. Itil, S. Ferracuti, A. Freedman, et al. Computer-analyzed EEG (CEEF) and dynamic brain mapping in AIDS and HIV-related syndrome: a pilot study. *Clin. Electroencephal.* 21:140 (1990).

161. M.A. Pagano, P.E. Cahn, M.L. Garau, et al. Brain-stem auditory evoked

potentials in human immunodeficiency virus-seropositive patients with and without acquired immunodeficiency syndrome. *Arch. Neurol.* 4:166 (1992).

162. H.-J. Welkoborsky, and K. Lowitzsch. Auditory brain stem responses in patients with human immunotropic virus infection of different stages. *Ear Hearing* 132:55 (1992).

163. G.M. Goodwin, A. Chiswick, V. Egan, et al. The Edinburgh cohort of HIV-positive drug users: auditory event-related potentials show progressive slowing in patients with Centers for Disease Control stage IV disease. *AIDS* 4:1243 (1990).

164. C. Ollo, R. Johnson, Jr., and J. Grafman. Signs of cognitive change in HIV disease: an event-related brain potential study. *Neurology* 41:209 (1991).

165. R. Rothenberg, M. Woelfel, R. Stoneburner, et al. Survival with the acquired immunodeficiency syndrome: experience with 5,833 cases in New York City. *N. Engl. J. Med.* 317:1297. (1987).

166. R.W. Klecker, J.M. Collins, R. Yarchoan, et al. Plasma and cerebrospinal fluid pharmacokinetics of 3'-azido-3'-deoxythymidine: a novel pyrimidine analog with potential application for the treatment of patients with AIDS and related diseases. *Clin. Pharmacol. Ther.* 41:407 (1987).

167. R. Yarchoan, K.W. Weinhold, H.K. Lyerly, et al. Administration of 3'-azido-3'-deoxythymidine, an inhibitor of HTLV-III/LAV replication, to patients with AIDS or AIDS-related complex. *Lancet* 1:570 (1986).

168. M. Hollweg, R.-R. Riedel, F-D. Goebel, U.Schick, and D. Naber. Remarkable improvement of neuropsychiatric symptoms in HIV-infected patients after AZT therapy. *Klin. Wochensch.* 69:409 (1991).

169. F.A. Schmitt, J.W. Bigley, R. McKinnis, et al. Neuropsychological outcome of zidovudine (AZT) treatment of patients with AIDS and AIDS-related complex. *N. Engl. J. Med.* 319:1573 (1988).

170. A. Brunetti, G. Berg, G. DiChiro, et al. Reversal of brain metabolic abnormalities following treatment of AIDS dementia complex with 3'-azido-2',3'-dideoxythymidine (AZT, zidovudine): a PET-FDG study., *J. Nucl. Med.* 30:581 (1989).

171. J.J. Sidtis, C. Gatsonis, R.W. Price, et al. Zidovudine treatment of the AIDS dementia complex: results of a placebo-controlled trial. *Ann. Neurol.* 33:343 (1993).

172. P.A. Pizzo, J. Eddy, J. Falloon, et al. Effect of continuous intravenous infusion of zidovudine (AZT) in children with symptomatic HIV infection. *N. Engl. J. Med.* 319:889 (1988).

173. K.M. Butler, R.N. Husson, R.M. Balis, et al. Dideoxyinosine in children with symptomatic human immunodeficiency virus infection. *N. Engl. J. Med.* 324:137 (1991).

174. E.R. Stiehm, Y.J. Bryson, L.M. Frenkel, et al. Prednisone improves human immunodeficiency virus encephalopathy in children. *Pediatr. Infect. Dis. J.* 11:49 (1992).

175. F.T. Saulsburg, K.A. Bringelsen, and D.E. Normansell. Effects of prednisone on human immunodeficiency virus infection. *South. Med. J.* 84:431 (1991).

176. T.P. Bridge, P.N.R. Heseltine, E.S. Parker, et al. Results of extended peptide T administration in AIDS and ARC patients. *Psychopharmacol. Bull.* 27:237 (1991).

177. B.J. Dezube, A.B. Pardee, B. Chapman, et al. Pentoxifylline decreases tumor necrosis factor expression and serum triglycerides in people with AIDS. *J. AIDS* 6:787 (1993).

CELLULAR AND MOLECULAR PATHOLOGY OF NOVEL CEREBRAL DISEASES IN AIDS

Peter L. Lantos

Department of Neuropathology
Institute of Psychiatry
London SE5 8AF United Kingdom

INTRODUCTION

Soon after the beginning of the acquired immunodeficiency syndrome (AIDS) epidemic, it was realized that the nervous system is a principle target of the human immunodeficiency virus-1 (HIV-1) infection. Neurologic complications in 50 unselected patients, some of whom had undergone postmortem examination, included opportunistic infections, lymphomas, and vascular diseases.[1] Subsequent neuropathologic studies on large cohorts have confirmed the important role of the nervous system in AIDS: neural tissues have been affected in the overwhelming majority of patients. Indeed, no parts of the nervous system have been spared: the brain and spinal cord, peripheral nerves and muscles have all been involved (for review see refs. 2, 3). Multinucleated giant cells, thought to be pathognomonic of HIV-1, were described in the brain,[4] and subsequently HIV-1 itself has been demonstrated by immunocytochemistry, electron microscopy, *in situ* hybridization and polymerase chain reaction (PCR) in the brain (for review, see refs. 3, 5).

The neuropathologic investigations have yielded three important observations. First, diseases affecting the central nervous system (CNS) fall into two distinct groups. The first group contains opportunistic infections, neoplasms and vascular complications, secondary diseases which develop as a consequence of immunosuppression caused by HIV-1. The spectrum of these diseases is not greatly different from the range of pathologies associated with other immunocompromised states. Viral, protozoan, bacterial and fungal infections may all develop, and although there are geographic differences in incidence, cytomegalovirus and toxoplasmosis occur most frequently with an average of 15.8% and 13.6% of cases, respectively, followed by cryptococcus (7.6%), progressive multifocal leucoencephalopathy (4.0%), and herpes simplex (1.6%). Of the neoplasms, primary and secondary lymphomas may affect the CNS in 5.5% and 2.1% of cases, respectively.[6] These are B cell lymphomas, often undifferentiated with the usual angiocentric pattern and diffuse, extensive invasion of the brain. Kaposi's sarcomas, whether primary or secondary, are extremely rare in the nervous system. Interestingly, an increased incidence of astroglial tumors has recently been reported.[7] The vascular complications, infarcts and hemorrhages, result from complex focal and generalized factors. The second group of diseases is associated primarily with HIV-1, although the causal role of the virus, with the exception of the first two disease entities, remains to be established. These have been defined in a consensus report and include: HIV-encephalitis, HIV-leucoencephalopathy,

Technical Advances in AIDS Research in the Human Nervous System
Edited by E.O. Major and J.A. Levy, Plenum Press, New York, 1995

vacuolar myelopathy and vacuolar leucoencephalopathy, lymphocytic meningitis, diffuse poliodystrophy and cerebral vasculitis, including granulomatous angiitis.[8]

The second important observation is that multiple pathologies are the rule rather than the exception in advanced AIDS. The nervous system may be afflicted by more than one disease: the brain not uncommonly may show HIV-encephalitis in combination with opportunistic infections and lymphomas. The third interesting finding is that the pathologic spectrum is not the same in different risk groups: the neuropathology varies in homosexual men, hemophiliacs, drugs abusers, and in children. An early finding of the low incidence of opportunistic infections, lymphomas and HIV-1-specific diseases in hemophiliacs[9] was confirmed in a larger comparative necropsy study[10] which found significantly higher prevalence of opportunistic infections (toxoplasmosis, cytomegalovirus) and progressive multifocal leucoencephalopathy, in nonhemophiliacs than in hemophiliacs. In contrast, fresh and old hemorrhages and cirrhosis of the liver were significantly more common in hemophiliacs. The most likely explanation for these differences is that hemophiliacs had died of intracerebral hemorrhage or cirrhosis at an early stage of the disease before the more advanced neuropathologic abnormalities associated with AIDS could have developed. More recently, neuropathologic differences were also observed between homosexual men and drug abusers in Edinburgh, Scotland. Giant cell encephalitis was more common in drug abusers (57% versus 25%), whereas both lymphomas and opportunistic infections developed more often in homosexual men. Since the amount of provirus, as demonstrated by PCR, did not correlate closely with the presence or severity of giant cell encephalitis, an explanation for these differences has yet to be found.[11] In children, a neuropathologic study of 174 cases from seven large medical centers in the U.S. revealed that microencephalopathy or brain atrophy was the commonest abnormality (65.5%), followed by HIV encephalitis (36.2%) and vascular pathology (17.2%), while opportunistic infections were relatively rare (9.7%). Thus, the CNS of children appears to be more often and more severely affected than that of adults.[12]

Recent investigations have focused on new cerebral diseases caused by HIV-1. The aim of this review is to define these novel cerebral diseases, and to describe the underlying cellular and molecular changes.

NOVEL CEREBRAL DISEASES ASSOCIATED WITH HIV-1

A consensus report by an international group of neuropathologists has attempted to introduce a neuropathologically-based terminology and to define diseases caused by HIV in the nervous system.[8] The following is a brief review of novel cerebral diseases in HIV-1 infection based on this nomenclature.

HIV-1 Encephalitis

This term should now replace various names previously in use, including AIDS-dementia complex, AIDS encephalopathy, subacute encephalitis with multinucleated giant cells, multinucleated giant cell encephalitis, etc. Macroscopically, HIV-1 encephalitis may or may not be associated with cerebral atrophy; in many cases of uncomplicated HIV-1 encephalitis, the brain may appear normal. Histologically, the encephalitis is characterized by multiple foci of cellular infiltrates composed of multinucleated giant cells, microglial cells, macrophages, and a varying number of lymphocytes. Astrocytosis is often seen. The presence of multinucleated giant cells is a diagnostic hallmark in the setting of other features of HIV encephalitis. These cells, formed by the fusion of macrophages, are the single most striking feature of HIV-1 encephalitis. The pattern of inflammation varies from case-to-case, but overall the white matter, deep grey matter and cortex are involved in this order of frequency. Macrophages, microglial cells and multinucleated giant cells may all be infected by HIV-1, and viral antigens and nucleic acids can be demonstrated by immunocytochemistry and *in situ* hybridization. The frequency of HIV-1 encephalitis varies from series-to-series, but the average incidence of 30.9%[6] seems reasonable and is accordance with our own experience. HIV-1 encephalitis may be complicated by opportunistic infections,most often by cytomegalovirus or toxoplasmosis. Coinfections of HIV-1 with JC virus have also been reported, with each virus infecting in a latent or productive fashion different cell populations to result in particularly severe encephalitis.[13]

HIV Leucoencephalopathy

In HIV leucoencephalopathy, the white matter bears the brunt of the disease: myelin loss, astrocytosis and the presence of macrophages and multinucleated giant cells characterize this diffuse damage. Without multinucleated giant cells, the presence of viral antigens or nucleic acids should be demonstrated by immunocytochemistry or *in situ* hybridization to confirm the diagnosis. The white matter of the cerebral hemispheres is usually extensively and symmetrically affected, but the cerebellar white matter may also be involved. The myelin loss appears as diffuse pallor on myelin stains, while histologically, there is evidence of the myelin lamellae being damaged and phagocytosed by macrophages. This disease, originally described as progressive diffuse leucoencephalopathy[14] has recently been further characterized, but doubts still exist as to whether this is a separate entity or part of a disease spectrum with an overlap with HIV encephalitis. Simple myelin pallor with or without astrocytosis in the absence of multinucleated giant cells and demonstrable HIV antigens or nucleic acids is a nonspecific change and in itself is not diagnostic of HIV leucoencephalopathy.

Vacuolar Myelopathy and Vacuolar Leucoencephalopathy

Petito et al.[15] originally described vacuolar myelopathy in AIDS patients, and noted the similarities with subacute combined degeneration of the spinal cord. Indeed, the posterior and lateral funiculi are chiefly involved, particularly at the level of the thoracic cord. Vacuolar myelopathy is the most common abnormality of the spinal cord in 18-30% of adult patients. It may be the sole abnormality of the spinal cord or it may occur in association with other diseases.[16]

The myelin damage becomes obvious on myelin stain by the pallor of the posterior and lateral funiculi. Histologically, there are vacuolar swellings of the myelin lamellae, the so-called vacuolar myelinopathy, and macrophages are replete with myelin debris within myelin sheaths. The macrophage response and the accompanying astrocytosis are usually proportional to the severity of the disease. Axonal damage varies according to disease severity from relatively well preserved axons in milder cases to occasional axonal spheroids in more severely affected cords. The severity of the disease was originally graded depending on the number of vacuoles, and the clinical deficits correlated well with the location and severity of the lesions.[15,16] However, vacuolar myelopathy is not a specific manifestation of AIDS and may occur in the absence of HIV infection.[17] The etiology is disputed: in addition to HIV infection of the spinal cord, metabolic cause, particularly B12 deficiency and infection by an opportunistic infection have been considered as causative factors.[16] A recent study indicates that vacuolar myelopathy in AIDS may not be due to direct HIV infection, but may be secondary to other factors, including abnormalities of folic acid or transcobalamine metabolism.[18] The same lesion may occasionally develop in the brain. This vacuolar leucoencephalopathy may occur as diffuse or focal myelin damage.

The pathogenesis of these vacuolar changes in the spinal cord has recently been investigated. In the spinal cord of HIV-positive patients, the predominant mononuclear cells are macrophages, present mainly in the posterior and lateral funiculi. These cells are more numerous than in HIV-negative controls and immunostain for class I and class II antigens as well as for interleukin 1 (IL-1) and tumor necrosis factor-α (TNF-α). The number of these activated macrophages is greatly increased in HIV infection in the spinal cord with or without vacuolar myelopathy, indicating that they are present before vacuolar myelopathy develops. Thus, a sequence of events is envisaged: activated macrophages release cytokines, such as TNF-α, which being toxic for myelin or oligodendrocytes, will damage myelin, whose debris will then be removed by macrophages, resulting in vacuole formation.[19]

Lymphocytic Meningitis

The clinical involvement of the meninges in the form of an aseptic meningitis is an early event of HIV-1 infection. Leptomeningeal thickening and focal accumulation of lymphocytes are not uncommonly seen at postmortem examination. However, this definition envisages significant lymphocytic infiltration of the leptomeninges and perivascular spaces without any demonstrable opportunistic pathogens.

Diffuse Poliodystrophy

Of the newly defined HIV-associated disease entities, this is clearly the most controversial and most elusive. The morphologic definition simply requires diffuse astrocytosis and microglial activation in the cerebral grey matter. The term was originally conceived to describe diffuse damage to the cerebral cortex, basal ganglia, and brainstem nuclei.[20] While there is little doubt that these abnormalities often occur in AIDS, and that grey matter pathology may occur independently of lesions in the white matter, the concept of poliodystrophy as a separate nosologic entity has not been universally accepted. In any grey matter pathology, the potential damage to the neurons should be established, yet the present definition of poliodystrophy does not address the question of neuronal loss.

Cerebral Vasculitis

Perivascular cuffing by mononuclear cells, lymphocytes, and pigment-containing macrophages, is often noted in AIDS brains. The lymphocytic cuffing is usually associated with lymphocytic leptomeningitis. However, this should not be confused with true cerebral vasculitis in which the vascular wall is infiltrated by lymphocytes.[21] In granulomatous angiitis, the vascular infiltrate may contain lymphocytes, plasma cells, macrophages, and multinucleated giant cells.[22] The pathogenetic relationship between these vascular diseases and HIV-1 infection remains to be established.

CELLULAR AND MOLECULAR PATHOLOGY OF THE BRAIN IN HIV-1 INFECTION

Neuronal Changes

Neuronal Loss. There is now increasing evidence to show that HIV-1 infection of the brain is associated with neuronal loss. In a preliminary morphometric analysis, neuronal density and perikaryal volume were assessed in Brodmann's area 11 of the fronto-orbital region of 18 unselected AIDS brains and the results compared with controls. Neuronal density was reduced by 18% and perikaryal volume by 31%.[23] However, since the area of neuronal profiles did not change significantly, this volume decrease probably reflected the change in neuronal density. As several patients were demented, the authors speculated that the significant neuronal loss was partly responsible for dementia. The brains in this study were unselected and had been affected by the usual range of diseases associated with AIDS, including opportunistic infections, lymphomas, and HIV-1 encephalitis. Therefore, it is difficult, if not impossible, to establish the pathogenetic role of HIV-1 in neuronal loss. Another study has, however, addressed the issue by analyzing neuronal populations in the superior frontal gyrus of those AIDS patients who had only either HIV-1 encephalitis or minimal pathology (perivascular cuffing or mild astrocytosis) in the brain. Using two independent methods, computer-assisted image analysis and a novel robust stereologic method, called the disector,[24] the results unequivocally showed a significant neuronal loss of 38% which occurred irrespective of whether encephalitis was present or not.[25] Therefore, this was the first study which demonstrated neuronal loss in the absence of any significant pathology. Further studies by the same group have demonstrated various degrees of neuronal loss in the neocortex: 30% loss in the primary visual cortex and 18% in the superior parietal lobule, while the inferior temporal gyrus did not show any significant change.[26] Reduction in the number of cortical neurons (200-500 μ^2) was also observed in the midfrontal, superior temporal and inferior parietal regions in brains with HIV encephalitis.[27] The discrepancy between the finding in the superior and inferior temporal gyri is not surprising in the light of investigations of aging changes; they have indicated that the inferior temporal gyrus is least affected by neuronal loss.[28]

A striking difference was found between the fronto-orbital cortex (Brodmann's area 11) and the superior parietal lobule (area 7): while in the former there was significant loss of neurons, accompanied by reduced perikaryal volume fraction, in the latter no neuronal damage was noted. Interestingly, neuronal loss did not correlate significantly with the development of dementia and HIV-specific neuropathology.[29] However, neuronal loss has not been found by quantitative morphometry in Brodmann areas 4, 9 and 40 in a prospective study using neuroimaging and psychometric evaluation of 6 AIDS patients and 6 controls.[30] These analyses clearly show that neuronal populations are not uniformly affected throughout the neocortex. This selective vulnerability, different from the pattern seen in neurodegenerative diseases, was confirmed by an immunocytochemical study. Parvalbumin and neurofilament immunoreactive neurons were quantified in the frontal cortex and hippocampus in cases of HIV encephalitis. While the density of both types of neurons appeared to be independent of the severity of HIV encephalitis in the hippocampus, there was a trend toward decreased density of parvalbumin-positive neurons reaching significance only in the CA3 layer.[31] These findings show that HIV encephalitis differentially affects specific populations of neurons. In all these investigations, neuronal populations have been assessed in fully developed AIDS and to date, only one study addressed the question of neuronal damage in the early stage of HIV-1 infections. Everall et al.[32] estimated neuronal density in the superior frontal gyrus of 14, HIV-infected, but symptom-free individuals and 15 HIV-negative controls. All were intravenous drug users and none had HIV-associated neuropathology. In contrast to AIDS patients, there was no difference in neuronal density between the HIV-positive and control groups, indicating that neuronal fallout occurs late during HIV infection.

Neuronal loss has been reported not only in the neocortex, but also in other areas of the brain, including the cerebellum,[33,34] inferior olivary nucleus,[34] substantia nigra,[35] and putamen,[36] but surprisingly not in the hippocampus.[37] Interestingly, neuronal loss in the putamen, as shown by pattern analysis, does not occur randomly, as the arrangement pattern is altered, indicating that neurotoxicity may be selective by affecting certain vulnerable, as yet unidentified neuronal populations.[38] Treatment with zidovudine (AZT) influences neuronal populations: neuronal density significantly increased by 22% in the CA1 area of the hippocampus of untreated patients, compared with the treated and control groups.[39] The cause of increased neuronal numerical density is uncertain, but thought to represent changes in the neuropil which may reflect primary dendritic damage.

Dendritic and Synaptic Changes. Neuronal damage is also reflected by dendritic and synaptic abnormalities developing in HIV infection. Qualitative and quantitative immunocytochemical analyses of synaptic density in the frontal region, using synaptophysin, revealed synaptic loss in cases of HIV encephalitis.[40]

Using a modified Golgi impregnation technique, in the midfrontal region, the apical dendrites became dilated, vacuolated and tortuous, and both their length and branching pattern were reduced in HIV encephalitis. Similar changes were observed in the basal and oblique dendrites, but to a lesser extent. Quantitative assessment revealed a 40-60% decrease in spine density throughout the entire length of the dendrites. Moreover, aberrant spines were noted in relation to abnormal second-order dendritic branches in laser confocal microscopy. However, no morphologic or quantitative differences were found between HIV-seropositive cases without encephalitis and controls, indicating that these severe dendritic changes occur only as a result of HIV encephalitis and not of HIV infection *per se*.[40] From these findings, the authors concluded that primary dendritic damage plays an important role in HIV encephalitis in contrast to other neurodegenerative diseases in which the primary pathology is presynaptic. Since, from the pathogenetic view, it is of considerable importance whether these changes occur with or without encephalitis, the results of a recent quantitative assessment of dendritic spines in the brains of cynomolgus monkeys infected by SIV_{mac251} gave additional insight. The spine count was consistently and significantly decreased in short-term infection and it was further reduced in the later stage of infection. This change occurred in the absence of encephalitis, indicating that severe neuronal damage, which may have profound clinical implications, may develop without infiltration by macrophages and microglia.[41]

The mechanism of neurotoxicity will be covered elsewhere, but it has recently been established that the administration of purified gp120 causes dystrophic dendritic changes in pyramidal neurons throughout the cerebral cortex and may lead to behavioral retardation.[42]

Spongiform Change. Spongiform encephalopathy has been reported in AIDS patients.[43,44] Both the fine vacuolation and the coarser sponginess (*status spongiosus*) were observed in the grey matter, accompanied by focal loss of neurons. The pathogenesis of vacuole formation could not be ascertained, but electron microscopy revealed that some of the vacuoles were, in fact, remnants of dendrites. These findings pose an interesting question. Does immunosuppression by HIV activate the highly atypical pathogen of transmissible spongiform encephalopathies to result in yet another opportunistic infection, and thus widen the spectrum of HIV-associated neurologic diseases? Prion proteins, however, could not be detected by Western blot analysis in the brains of AIDS patients with spongiform change.[45] Moreover, immunostaining with an antibody to prion prion yielded negative results in AIDS brains with spongiform degeneration (Lantos, unpublished observation).

Oligodendrocytes

Considering the frequency and severity of white matter damage in HIV infection, very little is known about oligodendroglial changes. While the often observed white matter pallor may be a nonspecific phenomenon, frequently resulting from edema, vacuolar leucoencephalopathy and vacuolar myelopathy both involve destruction of myelin sheaths. In an immunocytochemical study, mild myelin damage was associated with an increase of oligodendrocytes, and only in severe myelin damage did their number decrease. These oligodendroglial changes may represent an attempt to repair myelin damage caused by HIV. Their reactive capacity will become exhausted only in severe myelin damage, but even at this later stage, there was no gross loss of oligodendrocytes.[46] HIV p24 antigen was detected in all cases of severe myelin damage, but less frequently in brains with milder myelin loss. These findings raise the possibility of a low-grade persistent or latent infection of oligodendrocytes. Investigating cytokine expression of macrophages in vacuolar myelopathy, Tyor et al.[19] stipulated that cytokines, including IL-1 and TNF-α locally produced by macrophages, will have toxic effects on myelin or oligodendrocytes. Kimura-Kuroda et al.[47] have demonstrated that gp120 inhibits myelination and reduces the length and arborization of oligodendroglial processes in primary cultures of the rat cerebral cortex. Moreover, there was a rapid loss of the myelin already produced. These results suggest that gp120 may cause not only a functional disorder of oligodendrocytes, but also demyelination *in vitro*; these deleterious effects on the oligodendrocyte-myelin unit can explain the myelin damage and loss seen in HIV infection.

Astrocytes

Astrocytes play a prominent role in HIV-1 infection of the CNS: HIV encephalitis, HIV leucoencephalopathy, and diffuse poliodystrophy are all associated with astrocytic changes, usually astrocytosis, a proliferation of these cells. An increased activity of astrocytes, as well as microglial cells, was noted in the frontal cortex in all, including asymptomatic HIV-infected cases. Although the degree of these glial changes apparently correlated with the severity of lesions in the white matter, diffuse increase of glial fibrillary acidic protein (GFAP)-positive cells occurred even in those cortical areas which covered mildly or moderately affected areas.[48] However, a recent combined, morphometric and immunohistochemical study has cast some doubt on the widely held view of astrocytic hyperplasia in AIDS. In the frontal and parietal cortex, although the total number of astrocytes did not change in AIDS brains compared with controls, the number of GFAP-positive astrocytes significantly increased, while the number of GFAP-negative cells accordingly decreased. However, the nuclear size increased in both GFAP-positive and negative cells, while the cytoplasmic size increased only in GFAP-positive astrocytes. These findings do not support astrocytic hyperplasia in AIDS, but indicate the production of GFAP by protoplasmic astrocytes and the hypertrophy of these cells.[49]

Whether astrocytes themselves are infected or not is controversial and has been disputed. Although nonproductive infection of normal and neoplastic astrocytic cell lines has been known to occur, productive *in vitro* infection of astrocytes in human fetal organotypic cultures has only recently been reported.[50] Chronically infected astrocytoma cells in culture with restricted virus production express different antigenic forms of *nef* which can then be distinguished by their subcellular localization.[51] Moreover, infection of astrocytes in the postmortem brain has also been demonstrated. *In vitro* infection is characterized by restriction of gene repression to regulatory mRNAs and proteins like *nef*. Using immunocytochemistry for *nef* and GFAP, and *in situ* hybridization with monospecific *nef* probes, both *nef* mRNA and protein have been demonstrated in the brain of children who died with AIDS-associated progressive encephalopathy. In some cases, up to 20% of the reactive astrocytes showed evidence of HIV infection.[52] *In situ* PCR has also confirmed the presence of HIV-positive astrocytes in the brain.[53] The central role astrocytes play in cerebral pathology has been further confirmed by recent experimental evidence. By interfering with cerebral β adrenergic receptors, gp120 may alter astrocytic reactivity and glial-neuronal interactions and thus upset the delicate network of cytokines which is responsible for preventing viral and other infections.[54] Moreover, in transgenic mice, astrocytic expression of gp120 induced extensive astrocytosis and microglial activation, and neuropathologic changes which resembled those seen in HIV infection in man.[55]

Another, as yet unexplored aspect of astrocytic pathology is the occurrence of astrocytomas in AIDS patients. Following single case reports,[56-58] four further cases have recently been reported.[7] However, the causal relationship between these gliomas and HIV infection remains controversial. The occurrence of astrocytomas in AIDS patients may be coincidental, reflecting their expected prevalence in the population. Nonetheless, potential pathogenetic factors abound, including activation of a dominant oncogene or inactivation of a tumor suppressor gene by a viral promoter, impairment of the host's immune defenses, production of growth factors and cytokines, etc.

Astrocytes are now considered to play an increasingly important role in the pathogenesis of neuronal pathology. Neuronal damage caused by gp120 *in vitro* can be prevented by vasoactive intestine polypeptide (VIP) and by peptide T, its five-amino acid sequence homolog. VIP induces astrocytes to increase oscillations in intracellular calcium and to release factors essential for normal neuronal activity. gp120 may compete with endogenous VIP for a receptor on astrocytes, thus interfering with neuronal function.[59] Alternatively, neurotoxicity, elicited by HIV-infected macrophages may be amplified through a cell-to-cell interaction with astrocytes. These macrophage-astrocyte interactions produce cytokines, including TNF-α and IL-1β, and arachidonic acid metabolites. These, in turn, cause astrocytic proliferation and neuronal damage. TNF-α can also damage myelin and oligodendroglia as well as regulate HIV-1 gene expression. The resulting astrocytosis amplifies these cellular processes, while HIV infection is maintained in microglial cells, macrophages, mutinucleated giant cells, and possibly in astrocytes.[60]

The cytokines and/or arachidonic acid metabolites released by astrocytes and by macrophages and microglial cells may act synergistically with glutamate to activate N-methyl-D-aspartate (NMDA) receptors which, in turn, increase intracellular calcium. Nitric oxide synthase (NOS) is then activated and the resulting excessive production of nitric oxide destroys neurons.[61]

Cell adhesion molecules on the surface of astrocytes, as well as of neurons, elicited by HIV-1-infected monocytes in primary cultures of human fetal CNS may be another factor in the complex mechanism of neural tissue damage. The cytopathic effect is likely to be determined by the release of viral antigens either within the site of adhesion itself or within close range of the astrocytic membrane.[62]

Microglial Cells and Macrophages

Microglial cells and macrophages, together with multinucleated giant cells, are infected and play a pivotal role in HIV-associated pathology in the CNS. They are the predominant cell type in HIV encephalitis, HIV leucoencephalopathy, and vacuolar leucoencephalopathy and myelopathy. Microglial activation is also a feature of the more elusive diffuse poliodystrophy. Many investigations, using immunocytochemistry and *in situ* hybridization, have convincingly demonstrated HIV antigens and nucleic acids in macrophages, microglial cells, and multinucleated giant cells (for review, see ref. 63). Electron microscopy also revealed retroviral particles in these cells. Moreover, in a double-labeling immunocytochemical assessment, using cell-specifc markers to identify various cell types, only macrophages and microglial cells, labeled with *Ricinus communis* agglutinin-1, were found to contain the envelope glycoprotein, gp41, in cases of HIV encephalitis.[64]

Microglial reaction appears early in HIV infection: a transient increase in the density of microglial cells was observed in HIV-positive, but non-AIDS patients; the same brains also contained HIV proviral DNA.[65] In these asymptomatic, HIV-positive brains, the microglial response may be diffuse or more localized, particularly around blood vessels, often with lymphocytes forming perivascular cuffs. Once HIV encephalitis develops, the microglial response becomes rampant with disseminated foci of macrophages, microglial cells, and multinucleated giant cells. Multinucleated cells have been shown to bear macrophage markers (for review, see ref. 63), and are likely to derive from them. The size of multinucleated giant cells ranges from 10 μm up to 60-70 μm and the number of nuclei may exceed 25-30: these are often arranged at the periphery of the cytoplasm, but not infrequently are distributed haphazardly or may even form "nuclear clusters". These cells are not evenly dispersed in the brain. In HIV encephalitis, gp41-positive microglial cells are most frequently demonstrated in the globus pallidus, while the corpus striatum and thalamus contain fewer labeled cells. Of the infratentorial sites, many immunostained cells are present in the ventral midbrain, particularly, the substantia nigra, and dentate nucleus. A lower level of infection is observed in the cerebral and cerebellar white matter, and gp41-positive cells are rare in the cerebral cortex. The distribution of these infected cells is reminiscent of the pattern of a multisystem atrophy, but preferential involvement of the deep grey matter, particularly the basal ganglia, remains to be explained. There is no evidence that microglial cells in the basal ganglia are different from those in other regions, nor can the hypothesis be confirmed that blood vessels in the basal ganglia have unique features which facilitate the entry of HIV into the brain.[66] A recent quantitative analysis has revealed a positive correlation between ventricular enlargement, as an index of cerebral atrophy, and diffuse increase of microglial cells in the frontal cortex, but not with reactive astrocytosis in the cortex and white matter, nor with macrophages in the white matter.[67] However, the significance of this finding is somewhat limited, since the results have not been correlated with neuronal loss, HIV encephalitis, or white matter changes.

Microglial cells and macrophages are also active in vacuolar leucoencephalopathy and myelopathy. They are seen in large numbers in areas of myelin damage and sometimes lipid-laden macrophages are present in the vacuoles (for review see ref. 16). Activated macrophages, positive for IL-1 and TNF-α, increased in the posterior and lateral funiculi in HIV-positive individuals before the development of vacuolar myelopathy, indicating that the presence of these cells, and the cytokines they may release, are a prerequisite for myelin damage.[19]

Neurotoxicity associated with microglial cells and macrophage activity remains, for the time being, the most likely pathogenetic mechanism of cerebral injury. HIV-infected microglial cells and macrophages may release or activate neurotoxic substances, including gp120, cytokines, prostaglandins, oxidative radicals and proteases (for review see refs. 59, 68). Quinolinic acid, a neurotoxin acting through the NMDA receptor, is also produced by HIV-infected and γ-interferon-stimulated macrophages. However, it has recently been shown that the production of quinolinic acid is more dependent on the simultaneous production of cytokines than HIV-1 infection of macrophages.[69] Moreover, these cells are known to proliferate in AIDS, they are infected with HIV and, being ubiquitous in the CNS, are often found in proximity to neurons. These features enable them to play a central role in the complex cellular events of neurotoxicity. However, an alternative mechanism envisages microglial activation and proliferation to be a secondary phenomenon to neuronal damage which may be caused by other pathogenetic events and not by microglia-associated neurotoxicity.[70]

Blood-Brain Barrier: The Cerebral Endothelium

Cerebrovascular lesions, often manifesting as gross infarcts and hemorrhages, have been known to occur in AIDS,[21] but the more subtle disorders of cerebral microcirculation, leading to the breakdown of the blood-brain barrier (BBB) has been only more recently investigated. The penetration of the BBB by HIV-1 occurs early during infection, well before neurologic abnormalities develop.[71] The microvasculature of AIDS patients who did not have opportunistic infections or neoplasms showed striking abnormalities, including mural thickening, increased cellularity and endothelial hypertrophy and pleomorphism. These microvascular abnormalities might be associated with an alteration of the BBB which, in turn, could contribute to the damage of the cerebral parenchyma. Moreover, HIV-infected cells around blood vessels could mediate vascular injury.[72]

Evidence of serum protein leakage across the BBB was found in an immunocytochemical study, using rabbit antisera to human serum, albumin, immunoglobulins, and complement component 3c.[73] Most brains with various lesions associated with HIV had immunostaining in some neurons, glial cells, including astrocytes, in glial-macrophage nodules, endothelial cells, and inflammatory cells in and near destructive lesions. Somewhat different results were found in another immunocytochemical investigation which used detection of fibrinogen and immunoglobulin G to test the permeability of the BBB in postmortem brains with and without HIV encephalitis and in nonimmunosuppressed controls.[74] Both AIDS groups had higher immunostaining for fibrinogen and immunoglobulin G than the control group, but they did not differ significantly from each other. All focal lesions with tissue necrosis, not surprisingly, contained extravasated serum proteins, while 95% of microglial nodules were negative. A diffuse breakdown of the BBB was observed in 50% of the patients with AIDS even in the absence of cerebral pathology, including HIV encephalitis, whereas focal lesions were associated with leakage of serum proteins only when necrosis was present.

The pathogenesis of this diffuse increase of permeability remains to be established, but cytokines are likely to play a role. The diffuse breakdown of the BBB could facilitate viral entry into the brain and initiate a chain of events leading to tissue damage. A morphometric analysis revealed significantly more serum protein immunoreactivity in the glial cells in the subcortical white matter in the brains of AIDS patients with dementia than in those who were not demented or in seronegative controls.[75] Cerebral endothelial cells of all AIDS patients had intense ICAM immunostaining, while seronegative controls were negative. Moreover, NOS was detected in the luminal aspect of the endothelium of all demented patients, 35% of nondemented brains, and 10% of seronegative brains. NADPH-diaphorase activity reflected endothelial NOS immunostaining. These findings suggest that cerebral endothelial expression of ICAM and nitric acid is likely to contribute to the dysfunction of the BBB in AIDS patients with dementia

The original report, demonstrating HIV infection of endothelial cells both by immunocytochemistry and *in situ* hybridization[76] has not been confirmed and remains controversial.

CONCLUSIONS

These recent investigations have clearly demonstrated that HIV-1 infection causes profound and wide-ranging changes in the brain. The novel cerebral diseases need further investigations to refine their nosologic definition. No cell type in the CNS escapes HIV-1: neurons, oligodendrocytes, astrocytes, microglial cells and endothelial cells are all affected. There is increasing evidence that in addition to macrophages, microglia and multinucleated giant cells, at least one type of neuroepithelial cell, the astrocyte, is also infected. HIV-1 infection may cause neuronal loss even in the absence of any other pathology: this loss does not occur evenly throughout the brain (thus, a selective vulnerability appears to be operational) and develops at a late stage of the disease. More subtle neuronal abnormalities include devastation of the dendritic tree which together with neuronal loss may considerably contribute to dementia. To establish the precise cellular and molecular mechanism of neurotoxicity in HIV-1 infection remains the single, most important problem facing neuroscientists.

ACKNOWLEDGEMENT

The author wishes to thank the MRC National AIDS Neuropathology Database and Central Brain Tissue Bank in the Department of Neuropathology, Institute of Psychiatry for their help, and Mrs. Elizabeth Kemp for her skillful secretarial assistance.

REFERENCES

1. W.D. Snider, D.M. Simpson, S.L. Nielsen, J.W.M. Gold, C.E. Metroka, and J.B. Posner. Neurological complications of acquired immunodeficiency syndrome: analysis of 50 patients. *Ann. Neurol.* 14:403 (1983).
2. I.P. Everall, and P.L. Lantos. The neuropathology of HIV: a review of the first 10 years. *Int. Rev. Psychiatry* 3:307 (1991).
3. L.R. Sharer. Pathology of HIV-1 infection of the central nervous system: a review. *J. Neuropathol. Exp. Neurol.* 51:3 (1992).
4. L.R. Sharer, E-S. Cho, and L.G. Epstein. Multinucleated giant cells and HTLV-III in AIDS encephalopathy. *Hum. Pathol.* 16:760 (1985).
5. J. Michaels, L.R. Sharer, and L.G. Epstein. Human immunodeficiency virus type 1 (HIV-1) infection of the nervous system: a review. *Immunodef. Rev.* 1:71 (1988).
6. K. Kure, J.F. Llena, W.D. Lyman, et al. Human immunodeficiency virus-1

infection of the nervous system: an autopsy study of 268 adult, pediatric, and fetal brains. *Hum. Pathol.* 22:7090 (1991).

7. A. Moulignier, K. Mikol, G. Pialoux, et al. Cerebral glial tumours: an HIV-related neoplasm or a coincidental finding. Report of 4 cases. *Clin. Neuropathol.* 12 (Suppl. 1):S12 (1993).

8. H. Budka, C.A. Wiley, P. Kleihues, et al. HIV-associated disease of the nervous system: review of nomenclature and propose for neuropathology-based terminology. *Brain Pathol.* 3:143 (1991).

9. P.L. Lantos, J.E. McLaughlin, C.L. Scholtz, C.L. Berry, and J.R. Tighe. Neuropathology of the brain in HIV infection. *Lancet* 1:309 (1989).

10. M.M. Esiri, F. Scaravilli, P.R. Millard, and J.N. Harcourt-Webster. Neuropathology of HIV infection in haemophiliacs: comparative necropsy study. *Br. Med. J.* 299:1312 (1989).

11. J. Bell, C. Arango, J. Ironside, et al. Different neuropathological findings in homosexual and drug abusers with AIDS. *Clin. Neuropathol.* 12 (Suppl. 1):S8 (1993).

12. P.B. Kozlowski, P.A. Anzil, C. Rao, et al. Central nervous system (CNS) in children with AIDS: a multicenter study of 174 cases. *Clin. Neuropathol.* 12 (Suppl. 1):S25 (1993).

13. R. Vazeux, M. Cumont, P.M. Girard, et al. Severe encephalitis resulting from coinfections with HIV and JC virus. *Neurology* 40:944 (1990).

14. P. Kleihues, W. Lang, P.C. Burger, et al. Progressive diffuse leukoencephalopathy in patients with acquired immune deficiency syndrome (AIDS). *Acta Neuropathol.* 68:333 (1985).

15. C.K. Petito, B.A. Navia, E-S. Cho, B.D. Jordan, D.C. George, and R.W. Price. Vacuolar myelopathy pathologically resembling subacute combined degeneration in patients with the acquired immunodeficiency syndrome. *N. Engl. J. Med.* 312:874 (1985).

16. C.K. Petito. Myelopathies, *in:* "The Neuropathology of HIV Infection," F. Scaravilli, ed., Springer, London (1993).

17. S. S. Kamin, and C.K. Petito. Idiopathic myelopathies in non-AIDS patients. *Hum. Pathol.* 22:816 (1991).

18. C.K. Petito, K.S. Cash, and M.F. Falangola. HIV antigen and amplified DNA in AIDS spinal cords correlate with macrophage infiltration, but not with vacuolar myelopathy. *J. Neuropathol. Exp. Neurol.* 52:271 (1993).

19. W.R. Tyor, J.D. Glass, N. Baumrind, et al. Cytokine expression of macrophages in HIV-1-associated vacuolar myelopathy. *Neurology* 43:1002 (1993).

20. H. Budka, G. Constanzi, S. Cristina, et al. Brain pathology induced by infection with the human immunodeficiency virus (HIV). A histological, immunocytochemical and electron microscopic study of 100 autopsy cases. *Acta Neuropathol.* 75:185 (1987).

21. H. Mizusawa, A. Hirano, J.F. Llena, and M. Shintaku. Cerebrovascular lesions in acquired immunodeficiency syndrome (AIDS). *Acta Neuropathol.* 76:451 (1988).

22. B.A. Yankner, P.R. Skolnik, G.M. Shoukimos, D.H. Gabuzda, R.A. Sobel, and D.D. Ho. Cerebral granulomatous angiitis associated with isolation of human T-lymphotropic virus type III from the central nervous system. *Ann. Neurol.* 20:362 (1986).

23. S. Ketzler, S. Weis, H. Haug, and H. Budka. Loss of neurons in the frontal cortex in AIDS brains. *Acta Neuropathol.* 80:92 (1990).

24. D.C. Sterio. The unbiased estimation of number and sizes of arbitrary particles using a disector. *J. Microsc.* 134:127 (1984).

25. I.P. Everall, P.J. Luthert, and P.L. Lantos. Neuronal loss in the frontal cortex in HIV infection. *Lancet* 337:1119 (1991).

26. I.P. Everall, P.J. Luthert, and P.L. Lantos. Neuronal number and volume alterations in the neocortex of HIV infected individuals. *J. Neurol. Neurosurg. Psychiatry* 56:481 (1993).

27. C.A. Wiley, E. Masliah, M. Morey, et al. Neocortical damage during HIV infection. *Ann. Neurol.* 29:651 (1991).

28. H. Henderson, B.E. Tomlinson, and P.H. Gibson. Cell counts in human cerebral cortex in normal adults throughout life using an image analysing computer. *J. Neurol. Sci.* 46:113 (1980).
29. S. Weis, H. Haug, and H. Budka. Neuronal damage in the cerebral cortex of AIDS brains: a morphometric study. *Acta Histopathol.* 85:185 (1993).
30. D. Seilhean, C. Duyckaerts, R. Vazeux, et al. HIV-1-associated cognitive/motor complex: absence of neuronal loss in the cerebral neocortex. *Neurology* 43:1492 (1993).
31. E. Masliah, N. Ge, C.L. Achim, L.A. Hanse, and C.L. Wiley. Selective neuronal vulnerability in HIV encephalitis. *J. Neuropathol. Exp. Neurol.* 51:585 (1992).
32. I. Everall, F. Gray, H. Barnes, M. Durigon, P. Luthert, and P. Lantos. Neuronal loss in symptom-free HIV infection. *Lancet* 340:1413 (1992).
33. F. Graus, T. Ribalta, J. Abos, et al. Subacute cerebellar syndrome as the first manifestation of AIDS dementia complex. *Acta Neurol. Scand.* 81:118 (1990).
34. H. Abe, S.Weis, and P. Mehraein. Degeneration of the cerebellar dentate nucleus and the inferior olivary nucleus in HIV-1 infection: a morphometric study. *Clin. Neuropathol.* 12(Suppl. 1):S7 (1993).
35. M.G. Reyes, F. Faraldi, C.S. Senseng, C. Flowers, and R. Fariello. Nigral degeneration in acquired immune deficiency syndrome (AIDS). *Acta Neuropathol.* 82:39 (1991).
36. I.P. Everall, P.J. Luthert, and P.L. Lantos. Cell population changes in the putamen and frontal cortex in HIV infection. *Neuropathol. Appl. Neurobiol.* 17:246 (1991).
37. E. Spargo, I.P. Everall, and P.L. Lantos. Neuronal loss in the hippocampus in Huntington's disease: a comparison with HIV infection. *J. Neurol. Neurosurg. Psychiatry* 56:487 (1993).
38. I. Everall, H. Barnes, E. Spargo, and P. Lantos. Evidence for selective neuronal loss in the putamen in HIV-infected patients using spatial analysis. *Clin. Neuropathol.* 12 (Suppl. 1):S10 (1993).
39. E. Spargo, I.P. Everall, and P.L. Lantos. Evidence that AZT is neuroprotective in the hippocampus in HIV infection. *Clin. Neuropathol.* 12 (Suppl. 1):S14 (1993).
40. E. Masliah, N. Ge, M. Morey, R. DeTeresa, R.D. Terry, and C.A. Wiley. Cortical dendritic pathology in human immunodeficiency virus encephalitis. *Lab. Invest.* 66:285 (1992).
41. M.M. Montgomery, P. Luthert, F. Taffs, and P. Lantos. Dendritic spine abnormalities in Cynomolgus monkeys infected with simian immunodeficiency virus. *Clin. Neuropathol.* 12 (Suppl.1):S5 (1993).
42. J.M. Hill, R.F. Mervis, R. Avidor, T.W. Moody, and D.E. Brenneman. HIV envelope protein-induced neuronal damage and retardation of behavioural development in rat neonates. *Brain Res.* 603:222 (1993).
43. J. Schwenk, F. Cruz-Sanchez, G. Gosztonyi, and J., Cervos-Navarro. Spongiform encephalopathy in a patient with acquired immune deficiency syndrome (AIDS). *Acta Neuropathol.* 74:389 (1987).
44. J. Artigas, F. Niedobitek, G. Grosse, W. Heise, and G. Gosztenyi. Spongiform encephalopathy in AIDS dementia complex: report of five cases. *J. Acq. Immun. Def. Syndr.* 2:374 (1989).
45. P.N. Goldwater, and J.C. Paton. Apparent noninvolvement of prions in the pathogenesis of spongiform change in HIV-infected brain. *J. Neuropathol. Exp. Neurol.* 48:184 (1989).
46. M.M. Esiri, C.S. Morris, and P.R. Millard. Fate of oligodendrocytes in HIV-1 infection. *AIDS* 5:1081 (1991).
47. J. Kimura-Kuroda, K. Nagashima, and K. Yasui. HIV-1 gp120 causes demyelination in a primary cultures of rat cerebral cortex. *Clin. Neuropathol.* 12 (Suppl. 1):S3 (1993).
48. A. Ciardi, E. Sinclair, F. Scaravilli, N.J. Harcourt-Webster, and S. Lucas. The involvement of the cerebral cortex in human immunodeficiency virus encephalopathy: a morphological and immunohistochemical study. *Acta Neuropathol.* 81:51 (1990).

49. S. Weis, H. Haug, and H. Budka. Astroglial changes in the cerebral cortex of AIDS brains: a morphometric and immunohistochemical investigation. *Neuropathol. Appl. Neurobiol.* 19:329 (1993).

50. W. Lyman, K. Weidenham, W. Hatch, W. Rashbaum, and J. Larocca. HIV-1 infection of human fetal CNS organotypic cultures alters cholinergic activation of phospholipase C. *Clin. Neuropathol.* 12 (Suppl. 1):S4 (1993).

51. B. Kohleisen, M. Neumann, R. Hermann, et al. Cellular localization of Nef expressed in persistently HIV-1-infected low-producer astrocytes. *AIDS* 6:1427 (1992).

52. B. Blumberg, L. Sharer, Y. Saito, et al. HIV-1 gene expression restricted to *nef* in astrocytes. *Clin. Neuropathol.* (in press).

53. A. Braun, and G. Nuovo. Demonstration of HIV-1 infected glia in brain tissue sections by PCR *in situ* hybridization. *J. Neuropathol. Exp. Neurol.* 52:270 (1993).

54. G. Levi, M. Patrizio, A. Bernardo, T.C. Petrucci, and C. Agresti. Human immunodeficiency virus coat protein gp120 inhibits the β-adrenergic regulation of astroglial and microglial functions. *Proc. Natl. Acad. Sci. USA* 90:1541 (1993).

55. S. Toggas, E. Masliah, E. Rockenstein, and L. Mucke. Neurotoxicity of viral proteins - HIV-1 gp120 effects in transgenic models. *Clin. Neuropathol.* 12 (Suppl.1):54 (1993).

56. D.D. Ho, T.R. Rota, R.T. Schooley, et al. Isolation of HTLV-III from cerebrospinal fluid and neural tissues of patients with neurologic syndromes related to the acquired immunodeficiency syndrome. *N.Engl. J. Med.* 313:1493 (1985).

57. J. Gasnault, F.X.Roux, and C. Vedrenne. Cerebral astrocytoma in association with HIV infection. *J. Neurol. Neurosurg. Psychiatry* 51:422 (1988).

58. V. Kasantikul, S. Kaoroptham, and M. Hanvanich. Acquired immunodeficiency syndrome associated with cerebral astrocytoma. *Clin. Neuropathol.* 11:25 (1992).

59. S.A. Lipton. HIV-related neurotoxicity. *Brain Pathol.* 1:193 (1991).

60. L.G. Epstein, and H.E. Gendelman. Human immunodeficiency virus type 1 infection of the nervous system: pathogenetic mechanisms. *Ann. Neurol.* 33:429 (1993).

61. V.L. Dawson, T.M. Dawson, G.R. Uhl, and S.H. Snyder. Human immunodeficiency virus type 1 coat protein neurotoxicity mediated by nitric oxide in primary cortical cultures. *Proc. Natl. Acad. Sci. USA* 90:3256 (1993).

62. M. Tardieu, C. Héry, S. Peudenier, O. Boespflug, and L. Montaignier. Human immunodeficiency virus type 1-infected monocytic cells can destroy human neural cells after cell-to-cell adhesion. *Ann. Neurol.* 31:11 (1992).

63. M.M. Esiri. Role of the macrophage in HIV encephalitis, *in*: "The Neuropathology of HIV Infection," F. Scaravillia, ed., Springer, London (1993).

64. K. Kure, W.D. Lyman, K.M. Weidenheim, and D.W. Dickson. Cellular localization of an HIV-1 antigen in subacute AIDS encephalitis using an improved double labeling immunohistochemical method. *Am. J. Pathol.* 136:1085 (1990).

65. F. Scaravilli, E. Sinclair, F. Gray, and A. Ciardi. PCR detection of HIV proviral DNA in the brain of asymptomatic HIV-positive patients: correlation with morphological changes. *Clin. Neuropathol.* 12(Suppl. 1):S13 (1993).

66. K. Kure, K.M. Weidenheim, W.D. Lyman, and D.W. Dickson. Morphology and distribution of HIV-1 gp41-positive microglia in subacute AIDS encephalitis. *Acta Neuropathol.* 80:393 (1990).

67. B.B. Gelman. Diffuse microgliosis associated with cerebral atrophy in the acquired immunodeficiency syndrome. *Ann. Neurol.* 34:65 (1993).

68. I. Everall, P. Luthert, and P. Lantos. A review of neuronal damage in human immunodeficiency virus infection: its assessment, possible mechanism, and relationship to dementia. *J. Neuropathol. Exp. Neurol.* 52:561 (1993).

69. B.J. Brew, L. Pemberton, L. Evans, and M. Heyes. Quinolinic acid production by macrophages infected with demented and non-demented isolates of HIV. *Clin. Neuropathol.* 12 (Suppl. 1):S1 (1993).
70. C.K. Petito. What causes brain atrophy in human immunodeficiency virus infection? *Ann. Neurol.* 34:128 (1993).
71. L. Resnick, J.R. Berger, P. Shapshak, and W.W. Tourtellotte. Early penetration of the blood-brain barrier by HIV. *Neurology* 38:9 (1988).
72. T.W. Smith, U. DeGirolami, D. Hénin, FT. Bolgert, and J-J. Hauw. Human immunodeficiency virus (HIV) leukoencephalopathy and microcirculation. *J. Neuropathol. Exp. Neurol.* 49:357 (1990).
73. R. Rhodes. Evidence of serum-protein leakage across the blood-brain barrier in the acquired immunodeficiency syndrome. *J. Neuropathol. Exp. Neurol.* 50:171 (1991).
74. C.K Petito, and K.S. Cash. Blood-brain barrier abnormalities in the acquired immunodeficiency syndrome: immunohistochemical localization of serum proteins in postmortem brain. *Ann. Neurol.* 32:658 (1992).
75. C. Power, P.A. King, J.C. McArthur, et al. Alterations in the blood-brain barrier occur in HIV-demented patients. *Clin. Neuropathol.* 12 (Suppl. 1):S13 (1993).
76. C.A. Wiley, R.D. Schrier, J.A. Nelson, et al. Cellular localization of human immunodeficiency virus infection within the brains of acquired immune deficiency syndrome patients. *Proc. Natl. Acad. Sci. USA*, 83:7089 (1986).

PERIPHERAL NEUROPATHY IN AIDS: NEW INVESTIGATIVE APPROACHES

John W. Griffin, Steven L. Wesselingh, and Justin C. McArthur

Department of Neurology and Neuroscience
The Johns Hopkins Hospital
600 North Wolfe Street
Baltimore, Maryland 21205

INTRODUCTION

An extensive group of neurologic diseases affect the peripheral nervous system (PNS) of individuals infected with HIV (for reviews, see refs.1-3). As in the central nervous system (CNS), some of these disorders are due to opportunistic infections such as cytomegalovirus (CMV) infection of spinal roots and peripheral nerves.[4,5] Others, including the inflammatory demyelinating neuropathies occasionally seen in early stages of HIV infection,[6,7] are undoubtedly autoimmune in origin. Toxic neuropathies are of increasing importance because of the prominence of peripheral neurotoxicity resulting from the use of the antiretrovirals, dideoxycytidine (ddC) and dideoxyinosine (ddI).[8-10] The major PNS complication of HIV infection is the predominantly sensory neuropathy (PSN) of AIDS.[2,11-19] PSN is a disorder of unknown pathogenesis that is usually seen in advanced stages of AIDS. It has become one of the most frequent causes of new cases of symptomatic neuropathy in the U.S., with more than 30,000 cases annually. The incidence of neuropathy in individuals with HIV infection appears to be rising substantially, related both to the neurotoxic effects of antiretrovirals and to the HIV infection itself.[20] While this may in part be due to increased attention to the disorder in prospective studies, it undoubtedly also reflects the increasing numbers of severely immunodeficient individuals surviving longer after AIDS (and reaching later stages of HIV infection) together with the increasing use of antiretroviral neurotoxins.

This chapter will provide an overview of the clinicopathologic picture of the predominantly sensory neuropathy of AIDS, and describe two technical developments that should prove useful in elucidating its pathogenesis in clinical investigations of HIV-associated neuropathies and in assessing responses to treatment.

PREDOMINANT SENSORY NEUROPATHY (PSN) OF AIDS

Clinical Manifestations of PSN

As the name implies, the symptoms of PSN are primarily sensory in nature. They include both loss of sensibility (negative symptoms) and spontaneous sensory phenomena such as paresthesias and neuropathic pain (positive symptoms).[11,15,18] The most distressing symptom for most patients is the

Technical Advances in AIDS Research in the Human Nervous System
Edited by E.O. Major and J.A. Levy, Plenum Press, New York, 1995

neuropathic pain. It is experienced most intensely on the soles of the feet, and is associated in some individuals with mechanical allodynia and hyperesthesia. On examination, the most frequent findings include an elevated vibratory threshold in the toes, a variable loss of pin and thermal sensibility, often associated with an unpleasant dysesthetic response to stimulation of the feet, and in some individuals, a mild degree of weakness and atrophy in the legs, most often involving the intrinsic muscles of the feet.[11] Typically, the tendon reflexes of the ankle are depressed or absent, but the tendon reflexes at the knees are often exaggerated,[11] presumably reflecting concomitant CNS involvement, particularly vacuolar myelopathy.[2,13]

The manifestations of the neurotoxic disorder produced by the licensed antiretrovirals ddI and ddC (didanosine, VIDEX, Zalcitabine, HIVID) and other nucleoside analogs under trial (d4T, Stravudine) are similar to those of PSN.[9,21,22] In initial studies with relatively high doses of these agents, the neuropathy developed in a subacute fashion,[21] but as recently demonstrated,[8,10] there is a cumulation of neurotoxicity over time, even with normal therapeutic doses, so that as many as 35% of patients develop at least a mild neuropathy after 6 months of therapy with the current low doses. The incidence of neuropathy is highest in individuals with the most advanced systemic disease and lowest CD4 counts. It is often difficult to distinguish from the PSN associated with AIDS alone. It is likely that these agents amplify subclinical PSN, suggesting that patients with preexisting neuropathies may be more susceptible than others to neurotoxic complications, analogous to the increased toxicity of vincristine in the setting of preexisting neuropathies such as Charcot-Marie-Tooth disease.

Pathology of PSN

The pathologic changes in PSN are dominated by distally predominant degeneration of sensory axons.[12,13] This degeneration involves both the central processes of the primary sensory neurons in the gracile tract of the dorsal columns[12,13,23] and the peripheral extensions in the long cutaneous nerves[13,16,24] (Fig. 1). This pattern corresponds to other "dying back" degenerations of the primary sensory nerve fibers.[25,26] The regions of the long sensory axons farthest from the nerve cell bodies -- that, is, the most distal regions -- degenerate first. In the central processes, this distally predominant degeneration is reflected in active Wallerian-like degeneration of nerve fibers and reduced fiber density in the rostral gracile tract, compared to the dorsal roots and the gracile tract at the lumbar and thoracic levels[12-14,23] (Fig. 2). Similarly, the nerve fiber density is greater in the lumbosacral plexus in sciatic, peroneal, and tibial nerves, than in the distal regions of these nerves or in the sural nerve.[13]

In addition to simple Wallerian-like degeneration,[13] axonal atrophy (a reduction in the caliber of large axons) is a prominent feature in at least some cases or painful sensory neuropathy.[27] Both large and small fibers, including unmyelinated fibers, are lost at the level of the sural nerve[13,28] (Fig. 3).

The pathogenesis of PSN remains the subject of speculation. PSN typically develops in the setting of advanced AIDS and often occurs in the context of recent weight loss.[15] For this reason, nutritional factors have been implicated in its pathogenesis.[29] However, it can develop when weight and nutritional balance appear normal, and it is not generally improved by vitamin supplementation, although no clinical trials have been carried out, a few individual did note some improvement with vitamin B_{12}.[29] If nutritional factors play a role, they are probably secondary contributors and not the primary mechanism.

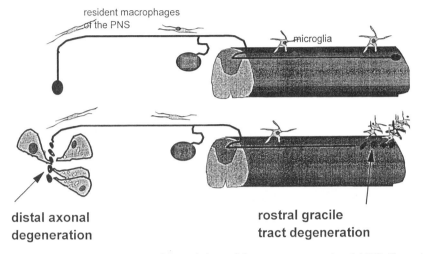

resident macrophages
of the PNS

microglia

**distal axonal
degeneration**

**rostral gracile
tract degeneration**

Figure 1. Diagrammatic representation of the pathology of the sensory neuropathy of AIDS, illustrating the distally predominant degeneration of both the peripheral and the central processes of the primary sensory neuron.

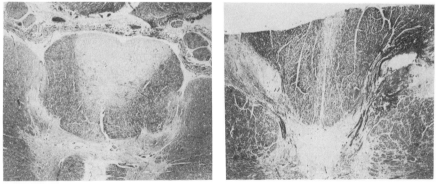

Figure 2. Comparison of the fiber densities in the dorsal columns of an individual with PSN. The left panel is from the lumbar cord and the right panel from the high thoracic cord. Note the greater extent of fiber loss in the gracile tract at the more rostral level.

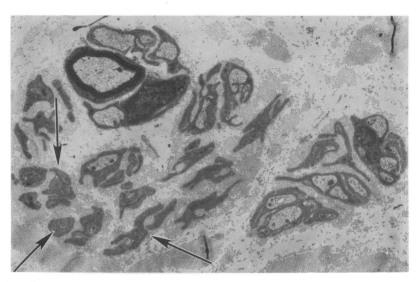

Figure 3. Electron micrograph illustrating the decrease in axons within the Schwann cell band of unmyelinated fibers (examples of denervated bands are identified by arrows).

On both epidemiologic and pathologic grounds, the possibility that PSN might frequently be due to CMV infection of peripheral nerve or dorsal root ganglia has been raised.[30,31] CMV infection can undoubtedly produce a painful neuropathy,[30,32] as recently reviewed,[2] and evidence of recent CMV has been adduced in several patients with painful sensory neuropathy,[30,32] while some cases of PSN may be due to CMV in the dorsal root ganglia or nerves. In addition, Cornford and coworkers have demonstrated a high frequency of patchy CMV infection of endothelial cells within the epineurium and, less frequently, the endoneurium, and found a correlation between the severity of CMV infection and the severity of neuropathy in individuals with and without pain.[5] In the Johns Hopkins series of 24 extensively studied cases of PSN, we excluded cases with CMV infection detectable by immunostaining.[13] These data indicate that, while CMV infection of nerve is frequently seen in the same patient population that develops PSN, perhaps reflecting the fact that both are associated with late stages of AIDS, PSN is not necessarily a consequence of CMV infection.[2]

In part because of the interest in the behavior of cells of macrophage lineage in HIV dementia, macrophages are undergoing study in PSN. In the normal PNS, there is a substantial population of resident macrophages as recently reviewed.[33-37] These cells bear analogies to both the stellate microglia and the perivascular macrophages of the normal CNS. Like the perivascular macrophages, they lie near blood vessels, but outside the endothelial cell basal lamina.[34,37,38] They are constitutively MHC Class II-positive and are likely to represent the major antigen-presenting cell of the PNS,[34,37] similar to the role of perivascular macrophages in the CNS.[39,40] Like the CNS perivascular macrophages,[41] the resident macrophages of the PNS are renewed from the bone marrow.[38] They are CD4-positive, but unlike the stellate microglia and the macrophages of the CNS, the macrophages in the nerves are only rarely productively infected by HIV, even in severe neuropathy,[14,42] although cells in the dorsal root ganglia are infected at a low level.[43]

Macrophages and stellate microglia in the CNS express a variety of activation markers, including high levels of MHC class II, complement receptor 3, and the cytokine tumor necrosis factor-α (TNF-α).[44,45] The level of TNF-α transcripts, as measured by solution phase reverse transcriptase polymerase chain reaction (RT-PCR), correlates significantly with the degree of dementia.[45] The reason for this prominent activation of macrophage-lineage cells in the CNS in HIV dementia could be due to local HIV infection or to abnormal regulation of these cells because of the immune abnormalities of AIDS.[45] In separating between these possibilities, studies of the PNS will be helpful because of the paucity of local productive HIV infection in the nerves. To the extent there is a similar degree of macrophage activation in the PNS as in the CNS, factors other than local HIV infection must be invoked.

In both the dorsal root ganglia[23,43] and in the peripheral nerves, there are abnormally prominent populations of activated macrophages. As in the CNS, these macrophages are prominently MHC class II- and TNF-α-positive.[14] Similarly, in the rostral gracile tracts, there are prominent activated macrophages that are intensely MHC class II- and TNF-α-positive.[14] The activation of macrophages in PSN is likely to be triggered by axonal and neuronal degeneration; previous studies have demonstrated that Wallerian-like degeneration of both axons and neuronal perikarya is sufficient to produce class II and TNF-α expression in the reactive macrophages and microglia.[46-48] In contrast to the prominence of macrophage responses, lymphocytes within the endoneurium are generally relatively scarce,[14] although epineurial lymphocytes have been emphasized.[5] Thus, in PSN the prominent macrophage responses in PSN may represent an exaggerated response to nerve fiber degeneration triggered by the relative absence of lymphocyte derived cytokines that normally modulate the macrophage response. For example, IL-4, IL-5 and IL-10 are able to deactivate macrophages and reduce TNF-α production. Because of the profound deficiency of T helper cells in the late stages of AIDS, normal constraints exercised by lymphokines on lymphocyte-independent macrophage responses may not be available. Exaggerated macrophage responses could amplify the neuropathic process in PSN.[14]

New Technical Approaches to PSN

The PNS is accessible to biopsy and direct physiologic investigation so that it offers intrinsic advantages over the CNS for pathogenetic studies. However, the tools for identifying early changes, for monitoring the spatiotemporal progression of nerve disease, and for detecting responses to therapy remain imperfect. Similarly, although the roles of cytokines and neurotrophins, as well as their interrelationships, are better understood in the PNS than in the CNS, their expression in human nerve disease has not been assessed, in part because the transcripts and gene products are active at extremely low levels, so that new methods for detection are required. The following section describes the current status of two newly developed methods applicable to HIV-associated neuropathies, the use of skin biopsies to study cutaneous innervation and the use of sensitive *in situ* hybridization techniques to examine cytokine and growth factor transcripts in neural cells and in target tissues.

Assessment of Cutaneous Innervation

The predominantly sensory neuropathy of AIDS underscores several of the difficulties in assessing the integrity of small fibers in the PNS. These fibers are "invisible' by standard electrodiagnostic methods, which "see" large, myelinated fibers predominantly. Quantitative sensory testing of small-fiber sensory modalities, such as warming and cooling sensibility and thermal pain thresholds, is a useful approach, and such tests have suggested the relatively early loss of warming and cooling sensation in PSN.[49] However, quantitative sensory testing is a psychophysical test that depends on alertness and motivation, and may be of limited value in the setting of serious systemic disease or dementia. Autonomic function tests such as heart period variability are objective and not limited by these restrictions; and abnormalities have been detected in some studies of individuals with AIDS.[50] However, by definition, they test autonomic rather than somatic sensory functions. In addition, normative data for severely ill individuals with systemic disease and weight loss are not available, so that the degree of specificity for AIDS neuropathy is uncertain.

Morphologic approaches to assessment of small fibers also have inherent limitations. Because of their size, quantitation of these fibers in nerve biopsies has required painstaking morphometry at the electron microscopic level.[13,51-53] This approach is notoriously expensive and labor-intensive, and the precision of measurement is limited by the inherent difficulties in identifying axons with certainty and distinguishing them from small Schwann cell processes in degenerating Schwann cell bands (Bungner bands). In addition, nerve biopsies assess only one cutaneous nerve, usually the sural, at a single site, and provide no information about terminal innervation and give data about only one point in time. Serial nerve biopsies, although occasionally done for special reasons, are not acceptable in most settings. Finally, sural nerve biopsies are invasive, produce discomfort, and in AIDS, where the medical focus is necessarily on life-threatening complications, they are often impractical.

An inherently appealing alternative to nerve biopsy is direct assessment of the cutaneous innervation by means of skin biopsy. Skin biopsies are simple, relatively painless, and can be easily performed even in ill AIDS patients. Multiple sites can be biopsied in a single session, so that the spatial distribution of cutaneous denervation can be assessed. In addition, biopsies can be done serially so that the natural history of the disease or the responses to treatment can be assessed. A number of previous approaches to assessing the innervation of skin have been described. Two extensive investigations of Meissner's corpuscles, complex touch receptors in the dermal papillae, were made by the Mayo Clinic Group,[54] using cholinesterase staining, and by Ridley[55,56] in London, using silver stains. Both series demonstrated a steep age-related decline in the density of Meissner's corpuscles. Ridley was able to demonstrate a decrease in density of innervation in peripheral nerve disease (examining the finger pads),[56] but in both series there was substantial interindividual variability, and the Mayo Clinic data defined intersite variation as a limiting problem. Meissner's corpuscles are largely restricted to glabrous (nonhairy) skin, as seen in the finger and toe pads, and are thus not appropriate for studies of the spatial distribution of cutaneous degeneration. Finally, the specialized sensory end-organs such as Meissner's corpuscles, are innervated by large cutaneous fibers, and provide no data about the status of the smallest fibers, such as the Aδ and C fibers.

Sensitive immunocytochemical approaches provide an alternative that is particularly promising.[57-60] At Johns Hopkins, McArthur and colleagues have initiated a study of skin biopsies in PSN and in the sensory neuropathy produced by ddI and ddC. Figure 4 illustrates the appearance of normal skin immuno-stained with antibodies to a neuronal marker, ubiquitin carboxy terminal hydrolase.[61] A striking feature of the cutaneous innervation, not appreciated before the availability of sensitive immunocytochemical approaches, is the dense epidermal innervation by unmyelinated axons. These axons are devoid of Schwann cell investment through most of their course within the epidermis, and many run to the stratum corneum. Examination of biopsies from sites on the foot, lower leg, and thigh suggest that the density of innervation will vary less than that of the specialized sensory end-organs of the skin, such as Meissner's corpuscles. The initial studies document that there is marked loss of these fine epidermal fibers in many patients with HIV sensory neuropathies as well as in ddC/ddI neuropathies.

Three issues require further technical development in order to make skin biopsies widely applicable to assess the spatiotemporal changes in nerve disease and the possible responses of nerve fibers to treatments such as the injection of nerve growth factors. First, appropriate systems of quantitation of dermal and epidermal fiber numbers must be developed. Second, it will be desirable to identify phenotypic changes in denervated skin -- that is, the loss or the new expression of markers as a consequence of denervation. Finally, identification of regenerating nerve fibers by their expression of growth-associated markers would provide an assay for early regenerative responses. Such measures would be particularly valuable in assessing potential therapeutic approaches and would undoubtedly find application in "small fiber" neuropathies, such as diabetes mellitus, in addition to PSN.

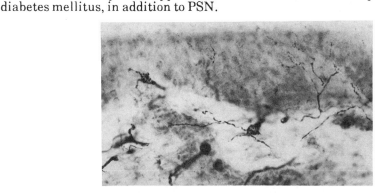

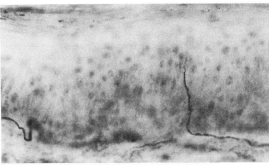

Figure 4. Immunocytochemical staining to demonstrate fine sensory axon terminals in the epidermis in a normal (upper panel) and in the distal leg of an individual with the sensory neuropathy of AIDS (lower panel).

Detection of Cytokines and Growth Factors by Reverse Transcriptase Polymerase Chain Reaction *in situ* Hybridization (RT/PCR-ISH)

In sensory nerve, neurotrophins synthesized by the innervated target cells contribute to long-term survival of specific fiber populations, even in adults. In nerve disease, they are required for regeneration of nerve fibers. One fiber population at risk in PSN, the unmyelinated sensory (C) fibers, are dependent on the neurotrophic, nerve growth factor (NGF), for their survival and successful regeneration in disease. NGF is taken up into axons and growth cones by means of a high-affinity receptor, trkA, and retrogradely transported in the axon to the nerve cell body. NGF produced by target cells is localized on the surface of the appropriate cells by a low-affinity NGF receptor, p75. The trkA on the axons can compete away the NGF bound on the target cells. Similarly, in nerve regeneration, denervated Schwann cells express p75 and bind NGF on their plasmalemmas, providing a preferred pathway for growing axons. Thus, one pathogenetic mechanism for PSN could be a failure of adequate production of neurotrophins such as NGF or the p75 receptor. Do the target cells in the skin produce normal amounts of NGF in AIDS? Is p75 appropriately synthesized and localized? These questions remain unanswered in human neuropathies because of the technical limitations of standard techniques for measuring growth factors.

A related issue is the production of cytokines in nerve disease. NGF production in denervated nerve is dependent on the cytokine interleukin-1 beta (IL-1β), produced, at least in large part, by activated macrophages.[62-64] Abnormalities in this cytokine-growth factor cascade would provide an attractive contributor to the pathogenesis of PSN.[2,14]

Studies of cytokine and neurotrophin expression in the PNS have been restricted by the same technical limitations that have operated in the CNS -- the limited sensitivity of immunocytochemical and standard *in situ* hybridization methods in detecting biologically important amounts of cytokines and growth factors. Wesselingh and coworkers have adapted the technique of RT/PCR ISH to studies of the brain, spinal cord, and peripheral nerves. The advantages and limitations of RT/PCR ISH are detailed elsewhere in this volume (see chapter by Nuovo). In the procedure that we have utilized, paraffin sections are adhered to glass slides, treated with an empirically determined concentration and duration of proteinase K, DNA is degraded by DNase treatment, and cDNAs are generated by reverse transcriptase. PCR amplification is performed in a cycling oven, and the PCR product is probed with a digoxigenin-labeled oligonucleotide specific to the internal sequence. The digoxigenin is then identified by anti-digoxygenin immunocytochemistry.

Comparisons to standard *in situ* hybridization, using the same digoxygenin-labeled probes, demonstrated the marked increased in sensitivity expected with amplification. In optimal preparations, there was no increase in nonspecific or background signal, as illustrated in Figure 5. The absence of hybridization to genomic DNA is reflected in the relative absence of nuclear staining, and the dense perikaryal staining. However, the potential for nonspecific hybridization requires routine performance of a series of controls, including the absence of reverse transcriptase, the absence of Taq polymerase, and the use of an irrelevant or nonsense internal probe. Using this technique, we have recently described the expression of TNF-α message in nerves from individuals affected with PSN and are extending this approach to studies of the relevant cytokines and growth factors in nerve and skin samples.

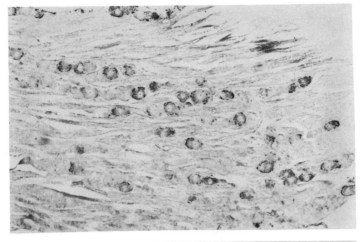

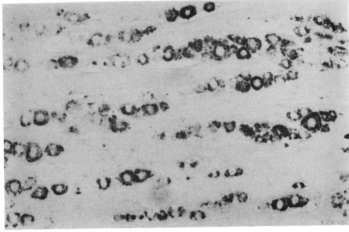

Figure 5. Comparison of nonamplified *in situ* hybridization (upper panel) and RT-PCR *in situ* hybridization (lower panel) in the dorsal root ganglion. The probe is for the neurofilament protein, NF-M, which is expressed in neurons. Note that the level of signal is greater, but that the cellular localizations are comparable.

CONCLUSIONS

PSN warrants intensive investigation both because of its morbidity and the need to develop effective treatments, and because its potential for providing unique insights into general mechanisms of disease and repair in the PNS. PSN is one of the few PNS disorders associated with a fatal disease. Thus, in contrast to most other neuropathies, autopsy examination of the entire PNS, with the potential for insights into the three-dimensional pathology and mechanisms of pathogenesis, is possible.

REFERENCES

1. D.R. Cornblath, J.C. McArthur, G. Parry, and J.W. Griffin. Peripheral neuropathies in human immunodeficiency virus infection, in: "Peripheral Neuropathy," P.J. Dyck, P.K. Thomas, K.W. Griffin, P.A. Low, and J. Poduslo, eds., W.B. Saunders, Philadelphia (1992).
2. J.W. Griffin, J.C. McArthur, J.D.Glass, and S.L. Wesselingh. Peripheral neuropathies in HIV infection; similarities and contrasts with the central nervous system, in: "HIV, AIDS, and the Brain," Raven Press, New York (1994).
3. G.J. Parry. Peripheral neuropathies associated with human immunodeficiency virus infection. Ann. Neurol. 23(Suppl):S49 (1988).
4. H.V. Vinters, M.K. Kwok, H.W. Ho, et al. Cytomegalovirus in the nervous system of patients with the acquired immune deficiency syndrome. Brain 112:245 (1989).
5. M.E. Cornford, H.W. Ho, and H.V. Vinters. Correlation of neuromuscular pathology in acquired immune deficiency syndrome patients with cytomegalovirus infection and zidovudine treatment. Acta Neuropathol. 84:516 (1992).
6. D.R. Cornblath, J.C. McArthur, P.G.E. Kennedy, A.S. Witte, and J.W. Griffin. Inflammatory demyelinating peripheral neuropathies associated with human T-cell lymphotropic virus type III infection. Ann. Neurol. 21:32 (1987).
7. J.W. Griffin, D.R. Cornblath, S.L. Wesselingh, et al. Pathology of HIV-associated Guillain-Barre syndrome and chronic inflammatory demyelinating polyneuropathy.   in press.
8. A.R. Berger, J..C. Arezzo, H.H. Schaumburg, et al. 2',3'-Dideoxycytidine (ddC) toxic neuropathy: a study of 52 patients. Neurology 43:358 (1993).
9. K.D. Kieburtz, M. Seidlin, J.S. Lambert, et al. Extended follow-up of peripheral neuropathy in patients with AIDS and AIDS-related complex treated with dideoxyinosine. J. Acq. Immun. Defic. Syndrome 5:60 (1992).
10. A. Blum, G. Dal Pan, CF. Raines, K. Mayjo, and J. McArthur. ddC-related toxic neuropathy: risk factors and natural history. Neurology (Abstract) (1993).
11. D.R. Cornblath, and J.C. McArthur. Predominantly sensory neuropathy in patients with AIDS and AIDS-related complex. Neurology 38:794 (1988).
12. N. Rance, J.C. McArthur, D.R. Cornblath, et al. Gracile tract degeneration in patients with sensory neuropathy and AIDS. Neurology 38:265 (1988).
13. J.W. Griffin, T.O. Crawford, W.R. Tyor, et al. Sensory neuropathy in AIDS. I. Neuropathology. Brain; in press (1994).
14. J.W. Griffin, W.R. Tyor, J.D. Glass, et al. Sensory neuropathy in AIDS. II. Immunopathology. Brain; in press (1994).
15. Y.T. So, D.M. Holtzman, D.I. Abrams, and R.K. Olney. Peripheral neuropathy associated with acquired immunodeficiency syndrome: Prevalence and clinical features from a population-based survey. Arch. Neurol. 45:945 (1988).
16. M.-P. Chaunu, H. Ratinahirana, M. Raphael, et al. The spectrum of changes on 20 nerve biopsies in patients with HIV infection. Muscle Nerve 12:452 (1989).
17. J.M. Leger, P. Bouche, F. Bolgert, et al. The spectrum of polyneuropathies in patients infected with HIV. J. Neurol. Neurosurg. Psychiatry 52:1369 (1989).
18. R.M. Levy, D.E. Bredesen, and M.L. Rosenblum. Neurological manifestations of the acquired immunodeficiency syndrome (AIDS): experience at UCSF and a review of the literature. J. Neurosurg. 62:475 (1985).
19. W.D. Snider, D.M. Simpson, S. Nielsen, et al. Neurological complications of acquired immune deficiency syndrome: Analysis of 50 patients. Ann. Neurol. 14:403 (1983).
20. H. Bacellar, J. McArthur, A. Munoz, et al. Temporal trends in incidence of

neurologic diseases in AIDS. *First Conference on Human Retroviruses and Related Infections*, Washington, D.C. (1993) (abstract).

21. T.C. Merigan, G. Skowron, S.A. Bozzette, et al. Circulating p24 antigen levels and responses to dideoxycytidine in human immunodeficiency virus (HIV) infections: A phase I and II study. *Ann. Intern. Med.* 110:189 (1989).

22. R.M.Dubinsky, R. Yarchoan, M. Dalakas, and S. Broder. Reversible axonal neuropathy from the treatment of AIDS and related disorders with 2',3'-dideoxycytidine (ddC). *Muscle Nerve* 12:856 (1989).

23. F. Scaravilli, E. Sinclair, J-C. Arango, et al. The pathology of the posterior root ganglia in AIDS and its relationship to the pallor of the gracile tract. *Acta Neuropathol.* 84:163 (1992).

24. V. Mah, L.M. Vartavarian, M.-A. Akers, and H.V. Vinters. Abnormalities of peripheral nerve in patients with human immunodeficiency virus infection. *Ann. Neurol.* 24:713 (1988).

25. P.S. Spencer, and H.H. Schaumberg. Central-peripheral distal axonopathy -- the pathogenesis of dying-back polyneuropathies, *in:* "Progress in Neuropathology, Vol. 3," H. Zimmerman, ed., Grune and Stratton, New York (1976).

26. J.B. Cavanagh. The significance of the "dying back" process in human and experimental neurological diseases. *Int. Rev. Exp. Pathol.* 3:219 (1964).

27. G.N. Fuller, J.M. Jacobs, and R.J. Guiloff. Axonal atrophy in the painful peripheral neuropathy in AIDS. *Acta Neuropathol.* 81:198 (1990).

28. G.N. Fuller, J.M. Jacobs,m and R.J. Guiloff. Subclinical peripheral nerve involvement in AIDS: an electrophysiological and pathological study. *J. Neurol. Neurosurg. Psychiatry* 54:318 (1991).

29. K.D. Kieburtz, D.W. Giang, R.B. Schiffer, and N. Vakil. Abnormal vitamin B$_{12}$ metabolism in human immunodeficiency virus infection. *Arch. Neurol.* 48:312 (1991).

30. G.N. Fuller, J.M. Jacobs, and R.J,.Guiloff. Association of painful peripheral neuropathy in AIDS with cytomegalovirus infection. *Lancet* 2:937 (1989).

31. G.N. Fuller, J.M. Jacobs, and R.J. Guiloff. Nature and incidence of peripheral nerve syndromes in HIV infection,. *J. Neurol. Neurosurg. Psychiatry* 56:372 (1993).

32. C. d'Ivernois, J.B. Winer, et al. Painful peripheral neuropathy and cytomegalovirus pneumonia in AIDS. *Lancet* 2:1239 (1989).

33. J.W. Griffin, R.R. George, C. Lobato, et al. Macrophage responses and myelin clearance during Wallerian degeneration: relevance to immune-mediated demyelination. *J. Neuroimmunol.* 40:153 (1992).

34. C. Nordstedt, S.E. Gandy, I. Alafuzoff, et al. Alzheimer beta/A4 amyloid precursor protein in human brain: Aging-associated increases in holo-protein and in a proteolytic fragment. *Proc. Natl. Acad. Sci. USA* 88:8910 (1991).

35. C.E. Bandtlow,M. Meyer, D. Lindholm, et al. Regional and cellular codistribution of interleukin 1 beta and nerve growth factor mRNA in the adult rat brain: possible relationship to the regulation of nerve growth factor synthesis. *J. Cell. Biol.* 111:1710 (1990).

36. V.H. Perry, M,.C. Brown, and S. Gordon. The macrophage response to central and peripheral nerve injury: a possible role for macrophages in regeneration. *J. Exp. Med.* 165:1218 (1987).

37. S. Monaco, J. Gehrmann, G. Raivich, and G.W. Kreutzberg. MHC-positive, ramified macrophages in the normal and injured rat peripheral nervous system. *J. Neurocytol.* 21:623 (1992).

38. K. Vass, W.F. Hickey, R.E. Schmidt, and H. Lassmann. Bone marrow-derived elements in the peripheral nervous system: An immunohistochemical and ultrastructural investigation in chimeric rats. *Lab. Invest.* (1993).

39. W.J. Streit, M.B. Graeber, and G.W. Kreutzberg. Expression of Ia antigen on perivascular and microglial cells after sublethal and lethal motor neuron injury. *Exp. Neurol.* 105:115 (1989).

40. M. Mato, S. Ookawara, and T. Saito-Taki. Serological determinants of fluorescent granular perithelial cells along small cerebral blood vessels in rodents. *Acta Neuropathol.* 72:117 (1986).
41. W.F. Hickey, and H. Kimura. Perivascular microglial cells of the CNS are bone marrow-derived and present antigen *in vivo*. *Science* 239:290 (1988).
42. D.D. Ho, T.R. Rota, R.T. Schooley, et al. Isolation of HTLV-III from cerebrospinal fluid and neural tissues of patients with neurologic syndromes related to the acquired immunodeficiency syndrome. *N. Engl. J. Med.* 313:1493 (1985).
43. M.M. Esiri, C.S. Morris, and P.R. Millard. Sensory and sympathetic ganglia in HIV-1 infection: immunocytochemical demonstration of HIV-1 viral antigens, increased MHC Class II antigen expression and mild reactive inflammation. *J. Neurol. Sci.* 114:178 (1993).
44. W.R. Tyor, J.D. Glass, P.S. Becker, et al. Cytokine expression in the brain during AIDS. *Ann. Neurol.* 31:349 (1992).
45. S.L. Wesselingh, C. Power, J.D. Glass, et al. Intracerebral cytokine mRNA in AIDS. *Ann. Neurol.*; in press (1993).
46. G. Stoll, H.-W. Mueller, B.D. Trapp, and J.W,. Griffin. Oligodendrocytes but not astrocytes express apolipoprotein E after injury of rat optic nerve. *Glia* 2:170 (1989).
47. G. Stoll, J.W. Griffin, C.Y. Li, and B.D. Trapp. Wallerian degeneration in the peripheral nervous system: Participation of both Schwann cells and macrophages in myelin degradation. *J. Neurocytol.* 18:671 (1989).
48. R.R. George, and J.W. Griffin. Contrasts between the CNS and the PNS in Wallerian degeneration: the dorsal radiculotomy model.
49. J.B. Winer, B. Bang, J.R. Clarke, et al. A study of neuropathy in HIV infection. *Quart. J. Med.* 302:473 (1992).
50. R. Freeman, and J.A. Cohen. Autonomic failure and AIDS, *in:* "Clinical Autonomic Disorders: Evaluation and Management," P.A. Low, ed., Little, Brown and Co. (1992).
51. J.M. Jacobs, and S. Love. Qualitative and quantitative morphology of human sural nerve at different ages. *Brain* 108:897 (1985).
52. F. Behse, F. Buchthal, F. Carlsen, G.G. Knappeis. Unmyelinated fibres and Schwann cells of sural nerve in neuropathy. *Brain* 98:493 (1975).
53. F. Behse, and F. Buchthal. Alcoholic neuropathy: clinical, electrophysiological, and biopsy findings. *Ann. Neurol.* 2:95 (1977).
54. C.F. Bolton, R.K. Winkelman, and P.J.Dyck. A quantitative study of Meissner's corpuscles in man. *Neurology* 16:1 (1966).
55. A. Ridley. Silver staining of nerve endings in human digital glabrous skin. *J. Anat.* 104:41 (1969).
56. A.Ridley. Silver staining of the innervation of Meissner corpuscles in peripheral neuropathy. *Brain* 196:539 (1991).
57. S.S. Karanth, D.R. Springall, S. Lucas, et al. Changes in nerves and neuropeptides in skin from 100 leprosy patients investigated by immunocytochemistry. *J. Pathol.* 157:15 (1989).
58. S.S. Karanth, D.R. Springall, D.M. Kuhn, M.M. Levene, and J.M. Polak. An immunocytochemical study of cutaneous innervation and the distribution of neuropeptides and protein gene product 9.6 in man and commonly employed laboratory animals. *Am.J. Anat.* 191:369 (1991).
59. C-J. Dalsgaard, M. Rydh, and A. Haegerstrand. Cutaneous innervation in man visualized with gene product 9.5 (PGP 9.5) antibodies. *Histochemistry* 92:385 (1989).
60. L. Wang, M. Hilliges, T. Jernbgerg, D. Wiegleb-Edstrom, and O. Johansson. Protein gene product 9.5-immunoreactive nerve fibres and cells in human skin. *Cell Tissue* 261 :25 (1990).
61. K.D.Wilkinson, K. Lee, S. Deshpande, et al. The neuron-specific protein PGP 9.5 is a ubiquitin carboxyl-terminal hydrolase. *Science* 246:6570 (1989).

62. D. Lindholm, R. Heumann, B. Hengerer, and H. Thoenen. Interluekin-1 increases stability and transcription of mRNA encoding nerve growth factor in cultured rat fibroblasts. *J. Biol. Chem.* 263:16348 (1988).
63. R. Heumann, D. Lindholm, C. Bandtlow, et al. Differential regulation of mRNA encoding nerve growth factor and its receptor in rat sciatic nerve during development, degeneration,and regeneration : Role of macrophages. *Proc. Natl. Acad. Sci. USA* 84:8735 (1987).
64. D. Lindholm, R. Heumann, M. Meyer, and H.Y. Thoenen. Interleukin-1 regulates synthesis of nerve growth factor in non-neuronal cells of rat sciatic nerve. *Nature* 330:658 (1987).

MODELS OF HIV-1 INFECTION AND NEUROTOXICITY IN THE HUMAN FETAL NERVOUS SYSTEM

OVERVIEW: MODELS OF HIV-1 INFECTION AND NEURO-TOXICITY IN THE HUMAN FETAL NERVOUS SYSTEM

Leon G. Epstein

Departments of Neurology, Pediatrics, Microbiology and Immunology
University of Rochester School of Medicine and Dentistry
Rochester, New York 14642

HIV infection of the nervous system is responsible for the clinical subcortical dementia in adult AIDS patients[1] and for the analogous progressive encephalopathy in children with AIDS.[2] Neuropathological studies have described inflammatory cell infiltrates composed largely of HIV-infected macrophages and multinucleated giant cells, white matter damage (edema), and neuronal loss or damage to the dendritic processes of neurons in the neocortex.[3-7]

Monocytes/macrophages/microglia are the only cells consistently shown to harbor productive infection *in vivo*.[3,8] New evidence has emerged demonstrating restricted HIV-1 infection in astrocytes *in vivo*.[9,10] (See also this volume, chapters by Erfle and Brack-Werner). Neurons *per se* show no evidence of direct infection by HIV-1 even by PCR-amplified *in situ* hybridization. HIV-1 infection of the rare neuron remains controversial (see this volume, chapter by Schmid).

These pathological and virological data, as well as several *in vitro* studies,[11-13] strongly suggest that HIV-1-infected macrophages, perhaps in concert with other neural cells, secrete one or more neurotoxins that indirectly damage neurons or myelin.[14] Recent evidence suggests that interactions between the HIV-1-infected monocyte/microglia and astroglia produce a cascade of cytokines and arachidonic acid metabolites, which act in an autocrine fashion to amplify the effect of a small number of productively infected cells.[13,14] The final common pathway causing neuronal death may be due to glutamate-mediated excitotoxicity, acting through the NMDA or other receptors.

Studies of HIV-1 infection require human neural tissue due to the host specificity of the virus. Adult nervous tissue from biopsies is difficult to obtain and neurons derived from such tissue do not survive in sufficient numbers *in vitro*. Moreover, viral-cell interactions are difficult to interpret in neuronal or astroglial tumor cell lines. This has led to the development of a number of methodologies and models utilizing human fetal tissue as monolayer cultures, or to form brain aggregates, or xenografts in rodent hosts[12,14,17] in order to investigate the pathogenetic mechanisms of tissue/cell damage due to HIV-1 in the nervous system. In her chapter, Dr. Pulliam describes many of the advantages of using brain aggregates including the presence of all neural cell types, a microenvironment containing growth factors and cytokines, and longer neuronal survival. The limitations, which apply to all models using fetal tissue, are the potential problems of differences in the properties of donor tissues, and concerns regarding extrapolating data obtained from human fetal tissue to fully developed adult nervous tissue. The xenograft model offers the possibility of studies of

Technical Advances in AIDS Research in the Human Nervous System
Edited by E.O. Major and J.A. Levy, Plenum Press, New York, 1995

57

longer duration. In this model, the neurons continue to differentiate and produce synapses and neuritic processes for several months. Additionally, the grafts develop a blood-brain barrier. The placement of HIV-1-infected human monocytes in this neural tissue produces the characteristic changes of astrocyte proliferation and neuronal cell loss (or damage). This may allow the characterization of specific neurotoxins *in situ*.

While HIV-1 infection of the nervous system is specific for the human host, the neurotoxins produced by HIV-1-infected cells may damage neuronal targets across species. Studies in which putative neurotoxins are delivered to regions of intact rodent brains may be necessary to determine which neurotransmitter pathways or subpopulations of neurons are susceptible to damage. Dr. Gelbard writes about experiments to determine the direct effect of putative neurotoxins or conditioned media delivered to the brain of neonatal mice, using Azlet mini-pumps.

Each of the chapters which follow describes the views of the author regarding HIV-1 neuropathogenesis, and reports on the methods used to generate their supporting data. Some of the highlights of these papers, and issues crosscutting them are offered.

Dr. Gendelman presents data to support the hypotheses that a small number of HIV-1-infected monocytes/microglia interact with astrocytes resulting in the secretion of high levels of the cytokines interleukin-1 beta (IL-1β) and tumor necrosis factor-α (TNF-α) as well as the production of arachidonic acid and its metabolites. An autocrine loop is established, producing more cytokines and amplifying the potentially neurotoxic effect of these cellular products. Furthermore, IL-1β probably causes astrocyte activation and/or proliferation. TNF-α stimulates the production of the intracellular protein NF-kB, which in turn upregulates HIV-1 transcription in infected brain macrophages and microglia.[18,19]

Dr. Gelbard, using primary cultures, explains that TNF-α, as well as platelet-activating factor (PAF) appear to be directly toxic to fetal neurons in a dose-dependent manner.[16] The neurotoxicity of TNF-α is reduced by CNQX which blocks the AMPA receptor,[16] while that of PAF is ameliorated by MK-801, which acts on the NMDA receptor.

These studies complement evidence from other investigators that neural damage caused by HIV-1 gp120 is mediated by excitatory amino acids.[15] Dawson et al. have suggested that nitric oxide is involved in this process.[20] Other groups have found that PAF acts directly as a potent modulator of excitatory synaptic transmission[21] and further, that arachidonic acid itself has a strong inhibitory effect on glutamate reuptake by astrocytes,[22] both of which would favor excitatory damage.

The most recent data, from Dr. Gendelman's laboratory, suggest that TGF-β released by astrocytes may, in fact, have a partial protective effect in negatively regulating cytokine (TNF-α) expression. These data are consistent with the findings of Wahl et al. that transforming growth factor-beta (TGF-β) colocalizes with HIV-1 *in situ* in human postmortem brain.[23] Further, Dr. Pulliam reports that while gp120 does not appear to be directly toxic to neurons in brain aggregates, it does damage a significant proportion of astrocytes leading her to hypothesize that the loss of the "protective" or supportive functions of astrocytes may play a role in secondary damage to neurons.

Several investigators touched on the emerging importance of the astrocyte in HIV-1 pathogenesis (see above). Dr. Tornatore provided compelling data that persistent, restricted HIV-1 infection occurs *in vivo* (see also ref. 9), and that primary human fetal brain cultures can be used to study the molecular mechanisms underlying the restriction of HIV-1 replication (by a rev block), and the reactivation of HIV-1 infection in astrocytes by cytokines such as TNF-α acting through the cellular transcription factor NF-kB.

Clearly the data obtained from these different models are sometimes contradictory. Some explanations are offered including the specificity of the host target tissue or HIV-1 strain. It is the opinion of this author that only by using all of the above-mentioned complementary models will a complete composite picture be formed. Toxic or protective products of specific cell types can only be isolated and identified using *in vitro* studies, while the effects of such products of specific cell populations will require studies in intact rodent brains. Issues regarding the ameliorating or toxic potential of therapeutic compounds, as well as the interactions of such compounds with HIV-1 may be best evaluated using intact human neural tissue in an aggregate or xenograft model.

Acknowledgements

The Laboratory of Molecular Neurovirology at the University of Rochester is supported in part by the U.S. Public Health Service grants AI32305 and P01-NS31492.

REFERENCES

1. B.A. Navia, B.D. Jordan, and R.W. Price. The AIDS dementia complex. I. Clinical features. *Ann. Neurol.* 19:517 (1986).
2. L.G. Epstein, L.R. Sharer, J.M. Oleske, et al. Neurologic manifestations of human immunodeficiency virus infection in children. *Pediatrics* 78:678 (1986).
3. L.R. Sharer. Pathology of HIV-1 infection of the central nervous system. A review. *J. Neuropathol. Exp. Neurol.* 51:3 (1992).
4. S. Ketzler, S. Weis, H. Haug, and H. Budka. Loss of neurons in the frontal cortex in AIDS brains. *Acta Neuropathol* 80:92 (1990).
5. C.A. Wiley, E. Masliah, M. Morey, et al. Neocortical damage during HIV infection. *Ann. Neurol.* 29:651 (1991).
6. E. Masliah,. C.L. Achim, N. Ge. Spectrum of human immunodeficiency virus-associated neocortical damage. *Ann. Neurol.* 32:321 (1992).
7. I.P. Everall, P.J. Luthert, and P.L. Lantos. Neuronal number of volume alterations in the neocortex of HIV-infected individuals. *J. Neurol., Neurosurg. & Psychiatry* 56:481 (1993).
8. J. Michaels, L.R. Sharer, and L.G. Epstein. Human immunodeficiency virus type 1 (HIV-1) infection of the nervous system: a review. *Immunodef. Rev.* 1:71 (1988).
9. Y. Saito, L.R. Sharer, L.G. Epstein, et al. Overexpression of Nef as a marker for restricted HIV-1 infection of astrocytes in post-mortem pediatric central nervous system. *Neurology* 44:474 (1994).
10. C. Tornatore, R. Chandra, J. Berger, and E. Major. HIV-1 infection of subcortical astrocytes in pediatric central nervous system. *Neurology* 44:481 (1994).
11. D. Giulian, K. Vaca, and C.A. Noonan. Secretion of neurotoxins by mononuclear phagocytes infected with HIV-1. *Science* 250:1593 (1990).
12. L. Pulliam, B.G. Herndier, N.M. Tang, and M.S. McGrath. HIV-infected macrophages produce soluble factors that cause histological and neurochemical alterations in cultured human brains. *J. Clin,. Invest.* 87:503 (1991).
13. P. Genis, M. Jett, E. Bernton, et al. Cytokines and arachidonic metabolites produced during human immunodeficiency virus (HIV)-infected macrophage-astroglia interactions: implications for the neuropathogenesis of HIV disease. *J. Exp. Med.* 176:1703 (1992).
14. L.G. Epstein, and H.E. Gendelman. Human immunodeficiency virus type 1 infection of the nervous system: pathogenetic mechanisms. [Review] *Ann. Neurol.* 33:429 (1993).
15. S.A. Lipton. Models of neuronal injury in AIDS: another role for the NMDA receptor? *Trends Neurosci.* 15:75 (1992).
16. H.A. Gelbard, K. Dzenko, D. Diloreto, et al. Neurotoxic effects of tumor necrosis factor in primary human neuronal cultures are mediated by activation of the glutamate AMPA receptor subtype: Implications for AIDS neuropathogenesis. *Dev. Neurosci.* (in press) (1994).
17. T.A. Cvetkovich, E. Lazar, B.M. Blumberg, et al. Human immunodeficiency virus type 1 infection of neural xenografts. *Proc. Natl. Acad. Sci. USA* 89:5162 (1992).

18. C. Tornatore, A. Nath, K. Amemiya, and E.O. Major. Persistent human immunodeficiency virus type 1 infection in human fetal glial cells reactivated by T-cell factor(s) or by the cytokines tumor necrosis factor alpha and interleukin-1 beta. *J. Virol.* 65:6094 (1991).

19. L. Vitkovic, T. Kalebic, A. de Cunha, and A. Fauci. Astrocyte-conditioned medium stimulates HIV-1 expression in a chronically infected promonocyte clone. *J. Neuroimmunol.* 30:153 (1990).

20. V.L. Dawson, T.M. Dawson, G.R. Uhl, and S.H. Synder. Human immunodeficiency virus type 1 coat protein neurotoxicity mediated by nitric oxide in primary cortical cultures. *Proc. Natl. Acad. Sci. USA* 90:3256 (1993).

21. G.D. Clark, L.T. Happel, C.F. Zorumski, and N. Bazan. Enhancement of hippocampal excitatory synaptic transmission by platelt-activating factor. *Neuron* 9:1211 (1992).

22. A.Volterra,D. Trotti, P. Cassutti, et al. High sensitivity of glutamate uptake to extracellular free arachidonic acid levels in rat cortical synaptosomes and astrocytes. *J.Neurochem.* 69:606 (1992).

23. A.M. Wahl, J.B. Allen, Nl. CcCarnety-Francis, et al. Macrophage- and astrocyte-derived transforming frowth gactor beta as a mediator of central nervous system dysfunction in acquired immune deficiency syndrome. *J. Exp. Med.* 173:981 (1991).

HIV-1-DERIVED NEUROTOXIC FACTORS: EFFECTS ON HUMAN NEURONAL CULTURES

Harris A. Gelbard, Kirk A. Dzenko, Leo Wang, Angela Talley, Harold James, and Leon Epstein

Department of Neurology
Pediatric Neurology Division
The University of Rochester Medical Center
Rochester, New York 14642

ABSTRACT

HIV-1 infection of the developing central nervous system (CNS) results in a primary encephalopathy that is clinically devastating. Although it is established that HIV-1 productively infects brain microglia and macrophages, the mechanism(s) for neuronal dysfunction remain controversial. We have recently demonstrated that cocultures of HIV-1-infected monocytes and primary human fetal astrocytes secrete high, but variable levels of the cytokines tumor necrosis factor alpha (TNF-α) and interleukin-1 beta (IL-1β) relative to control uninfected monocyte plus astrocyte cocultures.[1,2] Additionally, cocultures of HIV-1-infected monocytes and primary human fetal astrocytes secrete high levels of platelet-activating factor (PAF) (unpublished results). Both conditioned media from these cocultures and exogenous TNF-α, PAF, but not IL-1β are neurotoxic to primary cultures of human fetal neurons.[1,2] TNF-α-induced neurotoxicity is dose-dependent and can be blocked in part by AMPA receptor antagonists.[3] Studies suggest that the time course for this neurotoxicity is subacute, and occurs between 24-48 hours in this cell culture system. Furthermore, PAF-induced neurotoxicity is dose-dependent and can be blocked in part by NMDA receptor antagonists. Other studies demonstrate that TNF-α and PAF down-regulate the expression of neurotransmitter receptors such as the dopamine D_2 receptor, which may be dysfunctional in neuroAIDS. Taken together, these data suggest that TNF-α and PAF, produced by interactions between HIV-1-infected monocytes and astrocytes, may act as two candidate neurotoxins to produce neuronal dysfunction and death. Because these neurotoxins act in part through glutamate receptor systems, glutamate receptor antagonists may be useful in the pharmacotherapy of HIV-1-mediated encephalopathy.

INTRODUCTION

HIV-1 infection of the CNS in children results in neurologic abnormalities in 40-90% of children. Symptoms include developmental delays, cognitive deficits, and motor signs. Cognitive deficits may manifest themselves in older children as attention deficits,[4] suggesting the possibility of dopaminergic dys-

Technical Advances in AIDS Research in the Human Nervous System
Edited by E.O. Major and J.A. Levy, Plenum Press, New York, 1995

61

function. In contrast to adults, the neurologic abnormalities seen in children are largely due to a primary HIV-1 encephalopathy. In one series, only 5% of children had opportunistic infections of their CNS.[5] Thus, a model for HIV-1 infection of the developing nervous system may be the best approach to studying the effects of the virus on brain tissue, since it is unlikely that opportunistic infections may be present and confound our understanding of how the HIV-1 virus causes neurologic dysfunction of the brain.

How the HIV-1 virus causes neurologic disease remains controversial. The pathologic hallmarks associated with neurologic dysfunction in HIV-1 encephalopathy of brain tissue, in the absence of opportunistic infections of brain, include HIV-1-infected macrophages and multinucleated giant cells, profound astrocyte proliferation, and myelin pallor. There is neuronal loss in discrete areas of the retina, neocortex, and subcortex. There is also loss of synaptic density and vacuolation of dendritic spines in affected areas.[6-12] Additionally, Reyes et al.[13] have demonstrated neuronal cell loss in the substantia nigra, suggesting that dopaminergic pathways may be a target for HIV-1-mediated neurotoxicity.

The molecular mechanisms for neurologic dysfunction during HIV-1 infection of brain remain unclear. To date, no laboratory has convincingly indicated the presence of HIV-1 viral mRNA or p24 antigen in neurons or oligodendrocytes from postmortem brain tissue. Recent studies by Saito et al.[14] demonstrated "restricted" infection of astrocytes in postmortem brain and spinal cord from children with severe HIV-1 encephalopathy. The term "restricted" denotes that HIV-1 infection of astrocytes is marked by synthesis of several early regulatory gene products of HIV-1, including *nef*. Indeed, the only cell types that produce the entire HIV-1 virus in the brain are microglia and macrophages.[15] Thus, these cells are productively infected with HIV-1.

A question of paramount importance is how does HIV-1 cause neuronal dysfunction or cell loss when only a small number of brain microglia and macrophages support productive viral infection and some astrocytes may have "restricted" infection? At least one report demonstrated neuronal cell death after exposure of neurons to conditioned media from HIV-1-infected monocytoid cell lines.[16] A low molecular weight substance present in this conditioned media was found to be heat-stable, protease-resistant, and have agonist activity at the NMDA receptor. However, other laboratories were unable to reproduce this neurotoxicity, using conditioned media from HIV-1-infected macrophages.[17] A number of reports demonstrate that picomolar amounts of HIV-1 envelope protein gp120, in the presence of sublethal concentrations of glutamate, can be toxic to rat retinal ganglion cells *in vitro*.[18-21] The latter toxicity is associated with increased intracellular neuronal Ca^{2+} levels and was reversed by calcium channel or NMDA antagonists.[20,21] However, neuronal cell death in this system was abolished after depletion of macrophages from the primary cultures of neurons.[20] Taken together, these findings suggest the production of neurotoxic factors from HIV-1-infected macrophages is likely to require cell-to-cell interactions between astrocytes, macrophages and microglia, and neurons.[22]

In support of this idea, studies by Genis et al.[23] recently demonstrated that coculture of HIV-1-infected monocytes and human astrocytoma monoclonal cell lines induce cytokines and arachidonic acid metabolites from monocytes. These studies indicated that only conditioned media from HIV-1-infected monocytes cocultured with astroglial cells, but not HIV-1-infected monocytes alone or uninfected monocytes cocultured with astrocytes, maintains high levels of the cytokines interleukin-1 beta (IL-1β) and tumor necrosis factor alpha (TNF-α) as well as free arachidonic acid, leukotrienes, and platelet-activating factor (PAF). Furthermore, the HIV-1-infected monocyte appeared to be the main source of cytokine production. Importantly, only conditioned media from HIV-1-infected monocytes cocultured with astroglial cells, but not HIV-1 infected monocytes alone or uninfected monocytes cocultured with astrocytes, was toxic to cultured neurons in a dose-dependent fashion. One of the major criticisms of this system is that monoclonal astrocytoma cells represent nonphysiologic cell types, and that cell-to-cell interactions between HIV-1-infected monocytes and astrocytoma cells may produce neurotoxic factors in response to tumor antigens present on the astrocytoma cells.

For these reasons, we determined whether TNF-α and PAF, which are produced from HIV-1-infected monocytes in cell-to-cell contact with primary human fetal astrocytes, could be neurotoxic to primary cultures of human fetal neurons. As a measure of neuronal dysfunction, we have also studied the effects of sublethal doses of these substances on dopamine receptor expression in cells of neuronal origin. The results, taken together, provide fresh insights into the pathobiology of HIV-associated dementia and a conceptual framework for experimental therapeutics directed against neurotoxic factors elaborated by interactions between HIV-1-infected monocytes and astrocytes.

MATERIALS AND METHODS

Neuronal Cell Cultures

Human fetal brain tissue was obtained from second trimester elective therapeutic abortions in an ethical manner and in strict observation of the guidelines of the NIH and the University of Rochester. Neurons were obtained from the telencephalon with both cortical and ventricular surfaces of second trimester (13-16 weeks gestation) human fetal brain tissue according to a modified procedure of Banker and Cowan.[24] These neurons were explanted in a modified serum-free MEM hippocampal media containing N1 components and plated at a density of 10^5 cells/12 mm glass coverslip precoated with poly-L-lysine (70K-150K MW, Sigma, St. Louis, MO). Cells were cultured for 28 days under standard conditions until neurons were established. Under these conditions, neuronal cultures were >80% homogeneous as determined[25] by anti-human PGP 9.5 staining (Ultraclone, Ltd., Rossiter's Farmhouse, Wellow, Isle of Wight) and glial fibrillary acidic protein (GFAP)-positive staining comprised 15% of the total cell population.

Neuroblastoma Cell Cultures

Human neuroblastoma monoclonal SK-N-MC cells[26] were grown according to the above-cited protocol in MEM until 75% confluent, then treated with 10^{-6} to 5×10^{-7} M retinoic acid for 3 days to differentiate the cells into a neuronal phenotype. Cultures were then exposed to test reagents for 48 hours. Cells were trypsinized and prepared according to a modification of the method of Sidhu et al.[27] for use in radioreceptor assays.

Quantitation of Human Neuronal Viability

Coverslips with neurons were fixed at 48 hours after exposure to conditioned media from HIV-1-infected or uninfected monocyte-astrocyte-cocultures. Cells were fixed in 4% paraformaldehyde and incubated with Neurotag™ Red (a recombinant tetanus toxin C fragment conjugated to tetramethyl rhodamine isothiocyanate). This reagent stains soma and neuritic processes of neurons (Boeringer Mannheim Corp., Indianapolis, IN). Cell morphology of neurons on coverslips was examined by fluorescence microscopy. In some experiments, coverslips with neurons were fixed at 48 hours after exposure to various reagents at varying doses. Cells were fixed in 4% paraformaldehyde and incubated with PGP 9.5 antisera. Examiners (KAD, HAG, LGE) were blinded to the particular treatment used. All experimental and control treatments were performed in triplicate or more replicates. Digitized images of PGP 9.5-stained neurons in ≥ 15 microscopic fields were analyzed for the number of intact neuronal soma per $\overline{20X}$ field using an MCID densitometer (Imaging Research Inc., Ontario, Canada). Data were expressed as mean of neuronal cell count $\pm$SEM. Tests of statistical

Electron Microscopy

After exposure to various reagents, cultured human cortical neurons on 12 mm poly-L-lysine-coated coverslips were fixed in 4% glutaraldehyde for 15 minutes at 5°C, then transferred to 5% dextrose overnight at 5°C. Neurons were reacted with osmium for 15 minutes at 23°C followed by uranyl acetate for 15 minutes at 23°C. Coverslips were washed in graded ethanol (50 to 99%) and transferred to glass petri dishes. Neurons were washed once in acetone, followed by three changes in Durcupan (Chemie Fluka, Switzerland) every 2 hours.

Fixed neuronal cultures were separated from the coverslips in the following manner: beam capsules were filled with Durcupan. Coverslips were inverted on top of the Durcupan and pressed flush to the beam capsule. The assembly was cured at 70°C for 48 hours. After removal from the oven, the coverslip was glued with cyanoacrylate cement to a glass slide. After the glue dried, the slide was set on a hot plate for 5 to 15 seconds and the block was separated from the coverslip. Thin sections (80 nm) were cut with a diamond knife, contrasted with lead acetate, and then studied under a Zeiss 902 electron microscope.

Radioreceptor Assays

Dopamine D_2 receptor density in crude membrane pellets of SK-N-MC cells was determined by specific binding of the selective D_2 receptor antagonist ^3H-YM-09151-2 (0.25 nM, New England Nuclear, Boston, MA) in the presence and absence of excess (+)-butaclamol (6 µM) according to a modification of the method of Gelbard et al.[28]

Reagents

Recombinant TNF-α was obtained from Genzyme (Cambridge, MA). 1-0-Hexadecyl-2-0-acetyl-sn-glycero-3-phosphorylcholine (PAF) was obtained from Biomol Research Laboratories, Inc. (Plymouth Meeting, PA). (±)-α-amino-3-hydroxy-5-methylisoxazole-4-proprionic acid hydrobromide (AMPA HBr), 6-cyano-7-nitroquinoxaline-2,3-dione (CNQX), and dizocilpine (MK-801) were obtained from Research Biochemicals, Inc. (Natick, MA).

RESULTS

Neurotoxicity from HIV-1$_{ADA}$-Infected Monocyte and Astrocyte Co-culture Conditioned Media

Preliminary experiments using conditioned media from HIV-1-infected glial cell cocultures at a 1:10 dilution (v/v) on established human fetal neuronal cell cultures demonstrated profound neurotoxicity. Neuronal cultures exposed to the conditioned media from cultures of uninfected human monocytes and astrocytes or to HIV-infected or uninfected monocytes alone showed no neurotoxicity (data not shown). In contrast, neuronal cultures exposed to conditioned media from HIV-1$_{ADA}$-infected monocyte and human fetal astrocyte cocultures showed loss of neurons and their processes.[2] Under fluorescence microscopy, these cultures had little or no remaining cytoarchitecture identifying them as being neuronal in origin. Cellular debris was visible in all fields (data not shown).

PAF-Mediated Neurotoxicity

Recent studies suggest that regulatory relationships exist between PAF and the cytokines IL-1β and TNF-α.[29] Indeed, inhibitors of arachidonic acid metabolites such as dexamethasone and nordihydroguaiaretic acid decrease TNF-α production in HIV-1$_{ADA}$-infected monocyte and astroglial cocultures.[23] Furthermore, PAF is a potent stimulus for TNF-α production,[29] and is found at high levels in HIV-1-infected monocyte-glial cocultures.[23] Therefore, PAF may play an important role(s) in HIV-1-induced neurotoxicity. To test this, we exposed primary fetal neuronal cultures to PAF at concentrations equal to and greater than those present in coculture fluids. PAF (50-6,000 pg/ml) applied to primary fetal neuronal cultures was toxic to human fetal neurons in a dose-dependent manner after 48 hours of exposure (data not shown). The PAF-induced neurotoxicity was partially blocked by coincubation with 10 µM MK-801.[1] Interestingly, coincubation of 10 µM MK-801 ameliorated this neurotoxicity such that the neuronal cell count was 80% of control.

TNF-α-Mediated Neurotoxicity

We first examined the effect of increasing doses of TNF-α on neuronal number. At a dose of 20 pg/ml, TNF-α reduced neuronal cell number to 56% of control.[3] Neurons stained with PGP 9.5 were markedly reduced in number compared to controls (Figs. 1B and 1A, respectively). The uncompetitive NMDA receptor antagonist, MK-801, at a concentration of 10 µM, was ineffective in protecting against the neurotoxicity produced by 200 pg/ml of TNF-α (Fig. 1C). Using these conditions, neuronal cell number was 54% of control.[3] Neurons also appeared vacuolated and had greatly reduced neuritic processes (Fig. 1C). However, the AMPA receptor antagonist, CNQX, at a concentration of 10 µM, was able to ameliorate in part, the neurotoxicity produced by 200 pg/ml of TNF-α (Fig. 1D). Using these conditions, the neurons appeared to have dense neuritic processes with less cellular debris (Fig. 1D). At 1,000 pg/ml, TNF-α reduced neuronal cell number to 22% of control.[3]

Because CNQX was effective in reversing some of the neurotoxicity produced by TNF-α, we wondered wither TNF-α might exert some of its neurotoxic effects indirectly through AMPA receptors on cortical neurons in culture. Therefore, we examined whether sublethal concentrations of TNF-α could have synergistic toxicity with an AMPA receptor agonist. Neurons exposed to AMPA at a concentration of 100 µM for 48 hours, had no change in either morphology (Fig. 2C) or neuronal cell number.[3] Because CNQX can block other non-NMDA receptors (i.e., kainate receptors), we also examined the effects of the kainate receptor agonist, kainic acid, at a concentration of 30 µM on human cortical cultures. No change in morphology or neuronal cell number were observed (data not shown). There was also neurotoxicity observed when 50 pg/ml of TNF-α + 30 µM kainic acid were added to neuronal cultures for 48 hours (data not shown).

Because cultures of human fetal cortical neurons incubated with increasing doses of TNF-α (200-1,000 pg/ml) for 48 hours showed striking changes in neuronal cell number and morphology when visualized with phase microscopy (data not shown), we examined control neuronal cultures and neuronal cultures exposed to 200 pg/ml TNF-α for 48 hours using electron microscopy. Neurons in control cultures had numerous growth cones present (data not shown) as well as intact nuclear membranes, abundant cytoplasm, and well-organized intracellular organelles (Fig. 3A). In contrast, neurons exposed to 200 pg/ml of TNF-α had no growth cones, ragged, irregular nuclear membranes, chromatin clumping, scant cytoplasm (Fig. 3B), and abnormal appearing rough endoplasmic reticulum.[3]

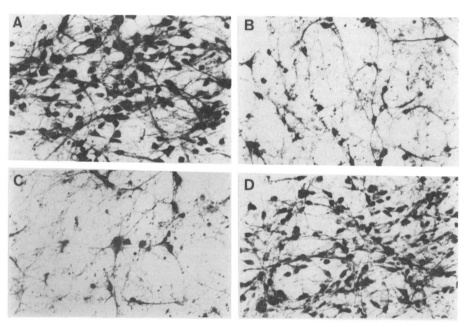

Fig. 1. Photomicrographs of cultures human fetal cortical neurons exposed to (A) control vehicle; (B) TNF-α (200 pg/ml); (C) TNF-α (200 pg/ml) + MK-801 (10 μM); or (D) TNF-α (200 pg/ml) + CNQX (10 μM) for 48 hours. Immunostained neuronal cell bodies and processes were identified with antisera to PGP 9.5 and photomicrographs were taken as described in Materials and Methods.

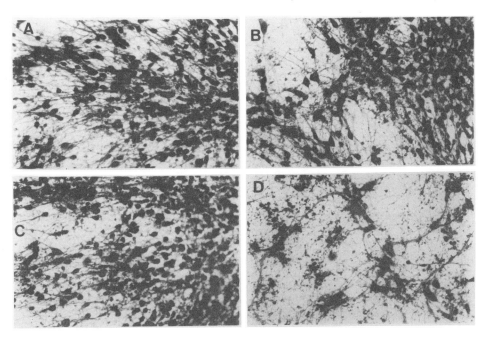

Fig. 2. Photomicrographs of cultured human fetal cortical neurons exposed to (A) control vehicle; (B) TNF-α (50 pg/ml); (C) AMPA (100 μM); and (D) TNF-α (50 pg/ml) + AMPA (100 μM) for 48 hours. Immunostained neuronal cell bodies and processes were identified with PGP 9.5 and photomicrographs were taken as described in Materials and Methods.

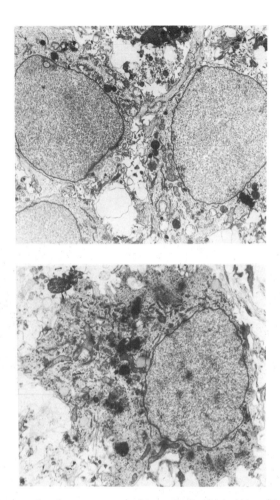

Fig. 3. Electron micrographs of neurons exposed to control. vehicle (A) and to TNF-α (200 pg/ml) (B) for 48 hours. Primary cultures of second trimester human fetal neurons were prepared as described in Materials and Methods. Neuronal cultures were fixed and prepared for electron microscopy as described in Materials and Methods. In (A) control neurons have intact nuclear membranes without evidence of chromatin condensation, as well as normal intracellular organelles (X 13,200). In (B) neurons exposed to TNF-α show irregular nuclear membranes, chromatin condensation, and abnormal appearing intracellular organelles (X13,200).

Dopamine D2 Receptor Expression in SK-N-MC Cells Exposed to TNF-α

The human neuroblastoma cell line SK-N-MC, when differentiated with retinoic acid to a neuronal phenotype, expresses increased levels of dopamine D2 receptors (unpublished data). Because autopsy findings suggest that dopaminergic cells may be lost in patients with AIDS,[13] and that some patients with AIDS had Parkinsonian symptoms after treatment with dopamine D2 receptor antagonists,[30] we examined whether one of the candidate neurotoxins, TNF-α, could affect the expression of dopamine D2 receptors. Accordingly, we exposed SK-N-MC cells to TNF-α, at a dose of 200 pg/ml for 48 hours, then assayed for D2 receptor specific binding. In a series of three replicate experiments, D2 receptor-specific binding was $63 \pm 14\%$ of control.

DISCUSSION

These results provide new insights into HIV-1-mediated neurologic dysfunction and neuronal cell death. Because HIV-1 encephalopathy is not characterized by direct neuronal infection, other mechanisms for neuronal dysfunction and cell death have to be investigated. Based on available experimental findings, the conceptual framework for HIV-1-mediated encephalopathy rests on aberrant cell-to-cell communication.[22,23] Other investigators have suggested that HIV-1 infection of the CNS ultimately results in activation of the NMDA subtype of the glutamate receptor with subsequent excitotoxic damage and death to the neuron.[20] Exactly how this is mediated remains controversial. Although the HIV-1 coat protein, gp120, has been shown to be neurotoxic in combination with subtoxic concentrations of glutamate, this toxicity is greatly ameliorated after depletion of macrophages from neuronal cultures.[20] Thus, other soluble neurotoxic factors may be produced by interactions between HIV-1-infected macrophages, astrocytes, and neurons.[22]

In support of this, the results presented here demonstrate that two candidate neurotoxins, PAF and TNF-α, produced by interactions between HIV-1, macrophages, and astrocytes, can be neurotoxic to human cortical neurons. This neurotoxicity is dose-dependent, and appears to involve activation of NMDA receptors (in the case of PAF) and non-NMDA, i.e., AMPA receptors (in the case of TNF-α). Furthermore, TNF-α, at low doses, can affect expression of the dopamine D_2 receptor, and may offer an explanation for the dopaminergic dysfunction seen in some patients with AIDS who are treated with neuroleptic agents.[30] Taken together, these results suggest that HIV-1-mediated encephalopathy is due to a number of neurotoxins that may be directly, or indirectly, produced by the HIV-1 virus. The ultimate activation of NMDA and non-NMDA receptors by these HIV-1-derived neurotoxins may provide a basis for future therapeutic approaches to this disease.

Acknowledgments

These studies were funded in part by AmFAR grant 500258-12-PG and 500278-14-PGR (H,.A.G.), the Strong Children's Research Fund (H.A.G.), and NIH Grants P01 NS31492-01 (H.A.G. and L.G.E.).

REFERENCES

1. H.A. Gelbard, K.A. Dzenko, R. White, L.G. Epstein. Human immunodeficiency virus-1-derived neurotoxic factors: effects of primary human fetal neuronal cultures. *Ann. Neurol.* 34:481 (1993).
2. K.A. Dzenko, R.J. White, P. Genis, et al. Increased secretion of cytokines and neurotoxins by co-cultures of HIV-1-infected macrophages and human fetal astrocytes. *Soc. Neurosci.* 19:1893 (1993).
3. H.A. Gelbard, K.A. Dzenko, K.A. diLoreto, et al. Neurotoxic effects of tumor necrosis factor alpha in primary human neuronal cultures are mediated by activation of the glutamate AMPA receptor subtype: implications for AIDS neuropathogenesis. *Dev. Neurosci.* (1994) (in press).
4. S.E. Cohen, T. Mundy, B. Karassik, et al. Neuropsychological functioning in human immunodeficiency virus type 1 seropositive children infected through neonatal blood transfusion. *Pediatrics* 88:58 (1991).
5. L.A. Civitello, P. Brouwers, and P.A. Pizzo. Neurological manifestations in 120 children with symptomatic human immunodeficiency virus infection. *Ann. Neurol.* 34:181 (1993).
6. I.P. Everall, P. J. Luthbert, and P.L. Lantos. Neuronal loss in the frontal cortex in HIV infection. *Lancet* 337:1119 (1991).
7. S. Ketzler, S. Weis, H. Haug, and H. Budka. Loss of neurons in the frontal cortex in AIDS brains. *Acta Neuropathol.* 80:92 (1990).

8. L.R. Sharer. Pathology of HIV-1 infection of the central nervous system (Review). *J. Neuropathol. and Exp. Neurol.* 51:3 (1992).
9. L.R. Sharer, L.G. Epstein, E.-S. Cho, et al. Pathologic features of AIDS encephalopathy in children: Evidence for LAV/HTLV-III infection of brain. *Hum. Pathol.* 17:271 (1986).
10. W.N. Tenhula, S.Z. Xu, M.C. Madigan, et al. Morphometric comparisons of optic nerve axon loss in acquired immunodeficiency syndrome. *Am. J. Ophthalmol.* 15:14 (1992).
11. C.A. Wiley, E.S. Masliah, M. Morey, et al. Neocortical damage during HIV infection. *Ann. Neurol.* 29:651 (1991).
12. C.A. Wiley, R.D. Schrier, J.A. Nelson, P.W. Lampert, and M.B.A. Oldstone. Cellular localization of human immunodeficiency virus infection within the brains of acquired immune deficiency syndrome patients. *Proc. Natl. Acad. Sci. USA* 83:7089 (1986).
13. M.G. Reyes, F. Faraldi, C.S. Senseng, C. Flowers, and R. Fariello. Nigral degeneration in acquired immune deficiency (AIDS). *Acta Neuropathol.* 82:39 (1991).
14. Y. Saito, L.R. Sharer, L.G. Epstein, et al. Overexpression of *nef* as a marker for restricted HIV-1 infection of astrocytes in postmortem pediatric central nervous tissues. *Neurology* (1994) (in press).
15. J. Michaels, L.R. Sharer, and L.G. Epstein. Human immunodeficiency virus type 1 (HIV-1) infection of the nervous system: A review. *Immunodef. Rev.* 1:71 (1988).
16. D. Giuliam, K. Vaca, and C.A. Noonan. Secretion of neurotoxins by mononuclear phagocytes infected with HIV-1. *Science* 250:1593 (1991).
17. E. Bernton, H. Bryant, M. Decoster, et al. No direct neuronotoxicity by HIV-1 virions or culture fluids from HIV-1-infected T cells or monocytes. *AIDS Res. Hum. Retroviruses* 8:495 (1992).
18. E.B. Dreyer, P.K. Kaiser, J.T. Offermann, and S.A.Lipton. HIV-1 coat protein neurotoxicity prevented by calcium channel antagonists. *Science* 248:364 (1990).
19. S.A. Lipton, N.J. Sucher, P.K. Kaiser, and E.B. Dreyer. Synergistic effects of HIV coat protein and NMDA receptor-mediated neurotoxicity. *Neuron* 7:1112 (1991).
20. S.A. Lipton. Human immunodeficiency virus-infected macrophages, gp120, and N-methyl-D-aspartate receptor-mediated neurotoxicity. *Ann. Neurol.* 33:227 (1993).
21. S.A. Lipton, and F.E. Jensen. Memantine, a clinically-tolerated NMDA open-channel blocker, prevents HIV coat protein-induced neuronal injury *in vitro* and *in vivo. Soc. Neurosci. Abstr.* 18:757 (1993).
22. L.G. Epstein, and H.E. Gendelman. Human immunodeficiency virus type I infection of the nervous system: pathogenetic mechanisms. *Ann. Neurol.* 33:429 (1993).
23. P. Genis, M. Jett, E.W. Bernton, et al. Cytokines and arachidonic acid metabolites produced during HIV-infected macrophage-astroglial interactions: Implications for the neuropathogenesis of HIV disease. *J. Exp. Med.* 176:1703 (1992).
24. G.A. Barker, and W.M. Cowan. Rat hippocampal neurons in dispersed cell cultures. *Brain Res.* 126:397 (1977).
25. C. Kent, and P.J. Clarke. The immunolocalisation of the neuroendocrine specific protein PGP 9.5 during neurogenesis in the rat. *Dev. Brain Res.* 58:147 (1991).
26. J.L. Biedler, L. Henson, and B.A. Spengler. Morphology and growth, tumorigenicity, and cytogenetics of human neuroblastoma cells in continuous culture. *Cancer Res.* 33:2643 (1973).
27. A. Sidhu, and P.H. Fishman. Identification and characterization of functional D_1 dopamine receptors in a human neuroblastoma cell line. *Biochem. Biophys. Res. Acta* 166:574 (1990).
28. H.A. Gelbard, M.H. Teicher, G. Faedda, and R.J. Baldessarini. Postnatal development of dopamine D_1 and D_2 receptor sites in rat striatum. *Dev. Brain Res.* 49:123 (1989).

29. P.E. Poubelle, D. Gingras, C. Demers, et al. Platelet-activating factor (PAF-acether) enhances the concomitant production of tumor necrosis factor-alpha and interleukin-1 by subsets of human monocytes. *Immunology* 72:181 (1991).
30. K.D. Kieburtz, L.G. Epstein, H.A. Gelbard, and J.T. Greenmayre. Excito-toxicity and dopaminergic dysfunction in the AIDS dementia complex: therapeutic implications. *Arch. Neurol.* 48:1281 (1991).

EXPERIMENTAL MODEL SYSTEMS FOR STUDIES OF HIV ENCEPHALITIS

Howard E. Gendelman,[1] Peter Genis,[1] Marti Jett,[2] and Hans S.L.M. Nottet[1]

[1]Departments of Pathology and Microbiology and Medicine
University of Nebraska Medical Center
600 South 42nd Street
Omaha, Nebraska 68198-5215
[2]Department of Molecular Pathology
Walter Reed Institute of Research
Washington, D.C. 20307

INTRODUCTION

HIV-1 enters the brain shortly after systemic infection, but in most individuals, the viral replication which follows, remains limited.[1,2] Most commonly, HIV entry into the brain shows no clinical abnormalities and HIV remains restricted in the central nervous system (CNS) for long periods of time.[3] Productive HIV replication in brain tissue occurs only as a late manifestation of disease. Acute meningitis or meningoencephalitis can occur weeks after viral infection and is characterized by headache, seizures, meningismus, photophobia and/or altered mental function but is usually self-limited and nonprogressive.[4] After a period of time, usually measured in years, following viral exposure, productive HIV replication in brain tissue heralds neurologic disease.[5,6] These events are associated with advanced immunosuppression.[6] Here, the CNS becomes a major reservoir for HIV,[7-9] and virus is almost exclusively expressed in cells of macrophage lineage (brain macrophages, microglia and multinucleated giant cells).[10-14] However, there is a discrepancy between the numbers of productively infected macrophages and the severity of tissue damage.[15] These observations suggest that indirect mechanisms for tissue damage, including the release of viral and/or cellular factors, mediate CNS tissue damage.[16-23]

Exactly how HIV enters the brain and preferentially infects macrophages are areas of intense debate. Presumably, neural cellular factors control the levels and spread of infection in brain macrophages and microglia. HIV tropism for macrophages is an essential requirement for HIV neuroinvasiveness. The origins of infection of brain macrophages likely reside from either an expansion of latently infected monocytes that carry HIV into the brain (the "Trojan horse" hypothesis) or by a spreading infection within *de novo* susceptible brain macrophages.[24,25] Virus may penetrate the brain through a disrupted blood-brain barrier,[26] likely initiated by a cellular dysregulation between brain capillary endothelial cells and HIV-infected blood monocytes. Alternatively, the cellular control mechanisms in brain responsible for HIV restriction might break down. This may occur through loss of an inhibitory or induction of a stimulatory viral replication factor. Ultimately, productively infected brain macrophages

Technical Advances in AIDS Research in the Human Nervous System
Edited by E.O. Major and J.A. Levy, Plenum Press, New York, 1995

will secrete metabolic, immune and/or viral-induced factors that precipitate neural injury. How the macrophage is triggered to produce such factors and their identity are critical to any understanding of HIV neuropathogenesis.[27] There is an emerging body of evidence suggesting that virus-infected macrophages do indeed secrete neurotoxins.[20-23] Secretory products from HIV-infected cells may thus alter neuronal viability, damage myelin and/or stimulate neurotransmitters resulting in neuronal dysfunction.

In order to discern the mechanism and identity of HIV-infected macrophage-induced neurotoxins, we developed experimental model systems that mimic some of the pathologic events associated with HIV encephalitis. We show that a disordered secretion of one or more cellular factors occurs within HIV-infected macrophages through interactions with astroglia and/or lipopolysaccharide (LPS). These factors include cytokines, arachidonic acid (AA) metabolites and PAF. They were collectively produced in the experimental systems and induced neuronal death.[27] HIV-infected monocytes produce increased levels of TNF after activation as compared to uninfected cells. Interestingly, mixtures of HIV-infected monocytes and human fetal astrocytes showed a diminished TNF response to LPS when compared to HIV-infected cells alone. This was due, in part, to the production of IL-10 and TGF-β. IL-10 produced from monocytes directly inhibited TNF production. These studies, *in toto*, suggest that HIV-infected macrophages can continuously disrupt neurologic function through different mechanisms and lead to brain dysfunction.

MATERIALS AND METHODS

Isolation and Culture of Monocytes

Monocytes were recovered from peripheral blood mononuclear cells (PBMCs) of HIV and hepatitis B-seronegative donors and leukopheresis and purified by countercurrent centrifugal elutriation. Cells suspensions were >98% monocytes, according to the criteria of cell morphology on Wright-stained cytosmears, by granular peroxidase, and by nonspecific esterase. Monocytes were cultured as adherent monolayers (1×10^6 cells/ml in 24-mm plastic culture wells) in Dulbecco's Minimum Essential Media (DMEM) (Sigma, St. Louis, MO) with recombinant human MCSF (FAP-809, Cetus Corp, Emeryville, CA) as previously described.[28] The human brain tumor-derived cell line U251 MG was obtained from D. Bigner.[29] The cells were grown as adherent monolayers in DMEM (Sigma) with 10% heat-inactivated fetal calf serum (FCS) (Sigma) and 50 μg/ml gentamicin and characterized as to their cell of origin.

Isolation and Propagation of Primary Human Astrocytes

Human fetal astrocytes were prepared from first or second trimester human fetal brain tissue obtained from elective abortions as previously described[30] and performed in full compliance with both NIH and the University of Nebraska Medical Center. Cells were cultured as adherent monolayers in DMEM (Sigma) with 10% FCS (Sigma). All culture reagents were screened and found to be negative for endotoxin contamination.

HIV Infection of Target Cells

Adherent monocytes cultured for 7 days were exposed to the monocyte-tropic HIV-1 strain at a multiplicity of infection (MOI) of 0.01 infectious virus particles/target cells. All viral stocks were tested and found free of mycoplasma contamination (Gen-probe II, Gen-probe Inc., San Diego, CA). Culture medium was half-exchanged every 2-3 days. Reverse transcriptase (RT) activity was determined in replicate samples of culture fluids added to a reaction mixture of 0.05% Nonidet P-40® (Sigma Chemical Co.), 10 μg/ml poly (A), 0.25 U/ml oligo (dT) (Pharmacia, Piscataway, NJ), 5 mM dithiothreitol (Pharmacia), 150 mM KCl, 15 mM MgCl$_2$, and ^{3}H-dTTP (2 Ci/mmol, Amersham Corp., Arlington,

Heights, IL) in pH 7.9 Tris-HCl buffer for 24 hours at 37°C. Radiolabeled nucleotides were precipitated with cold 10% trichloroacetic acid (TCA) and washed with 10% TCA and 95% ethanol in an automatic cell harvester (Skatron Inc., Sterling, VA) on glass filter discs. Radioactivity was estimated by liquid scintillation spectroscopy.[31,32]

Chemical Reagents

Dexamethasone was purchased from Sigma (St. Louis, MO) and indomethacin and nordihydroguaiaretic acid (NDGA) from Cayman Chemical Co. (Ann Arbor MI). All reagents were dissolved in ethanol and diluted with complete macrophage media. Final ethanol concentration in cell cultures was $\leq 0.1\%$. Lipopolysaccharide (LPS) was from Sigma.

Quantitation of Cytokine Activity

Culture fluids from control and HIV-infected monocytes were analyzed by ELISA for the human cytokines TNF-α and IL-1β (Quantikine Immunoassay, Research and Diagnostics Systems, Minneapolis, MN). TNF bioactivity was performed according to standard procedures.[33] Briefly, the murine L929 cell line was propagated in DMEM (Sigma), 5% FCS, 1% glutamine and 20 µg/ml gentamicin. Cells were retrieved in log phase and placed (0.5×10^5/well) into 96-well plates (Costar) with actinomycin D. Culture fluids were inoculated into cell monolayers and degree of cell lysis determined by crystal violet staining after a 24-hour incubation. LPS was from Sigma.

Analysis of [3H] Arachidonic Acid (AA) Metabolites Released by HIV-Infected Monocytes and Cocultures of HIV-Infected Monocytes and Astroglia

HIV-infected or control uninfected monocytes (5×10^6 cells/ml) cultured in 35-mm wells (Costar) in media containing 10% AB+ human sera were pulsed with [3H] AA (1.0 µCi/ml; 1 Ci = 37 GBq/American Radiolabeled Chemicals Inc., St. Louis, MO) for 18 hr. HPLC procedures followed previously published methods.[27]

Platelet-Activating Factor (PAF) Assay

PAF was measured in cell lysates in a radioimmunoassay according to the manufacturer's instructions (Amersham Chemical Co., Arlington Heights, IL).[27]

RESULTS

A Model Cell System That Mimics the Pathologic Findings of HIV Encephalitis

Our initial work and those of others have demonstrated that HIV infection of monocytes fails to alter constitutive phagocytic or monocyte effector cell function.[25,34] Indeed, following HIV-1 infection of monocytes, phagocytosis, antigen presentation, and cytokine production are similar if not identical to uninfected cells.[25] Moreover, neurotoxic activity was not demonstrated from HIV-1-infected monocyte culture fluids throughout the course of viral infection.[22] Therefore, if the HIV-1-infected brain macrophage produces neurotoxins, it would require cooperation of other cells in the brain or perhaps macrophage activators (opportunistic infection and/or immune stimuli).

Previous work performed in our laboratory has shown that the interactions between HIV-1-infected monocytes and PBMCs resulted in interferon alpha (IFN-α) production in PBMCs.[35] Could similar mechanisms occur in the CNS and be responsible for the observed cytokine response? Since both microglia (brain macrophages) and macroglia (astrocytes/oligodendrocytes) produce IL-1β and TNF-α after stimulation,[36] HIV-1-infected brain macrophages could stimulate an astrocyte cytokine response. Our earliest work seemed to support such a theory but the mechanism(s) involved in neural cytokine regulation was distinct from those observed with IFN-α. A variety of cytokines may produce neurotoxicity and as such contribute to the pathogenesis of CNS disease. Two cytokines, IL-1β and TNF-α, are associated with glial proliferation, neurotoxicity and demyelination. Interestingly, these cellular effects are all prominent features of HIV-related encephalopathy. TNF is found in postmortem brains of patients with HIV encephalitis. Moreover, TNF, at high concentrations, is a neurotoxin.[37,38] Human astrocytes proliferate in response to TNF-α and IL-1β,[39,40] and conditioned media from LPS-treated astrocytes stimulates HIV-1 gene expression in monocytic cells.[41]

These observations led us initially to investigate whether TNF-α and IL-1β were produced during the interactions between HIV-infected monocytes and astroglia. Monocytes were infected for 7 days with HIV-1$_{ADA}$ at a multiplicity of infection of 0.1. High levels of viral replication were determined as monitored by RT activity in culture fluids (6×10^6 cpm/ml) and formation of multinucleated giant cell syncytia. Mixtures of HIV-1$_{ADA}$-infected monocytes and astroglia U251 MG and HTB 148 produced a sustained TNF and IL-1 response. TNF-α and IL-1β protein and activity were seen only in coculture fluids of HIV-1-infected monocytes and glia (Table 1). Maximum levels were present 12-48 hours following cocultivation. In a series of 4 replicate experiments, maximum levels of TNF-α were 1,000 to 9,000 pg/ml (mean of 5,000) while IL-1β levels ranged from 400 to 5,000 pg/ml (mean of 900). The results were confirmed by assays of TNF activity. The underlying basis for this 10-fold difference was related to the levels of productive HIV infection. Peak cytokine levels occurred during the initial rise of RT activity, 3-5 days following virus infection, and diminished to baseline by day 10. TNF-α and IL-1β proteins were detected at only low levels <100 pg/ml in cocultures of uninfected monocytes and astroglia. The latter results suggest that the interactions seen between HIV-infected monocytes and astroglia are an extension of normal physiologic responses.

Analysis of the Cytokine-Producing Cell in Monocyte-Astroglia Cocultures

Cytokines produced during the interactions between HIV-infected monocytes and glia required viable mixtures of both cell types. When U251 MG or HTB 148 were mixed with 4% paraformaldehyde-fixed or freeze-thawed HIV-infected monocytes, cytokines were not detected. Pretreatment of HIV-infected monocytes with cycloheximide or actinomycin D before coculture determined if the infected monocyte was the primary cytokine producer. Cycloheximide and actinomycin D were titrated to inhibit HIV mRNA and protein synthesis (positive controls for this assay system). Analysis of TNF-α mRNA levels from cell lysates prepared from cycloheximide or actinomycin D-treated cocultures showed increased and decreased levels of TNF-α, respectively. However, both additions resulted in significant reductions in both TNF-α and IL-1β proteins. Previous reports show an up-regulation of TNF-α mRNA in monocytes following both LPS and cycloheximide treatment. These results coupled with the recently published demonstration of TNF-α and IL-1β protein in *in vivo* brain macrophages but not astroglia support the notion that the macrophage is the primary cytokine producer.

Table 1. Levels of TNF-α mRNA and protein coculture of HIV-infected mono-cytes and the U251 glial cell line.

Cell Treatments	TNF-α mRNA	TNF-α Protein (pg/ml)
Monocytes cultured with:		
medium	0	0
lipopolysaccharide (LPS)	+ +	2,250
medium with MCSF	0	0
HIV-infected monocytes cultured with:		
medium	0	0
endothelial cells	0	0
SK-N-MC (neuroblastoma)	0	0
HTB 148 glial cells	+ +	2,140
U251 glial cells	+ +	3,460
cycloheximide then U251 cells	+ + +	1,300
actinomycin D then U251 cells	+/-	90
U251 MG astroglial cells cultured with:		
uninfected monocytes	+ +	50
HIV-1$_{ADA}$	0	0
mycoplasma-infected monocytes	+ +	3,120
freeze-thawed HIV-infected monocytes	0	0
paraformaldehyde-fixed HIV-infected monocytes	0	0

TNF-α mRNA and protein in cell lysates and culture fluids of uninfected control, HIV-1$_{ADA}$-infected monocytes and/or U251 MG astroglial cells following 24 hour-incubations with the treatments listed. Monocytes cultured 7 days as adherent monolayers were exposed to HIV at an MOI = 0.01. One week after infection, virus-infected monocytes were cocultured with media or equal numbers of: endothelial cells, SK-N-MC (neuroblastoma) cells, HTB 148 glial cells, U251 MG astroglial cells, cycloheximide then U251 MG astroglial cells, and cycloheximide then U251 astroglial cells. The U251 MG astroglial cells were incubated with: uninfected monocytes, HIV-1$_{ADA}$, mycoplasma-infected monocytes, and freeze-thawed or paraformaldehyde-fixed HIV-infected monocytes. Cytokine mRNA levels were detected by coupled reverse transcription/PCR amplifications from cell lysates. The extracted RNAs were mixed with antisense primers and after reverse transcription, cDNA was amplified by PCR. The products of 25 cycles were analyzed by Southern blot hybridization. RNA was not detected (0), was readily (+ +) or detected at high levels (+ + +). Cytokine levels in culture fluids were determined by ELISA.

HIV-1 Infected Monocytes or Mixtures of HIV-Infected Monocytes and Primary Human Astrocytes Require Activation for Cytokine Production

To assay the possible physiologic relevance of our *in vitro* systems for HIV encephalitis, we determined whether cocultures of human fetal astrocytes and HIV-1 infected monocytes could produce similar effects as observed with virus-infected monocytes and astroglial cell lines. Surprisingly, TNF was not repro-ducibly detected in culture fluids of human fetal astrocytes and HIV-infected monocytes. When TNF was detected, it was low (< 100 U/ml) and poorly sus-tained. We reasoned that the U251 MG astroglial cell line supplied an activation stimulus for the HIV-infected monocytes that primary fetal astrocytes lacked. Therefore, we studied the effect of other stimuli of macrophage activation that could lead to an increased cytokine response in virus-infected monocytes.

Monocytes were infected for 7 days with HIV-1$_{ADA}$ at an MOI = 0.01 and then stimulated with LPS (0.1-10 ng/ml). This produced a marked increased in

TNF activity as compared to uninfected controls (Fig. 1). All LPS concentrations showed these effects for a 36-hour observation period. Interestingly, LPS treatment of cocultures of HIV-1$_{ADA}$-infected monocytes and human fetal astrocytes showed a decreased response to LPS when compared to HIV-1-infected cells alone (Fig. 2). This was an unexpected finding as both monocytes and astrocytes respond to cytokine production in both an autocrine and paracrine fashion. The expectation was that there would be an additive if not synergistic response to LPS treatment. This led us to investigate the production of a negative regulatory

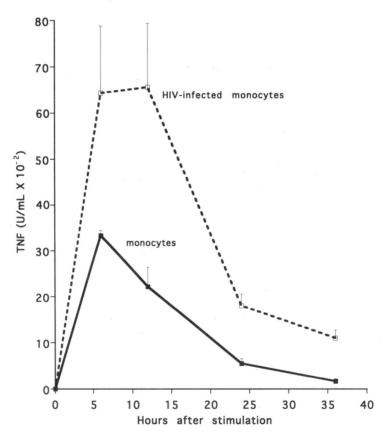

Figure 1. TNF activity in culture fluids of HIV-infected and control uninfected monocytes following LPS (1 ng/ml) stimulation. Adherent monocytes cultured for 7 days were exposed to HIV$_{ADA}$ at an MOI = 0.01. At 7 days of infection, HIV-infected and control uninfected monocytes were stimulated with 1 ng/ml LPS and TNF levels measured in culture fluids (for 36 hours) by bioactivity by lysis of actinomycin D-treated L929 cells.

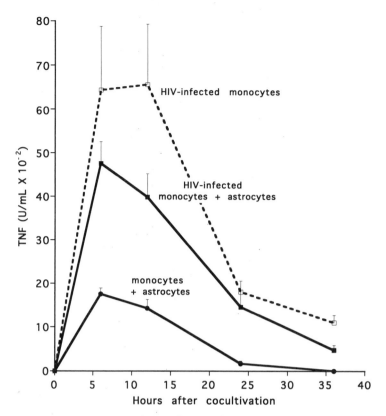

Figure 2. TNF activity in culture fluids of HIV-infected and control uninfected monocytes cocultured with primary human fetal astrocytes and stimulated with LPS (1 ng/ml). Adherent monocytes cultured for 7 days were exposed to HIV_{ADA} at an MOI = 0.01. At 7 days of infection, HIV-infected and control uninfected monocytes were stimulated with 1 ng/ml LPS. After 2 hours following LPS treatment, select monocytes were cocultured with astrocytes and TNF levels measured in culture fluids (for 36 hours) by bioactivity by lysis of actinomycin D-treated L929 cells.

factor that was synthesized by monocytes and/or astrocytes during cellular inter-actions. One such inhibitory factor, TGF-β was sought for several reasons: (a) it down-regulates TNF production in rodent astrocytes;[42] (b) is localized in brain tissue of HIV-infected patients with encephalopathy;[43] and (c) reportedly is in-duced in monocytes after HIV infection and in astrocytes after exposure to progeny HIV.[43] Levels (>2 ng/ml) of TGF-β were observed in a mixture of HIV-infected and control uninfected monocytes and human astrocytes but not in HIV-infected or control uninfected monocytes. These results, taken together, demon-strate that HIV-infected monocytes are more responsive to LPS-induced activation. The down-regulation of TNF activity following monocyte-astrocyte mixtures was possibly regulated, by the production of TGF-β. IL-10 produced from LPS-activated HIV-infected monocytes proved to be a more potent deactivator of TNFα than TGF-β2. Mechanisms could now be established for how HIV infection of brain macrophages modulates high levels of TNF activity and how this activity is controlled by intracellular interactions (Fig. 3).

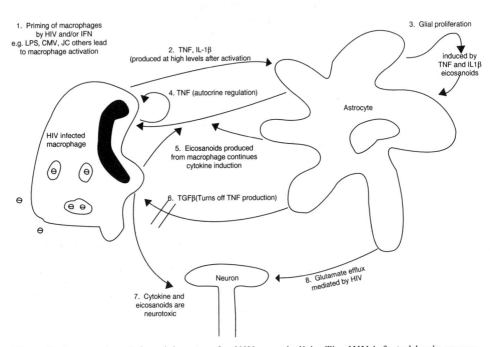

Figure 3. An experimental model system for HIV encephalitis. The HIV-infected brain macrophage is activated by immune and/or opportunistic infectious stimuli. Eicosanoids, PAF and cytokines are produced. This results in glia proliferation/activation and autocrine and paracrine production of TNF-α and IL-1β, factors. Factors that may include TGF-β2 and IL-10, produced by astrocytes and/or monocytes, turn off cytokine production. The arachidonic acid metabolites, PAF and cytokines produced during these cellular interactions, lead to neurotoxicity.

Arachidonic Acid (AA) Metabolites Induced During Coculture of HIV-Infected Monocytes and Astroglia: Implications for Cytokine Regulation

The control of cytokine production in activated HIV-infected monocytes was further investigated. For several reasons, AA metabolites were pursued as a likely regulatory pathway for neural injury and cytokine regulation. First, AA metabolites are up-regulated in monocytes after incubation with the viral envelope glycoprotein, gp120.[44] Second, these metabolic products can regulate TNF-α and IL-1β production in macrophages. TNF amplifies AA metabolites in response to IL-1 while PAF enhances TNF production.[45-47] Third, AA metabolites play important roles in developmental neurobiology and neuronal function.[48-51] Thus, we determined whether AA metabolites were produced during HIV-infected monocyte-astroglia interactions. Investigation of their physiologic role in neural cell injury was investigated in the companion report.

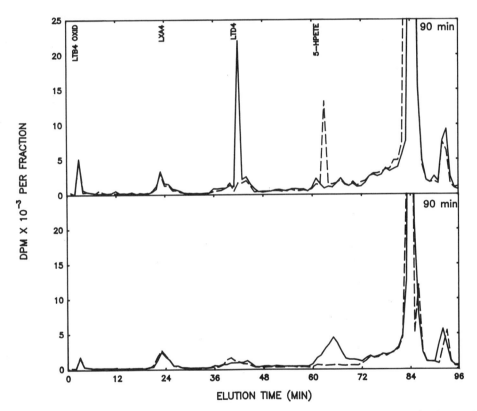

Figure 4. Arachidonic acid (AA) elution profiles of monocytes following HIV infection and cocultivation of HIV-infected monocytes and U251 astroglial cells. Ad-herent monocytes cultured for 7 days were exposed to HIV_{ADA} at an MOI = 0.01. At 7 days of infection, HIV-infected and control uninfected monocytes (5x10⁶ cells) were incubated with equal numbers of astroglial cells (U251 MG). At 90 minutes, generation of AA metabolites was determined. The metabolites were extracted, separated by HPLC, and analyzed quantitatively to determine DPM in the recovered fractions. The chromatograms were adjusted based on recovery of internal standards. Upper panel represents cocultures of HIV-infected (solid lines) or uninfected (broken line) monocytes and astroglial (U251 MG cells). The lower panel is HIV-infected (solid lines) and uninfected control (broken line) monocytes.

HPLC separation of AA metabolic products released from HIV-infected and control uninfected cells was evaluated along with replicate astroglia-monocyte cell mixtures. Cells were radiolabeled with [3H]-AA for 18 hours before coculture. The elution profiles of uninfected control (Fig. 4, bottom broken lines) and HIV-infected monocytes (Fig. 4, bottom solid lines) were virtually indistinguishable. However, HPLC analysis of the AA products released from HIV-infected monocytes after coculture with U251 MG astroglial cells (Fig. 4, top solid line) revealed signature profiles. Based on elution times of ^3H standard, the major products of the lipoxygenase pathway were LTB_4, LTD_4, and lipoxin A_4. Although increased amounts of 5-HETE methyl ester and lactone were in HIV-infected cells, the levels of these metabolites were indistinguishable between infected and uninfected (Fig. 4, top broken and solid lines) cell cocultures. Major increases were also seen in LTD_4 levels in infected cell cocultures. Levels of PAF were evaluated by a quantitative RIA (Fig. 5). Increased levels of PAF in cocultures of HIV-infected monocytes and astroglia were strongly associated with TNF-α production.

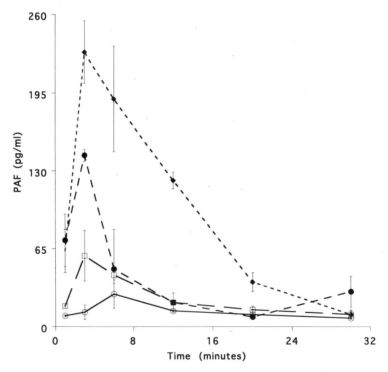

Figure 5. Monocytes cultured 7 days as adherent monolayers were exposed to HIV-1$_{ADA}$ at an MOI = 0.01. Seven days after infection, HIV-infected or control uninfected monocytes were cocultured 1:1 (monocytes/astroglial cells). At various times (in minutes) after coculture, HIV-infected monocytes, uninfected monocytes or monocyte cocultures were frozen on dry ice in ethanol and then, cell lysates were combined with ethanol washes of broken cells and extracted. PAF was eluted with approximately 70% recovery and quantitated by radioimmunoassay. The detectable levels of PAF in these assays were 30, 1, and 200 pg/ml. Levels of PAF in closed diamonds (HIV-1-infected monocytes and astroglial cells); closed circles (uninfected monocytes and astroglial cells); open boxes (HIV-infected monocytes); and open circles (uninfected monocytes). Error bars represent mean ± S.D.

To investigate a possible temporal relationship between AA metabolites and TNF-α, we added dexamethasone (inhibitor of phospholipase A), indomethacin (cyclooxygenase inhibitor), or NDGA (lipoxygenase inhibitor) to cocultures of HIV-infected monocytes and astroglia and measured TNF-α production (Table 2). Monocytes were infected with HIV at an MOI = 0.01 for 7 days before addition of U251 MG astroglial cells. The compounds were added together with equal numbers of astroglia. Both dexamethasone and nordihydroguaiaretic acid (NDGA) markedly reduced the levels of TNF-α in supernatant fluids of these cocultured cells. Interestingly, indomethacin increased TNF-α levels. This likely reflected shunting of the AA metabolites into the lipoxygenase pathway. This failure of NDGA to completely abrogate the TNF-α response suggests that PAF also participates in this cytokine response. Thus, AA metabolites and PAF both likely participate in the TNF-α induction demonstrated.

Table 2. Effect of arachidonic acid (AA) inhibitors on TNF-α levels following coculture of HIV-infected monocytes and astroglia.*

| | TNF-α Protein (pg/ml) | |
Hours after Coculture	12	48
Cell Treatments:		
Medium	3100	1760
Dexamethasone (10^{-5}M)	50	30
Indomethacin (0.4 µg/ml)	5030	5340
NDGA (5×10^{-5}M)	602	550

*Effect of AA inhibitors on TNF production. Monocytes cultured 7 days as adherent monolayers were exposed to HIV at an MOI = 0.01. One week after infection, virus-infected monocytes were cocultured with equal numbers of U251 MG astroglial cells. At the time of coculture, the cells were incubated with medium, dexamethasone (10^{-5}M), indomethacin (0.4 µg/ml) or NDGA (5×10^{-5}M). TNF-α production was measured by ELISA. Data represent means of duplicate determinations for 1 of 3 experiments performed.

DISCUSSION

CNS dysfunction is a common manifestation of HIV infection.[52] Indeed, progressive HIV disease is often associated with motor, sensory and cognitive disorders. Subacute encephalitis occurs in about one-third of infected patients. Characteristic morphologic features include a reactive astrocytosis and a predominance of microglia, microglial nodules, blood-derived macrophages and multinucleated giant cells in infected brain.[5,6] White matter pallor can progress to severe myelin loss in affected tissue. While HIV infection is clearly associated with these pathologic abnormalities, the relationship between tissue infection and disease manifestations remains uncertain. Despite HIV infecting brain macrophages and not neurons, there is profound neuronal loss in the cortex.[53-55] These observations support an emerging theory that indirect effects of viral replication including diffusible viral and/or cellular gene products produce neurotoxicity. Published reports suggest that brain dysfunction may be related to cell-encoded toxins generated from virus-infected macrophages.[15-21] Secretory products from HIV-infected cells may alter neuronal viability, damage myelin or stimulate neurotransmitters resulting in neuropathology. In support of this notion are recent studies demonstrating that disordered secretion of one or more cellular factors from HIV-infected macrophages produce neuronal death *in vitro*.[20,21]

In one report, HIV-infected U937 cells, a myelomonocytic cell line released toxic factors that destroyed cultured chick and rat neurons.[22] The monocyte-produced neurotoxin(s) were heat-stable and protease-resistant and acted via N-methyl-D-aspartate (NMDA) receptors.[21] It is possible that the results described in this report, namely the interactions between HIV-infected monocytes and astrocytes, represent an amplification of these previously reported findings. Indeed, activation/stimulation of HIV-infected macrophages might initiate these cellular responses that are then modified by the astrocytes. The ultimate result is the production of cytokines and neuronotoxins. The possible role of AA metabolites, low molecular weight heat-stable and protease-resistant factors, in these events, supports this contention. Indeed, TNF causes amplification of AA metabolites in response to IL-1 while PAF enhances TNF production.[56,57] An autocrine loop between AA metabolites and cytokines and *vice versa* could explain these glial cell interactions.

It is thus tempting to attribute the pathogenesis of HIV encephalopathy to secretory products produced from HIV-infected macrophages or through the interactions between HIV-1-infected macrophages and astrocytes. Perhaps interplay occurs between a number of toxic factors including cytokines, AA metabolites, and viral structural and/or regulatory proteins (gp120, tat, nef, etc.). TNF and IL-1 likely contribute to the *in vivo* neuropathology of HIV infection.[58] TNF regulates class I and II MHC antigens, and induces proliferation of astrocytes. Additionally, TNF can cause myelin damage and lysis in oligodendrocytes and can up-regulate HIV gene expression in monocytic cells.[41] Thus, TNF can facilitate production of inflammatory infiltrates in brain parenchyma and permit the penetration of virus-infected monocytes through the blood-brain barrier. These results suggest that cytokines, viral proteins, and lipidic compounds produced during glial cellular interactions all play roles in the neuropathogenesis of HIV disease.

Our efforts over the past decade have centered on the role of lentiviral infection within cells of macrophage lineage. We and other have demonstrated that macrophages, particularly in brain tissue, are a major reservoir and vehicle for dissemination of HIV. Macrophage-tropic viruses are present throughout the course of viral infection and are associated with CNS infection. Nevertheless, the role of HIV-infected brain macrophages in neurologic impairments has not been defined. Interactions between HIV-infected human monocytes and astroglial cell lines produce neuronotoxicity and glial proliferation. This was associated with high levels of IL-1β and TNF-α. Although the appearance of IL-1β and TNF-α response correlated with neuronal death, they alone do not explain progressive CNS injury after HIV infection. Lipidic compounds derived from membrane phospholipids, including products of the lipoxygenase system are now being considered as candidates for HIV-induced neurotoxins. AA metabolites are produced during cell-to-cell interactions between HIV-infected macrophages and astroglia, and can potentiate NMDA receptor current by increasing open channel probability. These metabolites with cytokines could act synergistically with endogenous glutamate to activate neuronal NMDA receptors ultimately stimulating the formation of nitric oxide or other final mediators toxic to neurons.[59] Other investigators demonstrated that gp120-stimulated monocytes release small, heat-stable, protease-resistant molecules that produce neuronal injury through stimulation of NMDA receptors.

Our present study uncovers a novel means of how HIV infection of brain macrophages might produce neural injury over long periods of time following infection. We showed that HIV-infected monocytes can produce increased levels of TNF after appropriate activation. Moreover, this macrophage activation can occur through one of several mechanisms, two of which were identified. These include cell-to-cell interactions between monocytes and astroglial U251 tumor cells and with LPS. Interestingly, studies of the interactions between HIV-infected monocytes and human astrocytes demonstrated both positive and negative regulatory responses for TNF. Control of TNF production occurred in part through IL-10 and possibly TGF-β. These data, taken together, provide fresh insights into the role of infected macrophages for HIV brain disease. The hyper-responsiveness of the HIV-infected macrophage to "activation" combined with negative regulatory control mechanisms can ultimately lead to subacute encephalopathy. In this way, opportunistic infection might trigger abnormalities in cytokine production with infected macrophages. Ultimately, the cytokines will positively regulate HIV infection in brain leading to production of TGF-β which acts to further control viral replication and tissue pathology.

Both astrocytes and macrophages produce TGF-β. The effects of TGF-β on macrophages are diverse and potent. TGF-β suppressed IFN-γ-induced expression of class II MHC and the production of IL-1, IL-6, and TNF in macrophages.[42]. Various immunoregulatory cytokines are produced in the CNS during HIV infection and all potentially serve as autocrine or paracrine mediators for viral replication and tissue injury. In such a way, both IL-10 and TGB-β could play an important negative regulatory function in the CNS cytokine network of virus-infected patients.[44] Indeed, TGF-β is localized to monocytes and astrocytes in areas of HIV brain pathology.[43] The production of TGF-β in brain likely permits recruitment of HIV-infected monocytes into brain providing a mechanism for efficient viral and disease spread.[43] These observations, taken together, provide strong evidence to support a new hypothesis that interactions between HIV-infected monocytes and astroglial cells are required to generate the neuropathogenesis of HIV disease.

ACKNOWLEDGMENTS

We thank Ms. Karen Spiegel for outstanding administrative and graphic support and unbridled dedication to work. Dr. H.E. Gendelman is a Carter-Wallace Fellow of the University of Nebraska Medical Center. These works were supported in part by 2 ROI HL43628-04A1, 1 PO1 NS 31492-01 awarded by the National Institutes of Health, the Nicholas B. Badami Fellowship, Carter-Wallace Fellowship, awarded by the Carter-Wallace, Inc., and the University of Nebraska Biotechnology Initiative, University of Nebraska Medical Center.

REFERENCES

1. L. Resnick, J.R. Berger, P. Shapshak, and W.W. Tourtellotte. Early penetration of the blood-brain barrier by HIV. *Neurology* 38:9 (1988).
2. L.E. Davis, B.L. Hjelle, V.E. Miller, et al. Early viral brain invasion in iatrogenic human immunodeficiency virus infection. *Neurology* 42:1736 (1992).
3. W.J. Atwood, J.R. Berger, R. Kaderman, C.S. Tornatore, and E.O. Major. Human immunodeficiency virus type 1 infection of the brain. *Clin. Micro. Rev.* 6:339 (1993).
4. D.D. Ho, M.G. Sarngaadharan, L. Resnick, et al. Primary human T-lymphotropic virus type II infection. *Ann. Intern. Med.* 103:880 (1985).
5. J. Michaels, L.R. Sharer, and L.G. Epstein. Human immunodeficiency virus type 1 (HIV-1) infection of the nervous system: a review. *Immunodef. Rev.* 1:71 (1988).
6. R.W. Price, and B.J. Brew. The AIDS dementia complex. *J. Infect. Dis.* 158:1079 (1988).
7. G.M. Shaw, M.E. Harper, B.E. Hahn, et al. HTLV-III infection in brains of children and adults with AIDS encephalopathy. *Science* 1:177 (1985).
8. J.A. Levy, J. Shimabukuro, H. Hollander, J. Mills, and L. Kaminsky. Isolation of AIDS-associated retroviruses from cerebrospinal fluid and brain of patients with neurological symptoms. *Lancet* 2:586 (1985).
9. D.D. Ho, T.R. Rota, R.T. Schooley, et al. Isolation of HTLV-III from cerebrospinal fluid and neural tissue of patients with neurologic syndrome related to the acquired immunodeficiency syndrome *N. Engl. J. Med.* 313:1493 (1985).

10. S. Koenig, H.E. Gendelman, J.M. Orenstein, et al. Detection of AIDS virus in macrophages in brain tissue from AIDS patients with encephalopathy. *Science* 233:1089 (1986).
11. C.A. Wiley, R.D. Schrier, J.A. Nelson, P.W. Lampert, and M.B.A. Oldstone. Cellular localization of human immunodeficiency virus infection within the brains of acquired immune deficiency syndrome patients. *Proc. Natl. Acad. Sci. USA* 83:7089 (1986).
12. R.N. Vazeux, N. Brousse, A. Jarry, et al. AIDS subacute encephalitis: identification of HIV-1-infected cells. *Am. J. Pathol.* 126:403 (1987).
13. M.H. Stoler, T.A. Eskin, S. Benn, R.C. Angerer, and L.M. Angerer. Human T-cell lymphotropic virus type III infection of the central nervous system: a preliminary *in situ* analysis. *J.A.M.A.* 256:2360 (1986).
14. D.H. Gabuzda, D.D. Ho, S.M. de la Monte, et al. Immunohistochemical identification of HTLV-III antigen in brains of patients with AIDS. *Ann. Neurol.* 20:289 (1986).
15. L.G. Epstein, and H.E. Gendelman. Human immunodeficiency virus type 1 infection of the nervous system: pathogenetic mechanisms. *Ann. Neurol.* 33:429 (1993).
16. H.E.Gendelman, and S. Gendelman. Neurological aspects of human immunodeficiency virus infection, *in:* "Neuropathogenic Viruses and Immunity," S. Specter, M. Bendinelli, and H. Friedman, eds., Plenum Press, New York (1992).
17. D.E. Brenneman, G.L. Westbrook, S.P. Fitzgerald, et al. Neuronal cell killing by the envelope protein of HIV and its prevention by vasoactive intestinal peptide. *Nature* 335:639 (1989).
18. E.B. Dreyer, P.K. Kaiser, J,.T. Offermann, and S.A. Lipton. HIV-1 coat protein neurotoxicity prevented by calcium channel antagonists. *Science* 248:364 (1990).
19. M.M. Sabatier, E. Vives, K. Mabrouk, et al. Evidence for neurotoxic activity of tat from human immunodeficiency virus type 1. *J. Virol.* 65:961 (1991).
20. L. Pulliam, B.G. Herndier, N.M. Tang, and M.S. McGrath. Human immunodeficiency virus-infected macrophages produce soluble factors that cause histological and neurochemical alterations in cultured human brains. *J. Clin. Invest.* 87:503 (1991).
21. D. Giulian, K. Vaca, and C.A. Noonan. Secretion of neurotoxins by mononuclear phagocytes infected with HIV-1. *Science* 250:1593 (1991).
22. E. Bernton, H. Bryant, M. Decoster, et al. No direct neuronotoxicity by HIV-1 virions or culture fluids from HIV-1 infected T cells or monocytes. *AIDS Res. Hum. Retroviruses* 8:495 (1992).
23. M. Tardieu, C. Hery, S. Peudenier, O. Boespflug, and l. Montagnier. Human immunodeficiency virus type 1-infected monocytic cells can destroy human neural cells after cell-to-cell adhesion. *Ann. Neurol.* 32:11 (1992).
24. R. Peluso, A. Haase, L. Stowring, M. Edwards, and P. Ventura. A Trojan horse mechanism for the spread of visna virus in monocytes. *Virology* 147:231 (1985).
25. H.E. Gendelman, J.M. Orenstein, L.M. Baca, et al. Editorial review: the macrophage in the persistence and pathogenesis of HIV infection. *AIDS (London)* 3:475 (1989).
26. L. Resnick, F. DiMarzo-Veronese, J., Schupbach, et al. Intra-blood-brain-barrier synthesis of HTLV-III specific IgG in patients with neurologic symptoms associated with AIDS or AIDS-related complex. *N. Engl. J. Med.* 313:1498 (1985).
27. P. Genis, M. Jett, E.W. Bernton, et al. Cytokines and arachidonic acid metabolites produced during human immunodeficiency virus (HIV)-infected macrophage-astroglia interactions: implications for the neuro-pathogenesis of HIV disease. *J. Exp. Med.* 176:1703 (1992).
28. H.E. Gendelman, J.M. Orenstein, M.A. Martin, et al. Efficient isolation and propagation of human immunodeficiency virus on recombinant colony-stimulating factor 1-treated monocytes. *J. Exp. Med.* 167:1428 (1988).
29. D.D. Bigner, S.H. Bigner, J. Ponten, et al. Heterogeneity of genotypic and

phenotypic characteristics of fifteen permanent cell lines derived from human gliomas. *J. Neuropathol. Exp. Neurol.* 40:201 (1981).

30. K.D. McCarthy, and J. deVellis. Preparation of separate astroglial and oligodendroglial cell cultures from rat cerebral tissue. *J. Cell. Biol.* 85:890 (1980).

31. H.E. Gendelman, L. Baca, H. Husayni, et al. Macrophage-human immunodeficiency virus interaction: viral isolation and target cell tropism. *AIDS (London)* 4:221 (1990).

32. D.C. Kalter, M. Nakamura, J.A. Turpin, et al. Enhanced HIV replication in MCSF-treated monocytes. *J. Immunol.* 146:298 (1991).

33. M.M. Hogan, and S.N. Vogen. Production of TNF by rIFN-γ-primed C3H/HeJ (*Lps^d*) macrophages requires the presence of lipid A-associated proteins. *J. Immunol.* 141:4196 (1988).

34. H.E. Gendelman, R.M. Friedman, S. Joe, et al. A selective defect of interferon-α production in human immunodeficiency virus-infected monocytes. *J. Exp. Med.* 172:1433 (1990).

35. H.E. Gendelman, L.M. Baca, C.A. Kubrak, et al. Induction of interferon alpha in peripheral blood mononuclear cells by human immunodeficiency virus (HIV)-infected monocytes: Restricted antiviral activity of the HIV-induced interferons. *J. Immunol.* 148:422 (1992).

36. J.E. Merrill, and I.S.Y. Chen. HIV-1, macrophages, glial cells, and cytokines in AIDS nervous system disease. *FASEB J.* 5:2391 (1991).

37. D.S. Robbins, Y. Shirzai, B. Drysdale, et al. Production of cytotoxic factor for oligodendrocytes by stimulated astrocytes. *J. Immunol.* 139:2593 (1987).

38. K.W. Selmaj, and C.S. Raine. Tumor necrosis factor mediates myelin and oligodendrocyte damage in vitro. *Ann. Neurol.* 23:339 (1988).

39. K.W. Selmaj, M. Farooq, T. Norton, C.S. Raine, and C.F. Brosman. Proliferation of astrocytes *in vitro* in response to cytokines. *J. Immunol.* 144:129 (1990).

40. L.Y. Chung, and E.N. Benveniste. Tumor necrosis factor-alpha production by astrocytes: induction by lipopolysaccharide, interferon-gamma and interleukin-1. *J. Immunol.* 144:2999 (1990).

41. L. Vitkovic, T. Kalebic, A. de Cunha, and A.S. Fauci. Astrocyte-conditioned medium stimulates HIV-1 expression in a chronically infected promonocyte clone. *J. Neuroimmunol.* 30:153 (1990).

42. A. Suzumura, M. Sawada, H. Yamamoto, and T. Marunouchi. Transforming growth factor-β suppresses activation and proliferation of microglia in vitro. *J. Immunol.* 151:2150 (1993).

43. S.M. Wahl, J.B. Allen, N. McCarney-Francis, et al. Macrophage- and astrocyte-derived transforming growth factor-β as a mediator of central nervous system dysfunction in acquired immune deficiency syndrome. *J. Exp. Med.* 173:981 (1991).

44. L.M. Wahl, M.L. Corcoran, S.W. Pyle, et al. Human immunodeficiency virus glycoprotein (gp120) induction of monocyte arachidonic acid metabolites and interleukin 1. *Proc. Natl. Acad. Sci. USA* 86:621 (1989).

45. C. Dubois, E. Bissonnette, and M. Rola-Pleszczynski. Platelet-activating factor (PAF) enhances tumor necrosis factor production by alveolar macrophages: Prevention by PAF receptor antagonists and lipoxygenase inhibitors. *J. Immunol.* 143:964 (1989).

46. P.E. Poubelle, D. Gingras, C. Demers, et al. Platelet-activating factor (PAF-acether) enhances the concomitant production of tumour necrosis factor alpha and interleukin-1 by subsets of human monocytes. *Immunology* 72:181 (1991).

47. J.A. Lindgren, T. Hokfelt, S-E. Dahlen, C. Patrono, and B. Samuelsson. Leukotrienes in the rat central nervous system. *Proc. Natl. Acad. Sci. USA* 81:6216 (1984).

48. P. Conti, M. Reale, R.C. Barbacane, M. Bongrazio, M.R. Panara, and S. Fiore. The combination of interleukin 1 plus tumor necrosis factor causes grater generation of LTB_4, thromboxanes, and aggregation on human macrophages than these compounds alone, *in*: "Prostaglandins in

Clinical Research: Cardiovascular System.' Alan R. Liss, Inc., New York (1989).

49. T. Shimizu, Y. Takusagawa, T. Izumi, N. Ohishi, and Y. Seyama. Enzymic synthesis of leukotriene B_4 in guinea pig brain. *Int. Soc. Neurochem.* 48:1541 (1987).

50. G.D. Nicol, D.K. Klingberg, and M.R. Vaska. Prostaglandin E_2 increases calcium conductance and stimulates release of substance P in avian sensory neurons. *J. Neurosci.* 12:1917 (1992).

51. M.A. Wasserman, E.F. Smith, D.C. Underwood, and M.A. Barnette. Pharmacology and pathophysiology of 5-lipoxygenase products, *in*: "Lipoxygenases and Their Products," S.T. Crooke and A. Wong, eds., Academic Press, Inc., San Diego (1991).

52. B.A. Navia, E.S. Cho, C.K. Petito, R.W. Price. The AIDS dementia complex. II. Neuropathology. *Ann. Neurol.* 19:525 (1986).

53. S. Ketzler, S. Weis, H. Haug, and H. Budka. Loss of neurons in the frontal cortex in AIDS brains. *Acta Neuropathol.* 80:92 (1990).

54. C.A. Wiley, E. Masliah, M. Morey, et al. Neocortical damage during HIV infection. *Ann. Neurol.* 29:651 (1991).

55. I.P. Everall, P.J. Luthert, and P.L. Lantos. Neuronal loss in the frontal cortex in HIV infection. *Lancet* 337:1119 (1991).

56. M.A. Collart, D. Belin, J-D. Vassalli, S. De Kossodo, and P. Vassalli. γ-Interferon enhances macrophage transcription of the tumor necrosis factor/cachectin, interleukin 1 and urokinase genes, which are controlled by short-lived repressors. *J. Exp. Med.* 164:2113 (1986).

57. S.H. Zuckerman, G.F. Evans, and L. Guthrie. Transcriptional and post-transcriptional mechanisms involved in the differential expression of LPS-induced IL-1 and TNF mRNA. *Immunology* 73:460 (1991).

58. W.R. Tyor, J.D. Glass, J.W. Griffin, et al. Cytokine expression in the brain during the acquired immunodeficiency syndrome. *Ann. Neurol.* 31:349 (1992).

59. V.L. Dawson, T.M. Dawson, G.R. Uhl, and S.H. Snyder. Human immunodeficiency virus type 1 coat protein neurotoxicity mediated by nitric oxide in primary cortical cultures. *Proc. Natl. Acad. Sci. USA* 90:32576 (1993).

CELL CULTURES FROM HUMAN FETAL BRAIN PROVIDE A MODEL FOR HIV-1 PERSISTENCE AND REACTIVATION IN THE CENTRAL NERVOUS SYSTEM

Eugene O. Major, Walter A. Atwood, Katherine E. Conant, Kei Amemiya, Judith Boston, and Renee G. Traub

Laboratory of Molecular Medicine and Neuroscience
National Institute of Neurological Disorders and Stroke
National Institutes of Health
Bethesda, Maryland 20892

INTRODUCTION

Cell cultures derived from human fetal tissues have been used for many years for the laboratory diagnosis of viral infections. In 1971, cultures prepared from human fetal brain were used in the isolation of a human polyomavirus, JCV, which was identified as the etiologic agent for the demyelinating disease, progressive multifocal leukoencephalopathy.[1,2] Since JCV infected the oligodendrocyte in the brain, it was thought that JCV also infected the oligodendrocyte or its precursor cell in cultures from fetal brain.[3,4] Laboratory investigations of the lineage of fetal brain-derived cells revealed that these precursor cells were difficult to identify and were in small numbers compared with other neural-derived cells, such as astrocytes and neurons.[4-6] Since JCV does not infect neurons in the brain or in cultures, astrocytes were implicated as the predominant cell type in these cultures in which JCV multiplied.[7] This observation was later confirmed both *in situ* in histopathological samples and in cell cultures with the establishment of astrocyte cell lines susceptible to JCV infection.[8,9] Although cultures from fetal brain tissue demonstrate a diverse population of cell types, it has been possible to prepare cultures highly enriched for astrocytes. It has been these astrocyte-pure cultures from human fetal brain that have served as cell substrates for studies of neurotropism of viral pathogens. With the observation that HIV-1 was neuroinvasive (a characteristic of the lentivirus family), and was demonstrated in patients with dementia, laboratory and clinical investigations began to determine whether HIV-1 was also neurotropic, i.e., able to infect neural-derived cells. Astrocyte cell cultures from human fetal brain were used to initiate these studies.

MATERIALS AND METHODS

Preparation of Cell Cultures from Human Fetal Brain

Brain tissue is initially placed into Eagle's Minimum Essential Medium (E-MEM) supplemented with 20% fetal bovine serum and 2 mg/ml penicillin/streptomycin and 5 mg fungizone until available for dissection.[10] Individual samples, from 8-12-week fetuses, are maintained and processed separately.

Technical Advances in AIDS Research in the Human Nervous System
Edited by E.O. Major and J.A. Levy, Plenum Press, New York, 1995

89

Tissue fragments are then washed in phosphate-buffered saline (PBS) with antibiotics following dissection of meninges and blood vessels. The brain is aspirated through small gauge needles, centrifuged at 500 rpm for 5 min, washed and then placed into poly-D-lysine-coated tissue culture plastic ware. The cultures are allowed to settle for 5-7 days before refeeding and subsequent culture of cell material that has not adhered to the flasks. The resulting cultures demonstrate a heterogeneous population of cells with a layer of flat cells with large nuclei and cytoplasm attached to the flask and multiple, process-bearing cells forming a top layer of cells. These cell types can be separated by placing the flask in an incubator on a rotary shaker set at 225 rpm for 2-4 hr. The top layer of process-bearing cells are dislodged from the adherent cells. This process can be repeated several times to completely free the bed layer of cells for subsequent passage by trypsinization.[11] The cell types can then be individually cultured and expanded for up to 20 cell generations, approximately 7-9 passages.

Identification of Cell Types by Immunofluorescent Analysis

Identification of the cell types is made by the presence of their intermediate filaments, glial fibrillary acidic protein (GFAP) for astrocytes, and neurofilament (NF) for neurons. Precursor cells to the myelinating oligodendrocyte can be detected by the expression of surface galactose ceramides.[5,12] The separated populations of cells are cultured on poly-D-lysine-coated glass coverslips. Cells are washed in PBS, fixed in methanol-acetone for 20 min at -20°C, and reacted with antibody to GFAP (Dako) or NF (H form, Boeringer- Mannheim). Although not done in these studies, detection of cell surface galactose ceramide is done by antibody staining to viable cells on coverslips followed by fixation in 90% ethanol, 10% acidic acid.[4]

Immunofluorescent Analysis of Cell Surface Antigens by Flow Cytometry

Human fetal astrocytes were prepared from primary cultures of fetal brain as described above. The purity of the astrocytes was assessed at greater than 98% by immunofluorescent staining of the cells with antibody to GFAP. Cells were washed three times with Hank's buffered saline solution (HBSS) containing 2% fetal calf serum and harvested by scraping. The cells ($1x10^6$) were then incubated with monoclonal antibodies directed at major histocompatibility complex (MHC)-encoded class I antigens (BB7.7), MHC-encoded class II antigens (anti-HLA-DR FITC), intracellular adhesion molecule-1 (ICAM-1; anti-CD54 FITC), CD4 (anti-CD4 FITC), CD8 (anti-CD8 PE), or with isotytpe matched negative control antibodies for 30 min on ice. The BB7.7 antibody was used as undiluted hybridoma supernatant and was detected with a goat anti-mouse IgG conjugated to FITC at a 1:50 dilution (Jackson Immunoresearch). All other antibodies were primary conjugates and were used at a 1:5 dilution as recommended by the manufacturer (Becton-Dickinson). To assess the effect of gamma-interferon (γ-IFN on MHC class I, II, and ICAM-1 expression, the cells were incubated with γ-IFN (500 U/ml) for 24 hr and then harvested as described above.

Preparation of Nuclear Extracts and Gel Shift Assays

Nuclear extracts were prepared from cultures of human fetal astrocytes as described elsewhere.[13,14] Oligonucleotide probes were synthesized on an Applied Biosystems 380A DNA synthesizer. The sequences of the oligonucleotides used are as follows:

NFkB probe: (5'-GGGACTTTCC-3')
Mutant NFkB probe: (5'-GTTACTTTAC-3')

Double-stranded oligonucleotides were end-labeled with ^{32}P-ATP and gel-purified. Labeled probes (30,000 CPM) were incubated with 1-0 ug of nuclear extract in the presence or absence of a 10-fold molar excess of either unlabeled homologous probe or unlabeled mutant probe. The DNA binding reactions also contained 10 mM Tris-HCl (pH 7.9), 50 mM NaCl, 5 mM MgCl2, 0.5 mM EDTA,

1 mM DTT, 10% glycerol (v/v), and 4 μg of the nonspecific competitor poly (dI-dC) (Pharmacia Inc). The reactions were carried out for 15 min at room temperature, and electorphoresed on 6% Tris-glycine polyacrylamide gels. The gels were dried and samples visualized by autoradiography with Kodak XAR-5 film with an intensifying screen. To assess the effect of tumor necrosis factor-α (TNF-α) induction of NF-kB, cultures were treated for 48 hr with TNF-α (10 ng/ml).

Transfection of DNA into Human Fetal Brain Cells

Plasmid DNA was introduced into cultured astrocytes using the calcium phosphate precipitation technique.[15] Plasmid pNL4-3 contains an infectious clone of the HIV-1 genome.[16] pBennCAT has the reporter gene for chloramphenicol acetyltransferase (CAT) directly linked to the HIV-1 regulatory sequences, LTR.[17] DNAs were precipitated in HEPES buffer, pH 7.1, 127 mM NaCl, 5 mM KCl, 0.7 mM Na_2HPO_4, 6 mM glucose, 21 mM HEPES (N-2-hydroxyethylpiperazine-N-2'-ethanesulfonic acid), with 125 mM $CaCl_2$ in the final concentration. The DNA precipitate usually remained on the cells for 4 hr. The cells were then washed with E-MEM with 15% glycerol to enhance DNA uptake from the cell membrane.

CAT Assay

Cellular extracts were prepared from transfected cells at 48 hr, frozen, and thawed five times. A liquid diffusion method was used to quantitate the activity of the enzyme in the extracts. The reaction mixture contained 100 mM Tris-HCl, pH 7.8, 1 mM chloramphenicol, 0.5 μCi [3H] acetyl CoA (Dupont NEN, Boston, MA) and 50-100 μg of cell extract. Protein concentration was measured by the method of Bradford. Each transfection was performed in duplicate or triplicate and repeated at least twice.

RESULTS

Phenotypic Characteristic of Human Fetal Brain Cultures

Cell cultures enriched for astrocytes are prepared form individual brain tissue samples. Astrocytes from human fetal brain can undergo multiple cell divisions, approximately 20 generations, before loss of expression of their intermediate filament, GFAP, and the beginning of senescence. Homogeneous astrocyte cultures from individual brain tissues (Fig. 1A and B) can reach cell concentrations of 100 million cells by passage 5 or 6. Consequently, multiple experiments can be conducted and repeated using sibling cultures which allows a normalization of assessment of viral gene expression. The neuronal population of cells from fetal brain do not demonstrate similar mitotic activity and are lost in cultures as the cells are trypsinized and passaged. Neurons, identified by the presence of their extended processes and cytoskeletal neurofilament (Fig. 2A and B) frequently imbed their processes in the layer of GFAP-positive cells (Fig. 3). Neurons survive for longer periods in culture if astrocytes are present, presumably due to the release of neurotrophic factors such as nerve growth factor (NGF) secreted by the astrocytes.[18] In cultures in which astrocytes and neurons were maintained in medium conditioned by pure astrocyte cultures, either from separated astrocyte preparations or an astrocyte cell line, SVG,[8] neuronal survival and neurite outgrowth were evident. Similar cultures in which NGF antibodies were present did not demonstrate such neurite outgrowth (Fig. 4A and B).

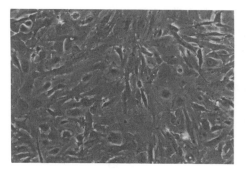
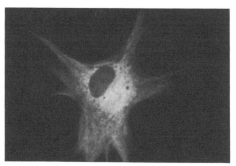

Figure 1. (A) Phase photomicrograph of a culture of human fetal astrocytes at passage 4 prepared from 12-week fetal tissues and separated from neurons and oligodendrocytes as described in Materials and Methods. (Magnification 320X.) (B) Human fetal astrocyte demonstrating glial fibrillary acidic protein as characteristic cytoskeletal intermediate filament. Indirect immunofluorescence assay used mouse monoclonal anti-GFAP and FITC-conjugated goat anti-mouse immunoglobulins. (Magnification 640X using epifluorescence microscopy.)

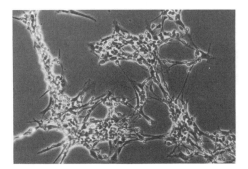
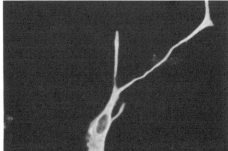

Figure 2. (A) Phase photomicrograph of human fetal neurons from the fetal brain described in Figure 1 and separated from astrocytes and oligodendrocytes. (Magnification 320X.) (B) Indirect immunofluorescence assay using mouse antibody to the human H-neurofilament protein which identified the cells in (A) and Figure 3 as neurons. (Magnification 640X.)

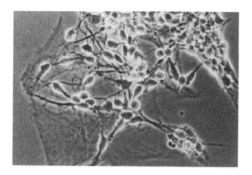

Figure 3. Phase photomicrograph of human fetal neurons with extended neurites which attach to and imbed in layer of astrocytes. (Magnification 640X.)

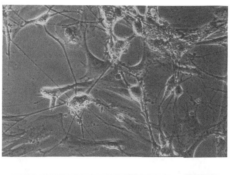

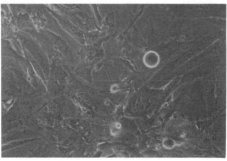

Figure 4. (A) Human fetal brain with both astrocytes and neurons cultured with medium conditioned by the SVG cell line[8] showing extensive neurite outgrowth, and (B) in similar medium with antibody to NGF maintained in the medium for 7 days showing limited neurite processes.

Detection of MHC Class I, II, and ICAM-1 on Human Fetal Astrocytes Before and After Induction with γ-Interferon

Expression of MHC class I and II antigens and expression of ICAM-1 was assessed on untreated and human fetal astrocytes prepared as described in the Materials and Methods. MHC class I antigen (Fig. 5A) and ICAM-1 (Fig. 5B) are constitutively expressed on the surface of these cells. Treatment of the cells with γ-interferon increased the concentration of these molecules on the cell surface. Expression of MHC class II antigen could only be detected on γ-interferon-treated astrocytes (Fig. 5C).

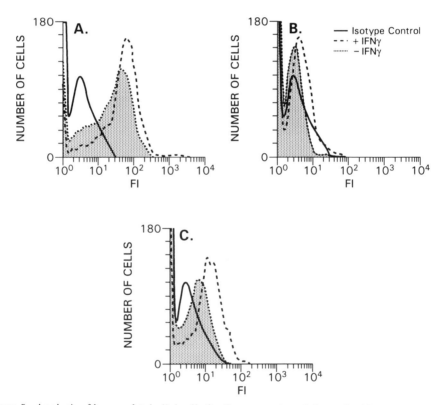

Figure 5. Analysis of human fetal glial cells for the expression of the major histocompatibility complex (MHC) class I in panel A; MHC class II in panel B; and ICAM-1 in panel C using flow cytometry. Cells were cultured in the presence or absence of γ-interferon (identified in legend).

Analysis of CD4 and CD8 Expression on Human Fetal Astrocytes

We and others have previously determined that HIV-1 was able to infect astrocytes from human fetal brain[19-24] which resulted in low level of infection in a small number of cells. Here we tested astrocyte cultures for the presence of the HIV-1 receptor, CD4, together with the marker for T cell suppressor cells, CD8, to determine if inefficient infectivity could be partly due to the absence of the viral receptor. The human monocyte line, A3.01, served as the positive control since these T cell-derived cultures expressed both surface markers and are highly susceptible to HIV-1 infection. Human fetal astrocytes did not express either CD4 or CD8 molecules (Fig. 6, lower panel) in contrast to other reports.[25] The A3.01 cells expressed high concentration of CD4 and lower levels of CD8, as seen in Figure 6 (upper panel). Astrocyte cultures were also tested for the presence of alternate receptors for HIV-1,[26,27] galactose ceremides, which also proved negative on these cells (personal communication, D. Cook and F. Gonzalez-Scarano). Evidence for a high molecular weight cell surface protein on fetal astrocytes that may serve as the HIV-1 receptor is presented in the chapter by Nath et al. in this volume (*vida infra*).

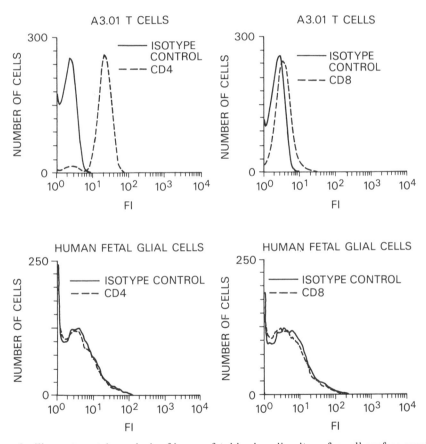

Figure 6. Flow cytometric analysis of human fetal brain cell culture for cell surface markers, CD4 and CD8. The human monocyte cell line, A3.01, was used as the positive control.[16] Relative concentration of cells is shown on the *y* axis, and the relative intensity of fluorescence is shown on the *x* axis.

Expression and Transactivation of the HIV-1 LTR in Primary Cultures and Cell Lines Established from Human Fetal Astrocytes

HIV-1 does infect astrocytes in these cultures which results in a noncytopathic but productive infection. HIV-1 infection in the few astrocytes that become infected leads to a latent infection.[19] In order to assess the efficiency of HIV-1 expression in these cultures, astrocytes were transfected with the plasmid, pBennCAT which contains the HIV-1 LTR placed upstream from the CAT reporter gene. Figure 7 shows that a moderate rate of CAT activity was detected in extracts prepared from primary astrocytes and POJ astrocytes, a cell line established using the JCV T protein.[19] A lower rate of CAT activity was obtained with extracts from transfected SVG cells. Transfection of these three cell cultures with pSVOCAT, a promoter-enhancerless CAT plasmid, resulted in only background activity. Transfection with pSV2CAT, however, yielded moderate-to-high amounts of CAT expression. All transfections were done in triplicate during several experiments with similar results. (Fig. 7A, B, and C).

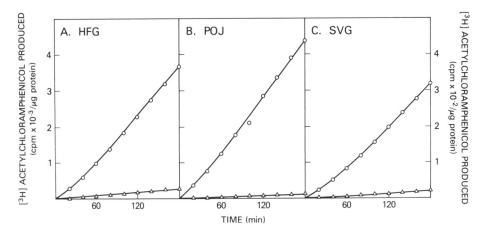

Figure 7. CAT activity in protein extracts from human fetal astrocytes in primary cultures (A) or in established cell lines (B) POJ, and (C) SVG. Cells were transfected with either pBennCAT (◆), pSV2 CAT (●), or cotransfected with pBennCAT and the proviral clone of HIV-1, pNL4-3 (O). The y axis on right shows higher activity than on the left.

In order to examine the ability of the HIV-1 LTR to be transactivated in astrocytes by its *tat* protein, cells were transfected with both pBennCAT and the infectious clone of HIV-1, pNL4-3. Greater levels of CAT activity were present in all cells compared with pBennCAT alone, as shown in Table 1. The POJ cells showed the highest level of activity followed by normal astrocytes and then the SVG cells. These results demonstrated that the HIV-1 LTR is functional in astrocytes even without the *tat* transactivating protein and responds to transactivation by increased levels of CAT activity. Also, the viral antigen, p24, was detected in all cells indicating efficient expression of structural genes in these cells as well.

Table 1. Expression and transactivation of the HIV-1 LTR in human fetal glial cell lines.

Transfected DNA	CAT Activity[a]		
		Cell Line	
	HFG	POJ	SVG
pNL4-3 + pBennCAT	5926 (424)[b]	7269 (320)	565 (303)
pBennCAT	509	247	39
pSVOCAT	5	7	5
pSV2CAT	2963	986	111
TRANSACTIVATION[c]	12X	29X	15X

[a]CAT activity reported in pmoles/incorporated/hr/mg protein.
[b]Numbers in parentheses after CAT activity represent level of p24 (pg/ml) 2 days after transfection.
[c]Determined by dividing sum of CAT activity of pNL4-3 + pBennCAT by pBennCAT.

NF-kB Protein from Human Fetal Astrocytes Binds the HIV-1 LTR

Latent infection in cultured human fetal astrocytes in characterized by lack of synthesis of viral antigens or their mRNA. However, HIV-1 can be reactivated from these cells by either cocultivation with T cells or by addition of the cytokines TNF-α or interleukin-1β to the culture medium.[14,19] Since reactivation of HIV-1 gene expression in other cell types is associated with increased binding of NF-kB to kB sequence sites in these HIV-1 LTR, we sought to determine if NF-kB proteins were present in these cells that could recognize and bind to the HIV-1 sequences. This protein binding would be predicted by the CAT assays which demonstrated HIV-1 LTR activity in these cells. In the gel shift experiment shown in Figure 8 (arrow), astrocyte cultures treated with TNF-α led to a specific increase in binding of nuclear proteins to the kB binding site on the HIV-1 LTR. This result has been further clarified in these cultures demonstrating that the proteins binding to the LTR are the heterodimers of the NF-kB protein, p50/p65 complex.[14,28] Human fetal astrocytes are also susceptible to other neurotropic human viruses such as the human polyomavirus, JCV, which causes lytic infection of the myelin-producing oligodendrocytes as well as astrocytes. Similar nuclear protein extracts from cultured astrocytes demonstrate protein-DNA interaction with the JCV regulatory sequences.[13] Several of these sequences are overlapping NF-1/c-jun recognition sites for these transcription factors. The experiment in Figure 9 shows also that nuclear protein extracts containing the proteins that bind the HIV-1 NF-kB site also contain DNA-binding proteins that recognize the NF-1/c-jun binding site of another human neurotropic virus.

Competitor	No Extract	HFG			HFG + TNFα		
NFKB	–	–	+	–	–	+	–
NFKBm	–	–	–	+	–	–	+

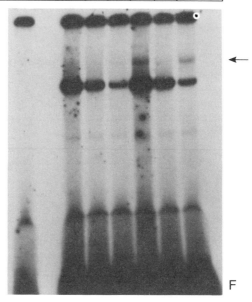

F

Figure 8. Competitive gel shift analysis of nuclear proteins extracted from human fetal glial cells (HFG) or from human fetal glial cells treated with TNF-α (HFG + TNF-α) binding to an oligonucleotide containing an NF-kB binding site from the HIV-1 LTR. Equivalent amounts of nuclear proteins were reacted with a ^{32}P-labeled oligonucleotide containing an intact NF-kB binding site (5'-GGGACTTTCC-3') either in the presence or absence of a 10-fold molar excess of unlabeled homologous competitor or mutant competitor (NF-KBm) (5'-GTTACTTTAC-3') for 15 min at room temperature. The resultant DNA/protein complexes were resolved on a 6% polyacrylamide Tris-glycine gel. The arrow indicates the position of a specific and inducible gel-shifted band. F indicates the migration of the free probe.

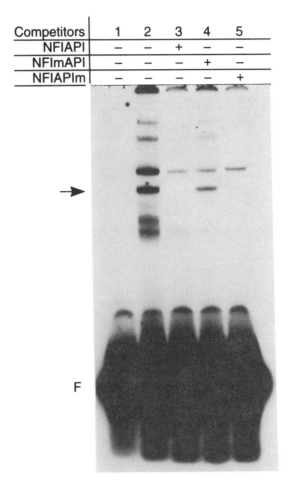

Figure 9. Competitive gel shift analysis of nuclear proteins isolated from human fetal glial cells binding to an oligonucleotide containing a NF1/AP1 binding site from the regulatory region of JC virus. Equivalent amounts of nuclear proteins were reacted with a ^{32}P-labeled NF1/AP1 oligonucleotide (5'-GGGATGGCTGCCAGFCAAGCATGAGCTCATACC-3') in the presence or absence of a 10-fold molar excess of unlabeled oligonucleotide mutated in either the NF1 binding site (5'-GGACAGCTGCCACTCAAGCATGAGCTCATACC-3') or the AP1 binding site (5'-GGGATGGCTGCCAGCCAAGCATGTGCTCATACC-3'). The resulting DNA/protein complexes were resolved on a 6% polyacrylamide Tris-glycine gel. The arrow indicates the position of the most prominent and specific gel-shifted band. F indicates the migration of the free probe.

DISCUSSION

Results from experiments using primary astrocytes have shown that the human fetal astrocyte has the necessary transcription factors for expression of the HIV-1 LTR. Cells that are transfected with pBennCAT, a recombinant DNA construct which contains the HIV-1 LTR upstream from the CAT gene demonstrate significantly greater CAT activity than do cells transfected with the control plasmid, pSVOCAT which does not possess an enhancer-promoter. Additionally, cotransfection of pNL4-3 with pBennCAT is associated with an additional increase in CAT activity due to the viral transactivating *tat* protein. These data are described in Table 1.

Using electrophoretic mobility shift assays, we have examined the binding of nuclear proteins to the HIV-1 LTR. Results suggest that the astrocytes express the transcription factor, NF-kB, as do other cells that allow HIV-1 expression.[29,30] The level of NF-kB is increased in astrocytes in response to various stimulants such as TNF-α. We have also demonstrated that NF-kB proteins increase binding to the HIV-1 LTR when stimulated with the phorbol ester, phorbol myristic acid (PMA).[28] Figure 8 shows the result of a gel shift assay demonstrating nuclear protein binding to an oligonucleotide homologous to the HIV-1 kB motif. The data compare the binding of nuclear proteins from unstimulated and TNF-α-treated astrocytes. The band which is competed away by excess unlabeled oligonucleotide but not by a mutant oligonucleotide represents protein bound specifically to the kB consensus sequence. This band is visibly increased when an extract from TNF-α-stimulated cells is used.

Not only does the primary astrocyte have the necessary transcription factors for expression of the HIV-1 LTR, the astrocyte also has the necessary cellular factors for multiplication of HIV-1 virions. Following either infection with virus or transfection with proviral DNA, cultures of fetal astrocytes demonstrate rapid synthesis of viral antigen, p24, and reverse transcriptase, leading to release of infectious progeny virions. This is a productive but noncytopathic infection since there is no evidence for syncytia formation or cell loss presumably due to the lack of the CD4 receptor on these cells to promote cell fusion as shown in Figure 5. Viral proteins and their mRNAs diminish during the next several weeks until neither can be detected in the astrocytes indicating establishment of a latent infection.[19] Cocultivation of these cells with uninfected lymphocytes leads to viral protein synthesis and infection of the lymphocytes. This is not due to residual virus in the cells or in the culture medium, since these culture fluids by themselves cannot initiate infection. Stimulation of latently infected astrocytes with the cytokines, TNF-α and interleukin-1β, and PMA also results in a rapid increase of HIV-1 mRNA and viral proteins. The cytokines may increase HIV-1 expression in part by increasing the NF-kB transcription factor which activates HIV-1 expression through binding to its cognate sequences on the LTR. Cytokines may also lead to changes in the expression of other necessary cellular cofactors such as proteins that may interact with the viral tat and rev regulatory proteins. It has been demonstrated that there are several factors which influence whether a cell is productively infected including those at the level of viral entry[31-33] and viral sequence variation.[34,35] Additionally, intracellular factors that regulate the fate of viral infection by interacting with viral sequences or with viral proteins most certainly are involved. We are currently investigating whether astrocytes do not demonstrate a permanent productive infection because they lack sufficient expression of these necessary cellular cofactors or because they express factors that specifically inhibit viral multiplication and therefore limit infection to a latent period which still remains responsive to extracellular stimuli, by cytokines present in the nervous system.

Consequently, HIV-1 infection of human astrocytes in culture can be divided into three stages as described in a summary figure, Figure 10. Phase I of the infection is productive, noncytopathic, followed by Phase II which is latent for long periods (from weeks to months), and then Phase III characterized as a reactivation period. It appears from experiments that these phases of HIV-1 infection can repeat as long as the cultures are maintained well. Cultures derived from human fetal brain can serve as an appropriate model to study the biology and molecular regulation of HIV-1 infection in the nervous system. Results from such studies will no doubt provide insights into the pathogenesis of HIV-1-associated encephalopathies and also into normal neural-derived cell functions as well.

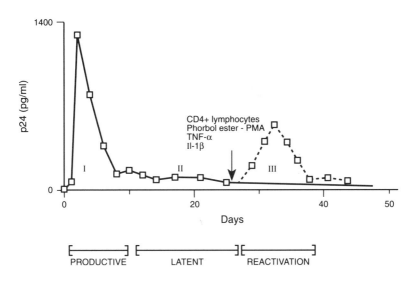

STAGES OF HIV-1 INFECTION IN HUMAN FETAL GLIAL CELLS

I HIV-1 infectious progeny are produced in a non-cytopathic infection

II Integrated proviral DNA is not expressed; neither viral proteins nor mRNA can be detected

III Viral synthesis can be reinitiated by cocultivation with CD4+ lymphocytes or specific cytokines

Figure 10. Graphic demonstration of the fate of HIV-1 infection in astrocyte cells prepared as independent cultures from human fetal brain.

REFERENCES

1. B.L. Padgett, C.M. Rogers, and D.L. Walker. JC virus, a human polyomavirus associated with progressive multifocal leukoencephalopathy: additional biological characteristics and antigenic relationships. *Infect. Immunol.* 15:656 (1977).
2. E.O. Major, K. Amemiya, C.S. Tornatore, S.A. Houff, and J.R. Berger. Pathogenesis and molecular biology of progressive multifocal leukoencephalopathy, a JC virus-induced demyelinating disease of the human brain. *Clin. Microbiol. Rev.* 5:49 (1992).
3. R.J. Frisque, J.D. Martin, B.L. Padgett, and D.L. Walker. Infectivity of the DNA from four isolates of JC virus. *J. Virol.* 32:476 (1979).
4. G.A. Elder, and E.O. Major. Early appearance of type II astrocytes in developing human fetal brain. *Dev. Brain Res.* 42:146 (1988).
5. P.G.E. Kennedy, and J. Fok-Seang. Studies on the development, antigenic phenotype, and function of human glial cells in tissue culture. *Brain* 109:12651 (1986).
6. R. Mirsky. The use of antibodies to define and study major cell types in the central and peripheral nervous system, *in:* "Neuroimmunology," J. Brockes, ed., Plenum, New York (1982).

7. E.O Major, and D.A. Vacante. Human fetal astrocytes in culture support the growth of the neurotropic human polyomavirus, JCV. *J. Neuropathol. Exp. Neurol.* 48:425 (1989).
8. E.O. Major, A.E. Miller, P. Mourrain, et al. Establishment of a line of human fetal glial cells that supports JC virus multiplication. *Proc. Natl. Acad. Sci. USA* 61:755 (1985).
9. C. Mandl, D.L. Walker, and R.J. Frisque. Derivation and characterization of POJ cells, transformed fetal glial cells that retain their permissivity for JC virus. *J.Virol.* 61:755 (1987).
10. E.O. Major, K. Amemiya, G. Elder, and S. Houff. Glial cells of the human developing brain and B cells of the immune system share a common DNA binding factor for recognition of the regulatory sequences of the human polyomavirus, JCV. *J. Neurosci. Res.* 27:461 (1990).
11. K.D. McCarthy, and J. de Vellis. Preparation of separate astroglial and oligodendroglial cultures from rat cerebral tissue. *J. Cell. Biol.* 85:890 (1980).
12. M.C. Raff, R. Mirsky, K.L.Fields, et al. Galactocerebroside is a specific cell-surface antigenic marker for oligodendrocytes in culture. (Letter) *Nature* 274:813 (1978).
13. K. Amemiya, R. Traub, L. Durham, and E.O. Major. Adjacent nuclear factor-1 and activator protein binding sites of the enhancer of the neurotropic JC virus: a common characteristic of many brain specific genes. *J. Biol. Chem.* 267:14204 (1992).
14. W. Atwood, C. Tornatore, R. Traub, K. Conant,and E.O. Major. Stimulation of HIV-1 gene expression and induction of NF-kB (p50/p65) binding activity in TNF-alpha treated human fetal glial cells. *AIDS Res. Hum. Retroviruses* 10:207 (1994).
15. F.L. Graham, and A.J.Van der Eb. A new technique for the assay of infectivity of human adenovirus 5 DNA. *Virology* 98:503 (1973).
16. A. Adachi, H.E. Gendelman, S. Koenig, et al. Production of acquired immunodeficiency syndrome-associated retrovirus in human and non-human cells transfected with an infectious molecular clone. *J. Virol.* 58:284 (1986).
17. H.E. Gendelman, W. Phelps, L. Feigenbaum, et al. Trans-activation of the human immunodeficiency virus long terminal repeat sequence by DNA viruses. *Proc. Natl. Acad. Sci. USA* 83:9759 (1986).
18. M. Eddleston, and L. Mucke. Molecular profile of reactive astrocytes - implications for their role in neurologic disease. *Neuroscience* 54:15 (1993).
19. C. Tornatore, A. Nath, K. Amemiya, and E.O. Major. Persistent human immunodeficiency virus type 1 infection in human fetal glial cells reactivated by T-cell factors or by the cytokines tumor necrosis factor-alpha and interleukin-1 beta. *J. Virol.* 65:6094 (1991).
20. C. Tornatore, K. Meyers, W. Atwood, K. Conant, and E.O. Major. Temporal characteristics of human immunodeficiency virus-1 transcripts in human fetal astrocytes. *J. Virol.* 68:93 (1994).
21. C. Cheng-Mayer, C. Weiss, D. Seto, and J.A. Levy. Isolates of human immunodeficiency virus type 1 from the brain may constitute a special group of the AIDS virus. *Proc. Natl. Acad. Sci. USA* 86:8575 (1989).
22. C.A. Wiley, R.D. Schrier, J.A. Nelson, P.W. Lampert, and M.B.A. Oldstone. Cellular localization of human immunodeficiency virus infection within the brains of acquired immune deficiency syndrome patients. *Proc. Natl. Acad. Sci. USA* 83:7089 (1986).
23. C. Tornatore, R. Chandra, J.R. Berger, and E.O. Major. HIV-1 infection of subcortical astrocytes in the pediatric central nervous system. *Neurology* 44:481 (1994).
24. Y. Saito, L.R. Sharer, L. Epstein, et al. Overexpression of *nef* as a marker for restricted HIV-1 infection of astrocytes in postmortem pediatric central nervous system. *Neurology* 44:474 (1994).
25. M. Ennas, D. Cocchia, E. Silvetti, et al. Immunocompetent cell markers in human fetal astrocytes and neurons in cultures. *J. Neurosci. Res.* 32:424 (1992).

26. J.M. Harouse, S. Bhat, S.L. Spitalnik, et al. Inhibition of entry of HIV-1 in neural cell lines by antibodies against galactosyl ceramide. *Science* 253:320 (1991).
27. S. Bhat, S.L. Spitalnik, G. Gonzalez-Scarano, and D.H. Silberberg. Galactosyl ceramide or a derivative is an essential component of the neural receptor for human immunodeficiency virus type 1 envelope glycoprotein gp120. *Proc. Natl. Acad. Sci. USA* 88:7131 (1991).
28. K. Conant, W. Atwood, R. Traub, C. Tornatore, and E.O. Major. An increase in p50/p65 NF-kB binding to HIV-1 LTR is not sufficient to increase HIV-1 expression in the primary human astrocyte. *Virology* (in press).
29. G. Nabel, and D. Baltimore. An inducible transcription factor activates expression of human immunodeficiency virus in T cells. *Nature (Lond.)* 326:711 (1987).
30. E.J. Duh, W. Maury, T. Folks, A. Fauci, and A.B. Rabson. Tumor necrosis factor-α activates human immunodeficiency virus type 1 through induction of nuclear factor binding to the NF-kappa B sites in the long terminal repeat. *Proc. Natl. Acad. Sci. USA* 86:5974 (1989).
31. C. Cheng-Mayer. Biological and molecular features of HIV-1 related tissue tropism. *AIDS* 4:S49 (1990).
32. R.J. Pomerantz, T. Didier, M. Feinbert, and D. Baltimore. Cells nonproductively infected with HIV-1 exhibit an aberrant pattern of viral RNA expression: a molecular model for latency. *Cell* 61:1271 (1990).
33. M. Robert-Guroff, M. Popovic, S. Gartner, et al. Structure and expression of tat, rev, and nef specific transcripts of human immunodeficiency virus type 1 in infected lymphocytes and macrophages. *J. Virol.* 64:3391 (1990).
34. F. Chiodi, A. Valentin, B. Keys, et al. Biological characterization of paired human immunodeficiency virus type 1 isolates from blood and cerebrospinal fluid. *Virology* 173:178 (1989).
35. J.A. Levy. Viral and cellular factors influencing HIV tropism, *in:* "Mechanisms and specificity of HIV entry into host cells," R. Duzgunes and F. Nejat, eds., Plenum, New York (1991).

USE OF HUMAN BRAIN CELL AGGREGATES FOR AIDS RESEARCH IN THE NERVOUS SYSTEM

Lynn Pulliam

University of California, San Francisco
San Francisco, California 94143
and
Veterans Administration Medical Center
4150 Clement Street (113A)
San Francisco, California 94121

INTRODUCTION

Since human immunodeficiency virus (HIV) is species-specific, how we study the neuropathogenesis of this infection is open to different approaches. Neuroscientists have historically utilized primary dissociated neural cells from rats and immortalized human neural cell lines (neuroblastoma and glioma) to study mechanisms associated with brain dysfunction. This is due in part to the technical difficulties involved in primary human neuronal cultures. While primary neural cells from rat can serve as a model for neural cell metabolism, species differences may limit the interpretation and extrapolation of the findings from neural cells to the human brain. Therefore, immortalized human cell lines have been widely used and have the advantage of being easy to maintain and able to produce abundant amounts for experimentation. However, the use of human neural tumor cell lines may not represent the normal environment.

My laboratory has established a human brain cell aggregate model that has been used to study HIV interactions in the central nervous system (CNS). It has the advantage of including all the cell types of the CNS in a three-dimensional shape; it has the disadvantage of each brain being inherently different as well as possibly reflecting fetal tissue rather than adult. In this chapter, I will briefly review the characterization of the human brain aggregate model, describe studies relating to HIV-associated neurotoxins using this model and compare results from several different models and offer explanations as to the divergent conclusions.

METHODS

Human brain cell aggregates are prepared from human fetal abortus brain between 16 and 18 weeks gestation.[1] Brain tissue is mechanically dissociated into single cells, and 1×10^5 cells/ml are put into DeLong flasks. A partial medium exchange is performed every other day. Cultures are rotated at all times and incubated at 37°C with 10% CO_2. Neural cells begin to aggregate with 2-3

Technical Advances in AIDS Research in the Human Nervous System
Edited by E.O. Major and J.A. Levy, Plenum Press, New York, 1995

105

days. The aggregates are comprised of neurons, astrocytes, oligodendrocytes with myelin, and microglial cells; the percentage of cell subtypes varies; however, aggregates commonly contain approximately 40% neurons, 40% astrocytes, 10% oligodendrocytes, and 10% microglial cells. These cells can be identified by immunostaining for cell-specific markers (Fig. 1).

Previously we reported that immunostaining for specific cell types was maximal after 10 days in culture.[1] Aggregates can be maintained as primary cultures with accompanying cell-specific immunostaining for 30 days.

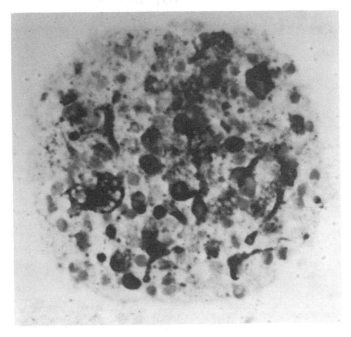

Figure 1. Human brain aggregate immunoperoxidase-stained with antibodies to glial fibrillary acidic protein (GFAP) to identify astrocytes, using the substrate DAB.

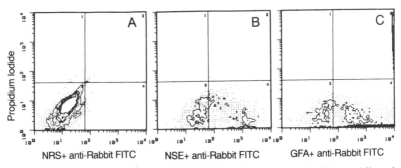

Fig. 2. Flow cytometry of human brain cells dissociated and stained with propidium iodide to indicate cell viability and antibodies to (A) normal rabbit serum (NRS, negative control); (B) neuron-specific enolase (NSE) to identify neurons; and (C) GFAP to identify astrocytes.

Another approach to more accurately quantify cell populations within brain cell aggregates is the dissociation of aggregates using an enzyme cocktail of trypsin and collagenase. Cells are then permeabilized, immunostained for specific cell types, stained with dyes for viability (propidium iodide) followed by flow cytometry (Fig. 2). Our laboratory has used antibodies to neuron-specific enolase (NSE) to indicate neurons and glial fibrillary acidic protein (GFAP) to identify astrocytes.

Myelin production increases over time in culture. Using a radioimmunoassay for myelin basic protein (MBP), we were able to recover up to 4 µg/mg protein at 20 days in culture. This approaches levels of MBP in human brain (white matter) of 6.2 µg/mg. Human brain aggregates continue to produce myelin while in culture. The enzyme cyclic nucleotide phosphohydrolase (CNP) occurs in high levels in myelin and oligodendrocytes, and has been used as a marker for demyelination/remyelination.[2] The highest levels of CNS we have obtained were after 40 days in culture; the level was approximately 175 nm/min/mg protein (Pulliam, unpublished data) compared to human white matter that averages CNP of 213 nm/min/mg protein.

The human brain aggregate system has a number of advantages over other *in vitro* systems. These include:

(a) The aggregates are three-dimensional and contain the major cells of the CNS within an extracellular matrix.

(b) The aggregates are primary neural cells that can be maintained as such without added nutrients (other than serum) for up to 40 days without loss of viability.

(c) The presence of human neurons allows for study of species-specific viruses or toxins that may affect neurons in an environment that includes other neural cells that may be protective. Primary neurons can be kept for up to 40 days.

(d) Brain cell aggregates can be treated like tissue specimens and sampled from the same flask over time. Each flask contains approximately one thousand brain aggregates.

(e) The aggregates can be dissociated at any time and stained with specific cell markers in addition to vital dyes to determine quantitative alterations in neural cell populations.

(f) The aggregates can be used to assess neurotoxicity of chemicals or other biological products in neural cells using vital dyes or biochemical analysis such as production of lactate dehydrogenase (LDH).

There are several disadvantages which should be kept in mind, and include:

(a) Every brain is inherently different. The area of the brain sampled cannot always be consistent.

(b) Results using human fetal brain tissue may not reflect adult brain tissue.

(c) Damage observed in human brain aggregates from a specific neurotoxin may reflect a cascade of events involving multiple neural cells rather than a direct hit.

AIDS Dementia

Dementia associated with AIDS may be caused by opportunistic infections; however, in the absence of these, the mechanism is still unknown. We are committed to neuropathology findings to gleam how this clinical and pathological condition ensues, and most importantly, what to look for in our *in vitro* models. Initially, the neuropathology described subcortical abnormalities, microglial nodules, astrocytosis and multifocal rarefaction in the white matter. However, these findings were not consistent with the level of clinical dementia. These reports were followed by studies demonstrating loss of neurons even though they were not directly infected. With the demonstration of HIV infection of microglia/macrophages in the brain, it followed that dementia might be associated with toxic factors or cytokines produced from these cells which may directly be toxic to neurons or initiate a toxic cascade that results in neuronal dropout or dysfunction. We turned our attention to studying this infection *in vitro*, using HIV infection of human macrophages and the human brain cell aggregates as a model for neural cell toxicity.

HIV-Induced Macrophage Neurotoxin

There have been several conflicting reports concerning a macrophage-induced neurotoxin produced from infection with HIV. Discrepancies in these results reflect the differences in the model systems which are noted in Table 1.

Table 1. Conflicting reports of potential HIV-infected macrophage neurotoxin.

	HIV Strain	Infected Cell	Indicator Cell
Guilian *et al.*, 1990	3B	U937, THP-1	Chick and rat neurons
Pulliam *et al.*, 1991	DV	Macrophage	Human brain aggregates
Bernton *et al.*, 1992	ADA, LAI	Macrophage	Rat neurons
Genis *et al.*, 1992	ADA, other strains	Monocyte Astrocyte	Rat brain explant

An initial report by Guilian et al.[3] used a lymphotropic HIV strain 3B to infect the promonocytic cell line U937 and the monocytic cell line THP-1. Soluble factors produced from these infections, but not an HIV-1-infected H9 lymphoid cell line, killed rat and chick neurons in culture. Furthermore, the N-methyl-D-aspartate (NMDA) antagonists kynurenic acid, MK-801, and 2-amino-5-phosphonovalerate (APV) blocked the toxic effects.

Our group used a macrophage-tropic HIV strain DV to infect primary human macrophages.[4] Soluble factors produced from this infection were incubated with human brain cell aggregates; neural cell damage resulted. Histologic examination revealed a peripheral rarefaction and loss of cell numbers. Immunocytochemistry showed a loss of neurons and selected astrocytes, oligodendrocytes and microglia. Electron microscopy confirmed these light microscopy results. It appeared that the toxin killed not only neurons but other neural cells. The damage did not appear immediate, but took at least 48 hours, and was independent of NMDA-sensitive receptors. Pursuing this finding, we cultured macrophages from patients with HIV infection. The degree of toxicity to human brain aggregates paralleled the proportion of macrophages expressing HIV p24. Recent data from our laboratory (unpublished) showed that neurotoxin production is not connected to the proportion of macrophages infected.

A third report by Bernton et al.[5] used several different strains of HIV including ADA, monocyte-tropic strains, and a lymphotropic strain LAI to infect human macrophages. Soluble factors from these infections were toxic to rat cortical neurons but were later found to be contaminated with mycoplasma. When experiments were repeated using mycoplasma-free HIV stock cultures, there was no toxicity to rat neurons. The investigators concluded that it was not the HIV but rather the mycoplasma that stimulated a toxic factor. This neurotoxic effect was also reversed by NMDA antagonists. The same group[6] reported that fluids from HIV-infected monocyte-glial cell interactions produced neurotoxins identified as arachidonic acid metabolites on rat brain explants. This interaction also resulted in the synthesis of tumor necrosis factor-alpha (TNF-α) and inter-leukin-1B (IL-1β) gene products. They concluded that a monocyte-astroglia interaction was necessary to cause toxicity.

Additional studies in our laboratory have shown that not all insults to macrophages cause neurotoxicity on human brain aggregates. Conditions that failed to cause neurotoxicity include: soluble factors produced from HIV$_{DV}$-infected T cells, LPS-stimulated macrophages, and hypoxia-induced macro-phages. We have also infected macrophages with several clinical strains isolated from patient macrophages; not all strains of HIV produced a soluble neurotoxin from macrophages suggesting neurotoxin-producing strains.

The neurotoxic factor(s) produced in our laboratory was greater than 1,000 and less than 10,000 MW. Our results suggest that some strains also produced a neurotoxin greater than 10,000 MW. This toxicity may be related to cytokine production by individual strains and is being further investigated.

gp120 Neurotoxicity

Brenneman and colleagues first reported that gp120 was toxic to rat hippo-campal neurons.[7] The effect was manifest as a 50% decrease in neuron-specific enolase (NSE) staining cells and was maximal at a dose of 1 pM gp120. Toxicity was diminished with the addition of vasoactive intestinal peptide. In separate studies, Dreyer and colleagues reported that gp120 was neurotoxic to rat retinal ganglion cells at a concentration of 200 pM.[8] Neurotoxicity was reversed by the calcium L-channel antagonist, nimodipine. Additional studies from Lipton's group showed that neurotoxicity associated with gp120 required the presence of endogenous glutamate.[9]

Table 2. Conflicting reports of gp120 neurotoxicity.

	Indicator Tissue	Neurotoxicity
Brenneman et al., 1988	Rat hippocampal neurons	Neuron
Dreyer et al., 1990	Rat retinal ganglion	Neuron
Pulliam et al., 1993	Human brain aggre-gates; human astrocytes	Astrocyte
Giulian et al., 1993	Chick ciliary neurons	Neuron

Our laboratory in collaboration with Dr. Raymond Swanson (Department of Neurology, University of California, San Francisco) treated rat hippocampal neurons with recombinant gp120$_{SF2}$ at a concentration of 1 nM (unpublished results). Rat hippocampal neurons developed NMDA receptor-sensitive neurons at approximately 14 days in culture. When gp120 was added before the neurons developed NMDA sensitivity, there was no toxicity (Fig. 3). Toxicity developed after neurons became NMDA-sensitive and could be diminished with the addi-tion of glutamate pyruvate transaminase. Alternatively, when HIV$_{DV}$-infected macrophage supernatant was incubated with rat neurons, there was toxicity regardless of NMDA sensitivity.

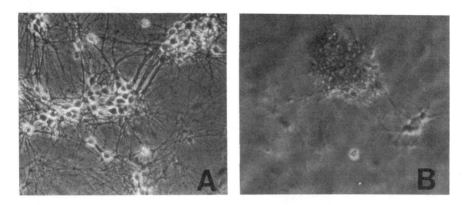

Fig. 3. Rat hippocampal neurons grown 10 days in culture and treated with (A) medium alone; neuron cultures treated with medium containing 1 nM gp120 appeared the same as the control; and (B) medium containing 20% HIV$_{DV}$-infected macrophage supernatant. The gp120-treated neurons did not appear toxic until NMDA was expressed at approximately 14 days in culture.

In an effort to test the toxicity of gp120 on human brain cells, our laboratory incubated recombinant gp120$_{SF2}$ and 3B at a low and high concentration (1 nM and 1 pM) with human brain cell aggregates.[10] Toxicity was manifest at the light microscopy level as a loose lacy appearance compared to control aggregates (Fig. 4).

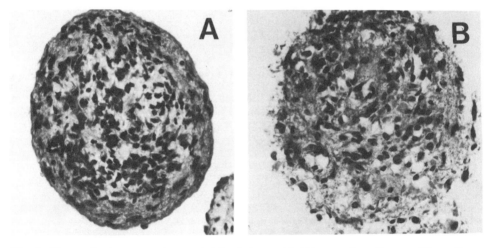

Fig. 4. Human brain aggregates treated for 5 days with (A) control medium or (B) medium containing 1 nM gp120$_{SF2}$.

Individual neural cells were also stained for the presence of CD4 antigen by incubation with fluorescein isothiocyanate (FITC)-conjugated OKT4 or Leu-3A. The ability of neural cells to bind gp120 was tested with a biotinylated form of gp120$_{SF2}$ (Fig. 5). Neural cells did not appear to have the CD4 antigen nor bind to gp120.

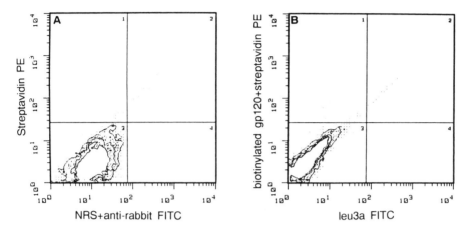

Fig. 5. Flow cytometry of human neural cells incubated with (A) normal rabbit serum conjugated to fluorescein and phycoerythrin (PE)-conjugated streptavidin or (B) biotinylated gp120 plus streptavidin PE and fluorescein-conjugated Leu-3A monoclonal antibodies.

These results strongly suggest that damage from gp120 treatment was not dependent on a CD4 receptor. Five human brain cell aggregate cultures were treated with gp120 for 7 days. Neuronal death was less than 5% as determined by flow cytometry staining with antibodies to NSE.[10] In four of five brain aggregate cultures, there was an increase in astrocyte death from 7 to 24% as determined by flow cytometry staining with antibodies to GFAP and propidium iodide staining for viability. Further confirmation of this finding was determined by the same gp120 treatments of human astrocyte monolayer cultures. Four of five different astrocyte preparations showed an increase in astrocyte death ranging from 5 to 40%. The other surprising finding was the apparent decrease in GFAP staining by flow cytometry suggesting a loss in intermediate filaments (Fig. 6).

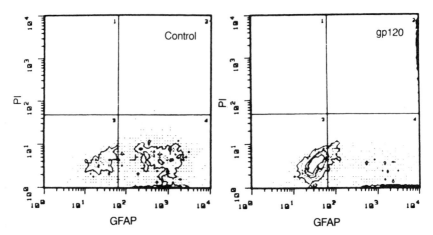

Figure 6. Flow cytometry of brain cell aggregates treated with 1 nM gp120$_{SF2}$ or untreated (control), dissociated into single cells and stained with antibodies to GFAP for the identification of astrocytes and propidium iodide (PI) for demonstration of viability.

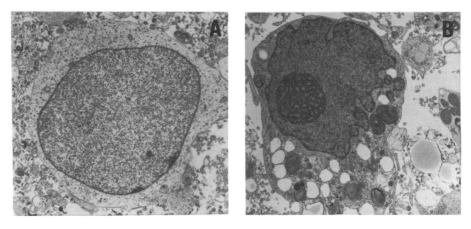

Fig. 7. Electron micrographs of cells within brain cell aggregates treated with 1 nM gp120$_{SF2}$ and consistent with astrocyte morphology but devoid of cytoplasmic intermediate filaments (A) (X43,750) or consistent with neuronal morphology with cytoplasmic vacuoles (B) (X43,750).

This finding was also apparent by ultrastructure (Fig. 7). Brain cell aggregates treated with gp120 contained cells reminiscent of astrocytes but not definitely identified since the cells were rounded and missing fibrils in the cytoplasm. Cells recognizable as neurons contained vacuoles in the cytoplasm.

All gp120-treated brain cultures showed astrocyte alterations manifest as either a decrease in GFAP and/or astrocyte death. Loss in intermediate fibrils is an unusual finding since most pathologic processes result in an increase of GFAP or gliosis. There are several reported circumstances where a loss in GFAP has been documented. A loss in GFAP staining with accompanying astrocyte loss was reported to precede demyelination in early herpes simplex virus infection.[11] A loss of GFAP has also been reported in hepatic encephalopathy where protoplasmic astrocytes lose GFAP in gray matter with a gliosis in the white matter.[12,13] Accumulation of intracellular calcium has been shown to cause a loss of astrocytic fibrils.[14] Finally, tumor necrosis factor has been shown to cause a marked decrease in GFAP mRNA after extended incubation (3-5 days).[15]. These combined data suggested that such astrocyte alterations may influence the protective properties that astrocytes perform for neurons which may subsequently influence the functions of neurons.

Human Brain Cell Aggregates Used As a Neurotoxicity Screen

The brain cell aggregate model has thus far been discussed in its use as a screen for neurotoxin (HIV-induced macrophage soluble factors) and protein damage (gp120).[16] Our laboratory has also used this model to screen for drug toxicity and agonists such as NMDA. As mentioned above, the expression of an NMDA receptor may be mandatory for neurotoxicity; therefore, it is necessary to demonstrate this receptor. Not all neural cell cultures will express this receptor. We screened for NMDA by incubating brain cell aggregates with 1 mM NMDA for 24 hours followed by staining with trypan blue for an increase in nonviable cells (trypan blue positive) compared to untreated control aggregates (Fig. 8). This technique is rapid and has correlated with extracellular LDH levels as an indicator of viability.

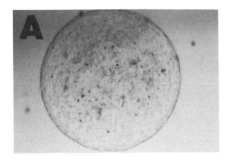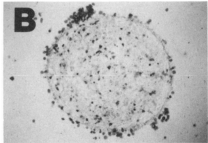

Fig. 8. Wet mounts of brain cell aggregates (A) untreated or (B) treated for 24 hours with NMDA. Both cultures were stained with trypan blue for several minutes. The aggregates treated with NMDA have numerous trypan blue-positive (nonviable) staining cells.

Human brain cell aggregates were used to test the neurotoxicity of the experimental drug trichosanthin (GLQ223, Pharmaceutical Development Group, Genelabs, Inc., Redwood City, CA). Direct treatment of brain cell aggregates with 2 mg/ml did not result in any morphological changes either by light micro-scopy or ultrastructure.[17] However, when trichosanthin was used to treat HIV-infected macrophages *in vitro* and these supernatants incubated with brain cell aggregates, there was marked morphological disruption (Fig. 9). These results emphasized the neurotoxic potential of any therapy targeted at HIV-infected cells. While drugs may not be directly toxic to neural cells, their interaction with virus-infected cells may cause the cells to release soluble factors that are toxic.

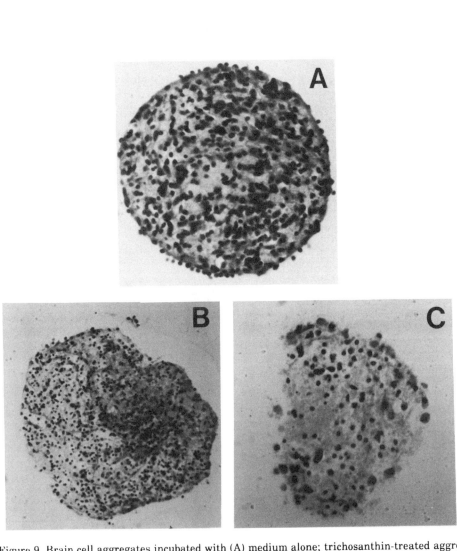

Figure 9. Brain cell aggregates incubated with (A) medium alone; trichosanthin-treated aggre-gates appeared the same; (b) 20% supernatant from HIV-infected macrophages; and (C) 20% supernatant from trichosanthin-treated HIV-infected macrophages.

CONCLUSIONS

It is clear that results may differ depending on the culture system and strain of virus utilized. Since the mechanism(s) associated with AIDS is still unknown, it is extremely important that hypotheses be tested on multiple systems. Several issues need to be considered when interpreting HIV neural cell experiments: (a) tumor or continuous cell lines versus primary cell cultures; (b) animal versus human neural cells; (c) single cell cultures versus mixed cell cultures including monolayers versus explants or aggregates; and (d) fetal versus adult neural cells.

REFERENCES

1. L. Pulliam, M.E. Berens, and M.L. Rosenblum. A normal human brain cell aggregate model for neurobiological studies. *J. Neurosci. Res.* 21:521 (1988).
2. T. Kurihara, and Y. Tsukada. The regional and subcellular distribution of 2',3'-cyclic nucleotide 3'-phosphohydrolase in the central nervous system. *J.Neurochem.* 14:1167 (1967).
3. D. Giulian, K. Vaca, and C.A. Noonan. Secretion of neurotoxins by mononuclear phagocytes infected with HIV-1. *Science* 250:1593 (1990).
4. L. Pulliam, B.G. Herndier, N.M. Tang, and M.S. McGrath. HIV-infected macrophages produce soluble factors that cause histological and neurochemical alterations in cultured human brains. *J. Clin. Invest.* 87:503 (1991).
5. E. Bernton, H. Bryant, M. Decoster, et al. No direct neuronotoxicity by HIV-1 virions or culture fluids from HIV-1 infected T cells of monocytes. *AIDS Res. Hum. Retroviruses* 8:495 (1992).
6. P. Genis, M. Jett, E.W. Bernton, et al. Cytokines and arachidonic metabolites produced during HIV-infected macrophage-astroglia interactions: implications for the neuropathogenesis of HIV disease. *J. Exp. Med.* 176:1703 (1992).
7. D.E. Brenneman, G.L.Westbrook, S.P. Fitzgerald, et al. Neuronal cell killing by the envelope protein of HIV and its prevention by vasoactive intestinal peptide. *Nature (Lond.)* 335:639 (1988).
8. E.B. Dreyer, P.K. Kaiser, J.T. Offermann, and S.A. Lipton. HIV-1 coat protein neurotoxicity prevented by calcium channel antagonists. *Science* 248:364 (1990).
9. S.A. Lipton, N.J. Sucher, P.K. Kaiser, and E.B. Dreyer. Synergistic effects of HIV coat protein and NMDA receptor-mediated neurotoxicity. *Neuron* 7:111 (1991).
10. L. Pulliam, D. West, N. Haigwood, and R.A. Swanson. HIV-1 envelope gp120 alters astrocytes in human brain cultures. *AIDS Res. Hum. Retroviruses* 9:439 (1993).
11. Y. Itoyama, T. Sekizawa, H. Openshaw, K. Kogure, and I. Goto. Early loss of astrocytes in herpes simplex virus-induced central nervous system demyelination. *Ann. Neurol.* 29:285 (1992).
12. R.A. Sobel, S.J. DeArmond, L.S. Forno, and L.F. Eng. Glial fibrillary acidic protein in hepatic encephalopathy. *J. Neuropath. Exp. Neurol.* 40:625 (1981).
13. H.A. Kretzschmar, S.J. DeArmond, and L.S. Forno. Measurement of GFAP in hepatic encephalopathy by ELISA and transblots. *J. Neuropath. Exp. Neurol.* 44:459 (1985).
14. S.J. DeArmond, M. Fajardo, S.A. Naughton, and L.F. Eng. Degradation of glial fibrillary acidic protein by a calcium-dependent proteinase: an electroblot study. *Brain Res.* 262:275 (1983).
15. K. Selmaj, B. Shafit-Zagardo, D.A. Aquino, et al. Tumor necrosis factor-induced proliferation of astrocytes from mature brain is associated with

down-regulation of glial fibrillary acidic protein mRNA. *J. Neurochem.* 57:823 (1991).
16. D. Giulian, E. Wendt, K. Vaca, and C.A. Noonan. The envelope glycoprotein of human immunodeficiency virus type 1 stimulates release of neuro-toxins from monocytes. *Proc.Natl. Acad. Sci. USA* 90:2769 (1993).
17. L. Pulliam, B.G. Herndier, and M.S. McGrath. Purified trichosanthin (GLQ223) exacerbation of indirect HIV-associated neurotoxicity *in vitro.* *AIDS* 5:1237 (1991).

INFECTION OF HUMAN FETAL ASTROCYTES WITH HIV

Avindra Nath and Meihui Ma

Departments of Medical Microbiology and Internal Medicine
University of Manitoba
Winnipeg, Manitoba, R3E OW3, Canada

INTRODUCTION

The ability of HIV to infect resident cell types within the brain has been a topic of intense discussion since the recognition of HIV-1 encephalopathy. Initial *in vitro* studies had suggested that glial cells (most likely astrocytes) from human fetal brain can be infected with HIV.[1,2] This was supported by the electron microscopic demonstration of HIV in human astrocytes *in vivo*.[3,4] However, several other researchers were unable to replicate these findings using conventional histopathological techniques. Only recently have four independent groups of investigators provided convincing evidence for astrocyte infection in pediatric and adult brain at postmortem using highly sensitive and novel techniques for viral detection.[5-9]

Astrocytes represent the most numerous cell type within the brain. They play very important functions in maintaining normal brain function (reviewed in ref. 10) (Fig. 1). They modulate neuronal survival and activity by regulating the extracellular environment and the release of neuroactive compounds. These cells interact with oligodendrocytes and influence myelin turnover via gap junctions and the release of various cytokines. Through interactions with microglia, astrocytes participate in immune responses in the brain. The vascular endothelium has an unique arrangement with astrocytes in establishing the blood-brain barrier (BBB). Astrocytes also communicate with one another via gap junctions. Thus, they form a network that can flow from one point to another, reaching distant sites. Hence, infection of even a small number of astrocytes could potentially have disastrous consequences for normal brain function.

AN IN VITRO MODEL FOR STUDYING ASTROCYTE INFECTION

Man is the only natural host for HIV. Hence the study of interactions of HIV with human brain tissue would be most applicable to understanding the pathogenesis of HIV encephalopathy. Use of primary brain tissue as opposed to malignant cell lines would be more closely representative of the *in vivo* situation. Adult brain tissue from patients undergoing surgery for epilepsy and fetal tissue represent the major sources of human brain tissue from which neural cells have been cultured. Both sources of tissue have certain advantages and disadvantages. Microglia and oligodendrocytes can be easily cultured from adult brain, but pure cultures of astrocytes are best obtained from fetal tissue. Since human fetal astrocytes continue to replicate in culture for about one month, large

Technical Advances in AIDS Research in the Human Nervous System
Edited by E.O. Major and J.A. Levy, Plenum Press, New York, 1995

numbers of cells can be obtained (Fig. 2). Methods for isolating these cells have been well established. Adult astrocytes do not replicate *in vitro*.

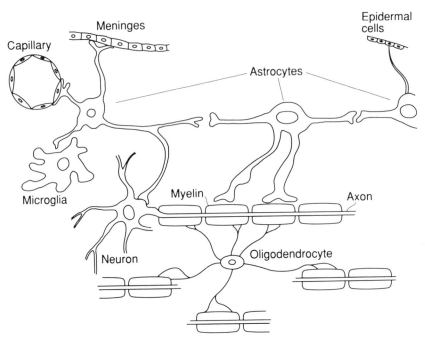

Figure 1. Interactions between the cells within the nervous system. The neurons pass signals to one another by releasing neurotransmitters. Oligodendrocytes form myelin that wraps around the axons and aids in the conduction of electrical impulses. Microglia are tissue macrophages that participate in phagocytosis and lymphokine secretion. Astrocytes send processes to the neuronal cell body and regulate the cellular environment. They influence both myelin turnover and ion conduction at the nodes of Ranvier. Astrocytes aid in formation of the blood-brain barrier by sending processes to capillaries. They also interact with the meningeal cells and with one another through gap junctions.

INFECTION OF ASTROCYTES IS STRAIN DEPENDENT

Several strains of HIV have been shown to infect astrocytes. Data from six different laboratories have shown that predominantly lymphotropic strains namely, HIV_{3B}, HIV_{SF2} (cytopathic and noncytopathic strains), HIV_{SF117}, HIV_{SF128A}, HIV_{RF}, HIV_{RUT}, HIV_{Eli} and HIV_{NL4-3} can infect human fetal astrocytes.[1,2,11-14] Furthermore, our laboratory has been unsuccessful in infecting astrocytes with monocytotropic strains HIV_{MO}[14] and HIV_{JRFL} (unpublished observations) as determined by p24 antigen detection in culture supernatants and polymerase chain reaction (PCR) for detection of proviral DNA. Using the above lymphotropic strains, approximately 0.1-1.0% of cells become infected. Although differences in the infectivity with different strains of HIV have been observed, the viral determinant responsible for these properties remains unknown. Viral strains used to infect astrocytes were initially isolated on lymphocytes and macrophages. Isolation of astrotropic strains of HIV, i.e., direct isolation of HIV from cerebrospinal fluid (CSF) or brain tissue on astrocytes in culture has yet to be attempted.

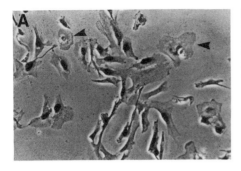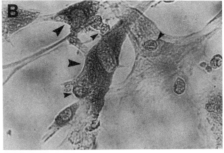

Figure 2. (A) Human fetal astrocytes in culture show incorporation of bromodeoxyuridine (bdu)[15] in the nuclei (staining dark). Two cells with microglial cell morphology do not show staining for bdu (arrow). (B) Human fetal astrocytes infected with chronically infected lymphoid cells with HIV_{SF2} show the lymphoid cells adhered to the astrocytes (small arrow) and the astrocytes staining for HIV antigen (large arrow) with a monoclonal antibody to gp41 by immunoperoxidase technique.

Infection of astrocytes with HIV leads to viral production during the first days of infection (productive phase). The level of viral production is much lower than that produced in lymphocytes (Fig. 2). Following this initial phase, the virus may either enter a latent phase where only proviral DNA can be detected (HIV_{NL4-3})[13] or a persistent phase where small amounts of virus can be detected in the culture supernatants (HIV_{3B}).[14] During these phases, coculture of the astrocytes with activated peripheral blood lymphocytes or CD4+ lymphoid cells results in cytopathic effects in the lymphocytes (syncytia formation and cell degeneration) caused by establishment of a productive HIV infection. HIV genome expression can also be up-regulated by cytokine stimulation.[13] No evidence of morphologic or cytopathic changes have been determined in the infected cells by microscopy or measurement of lactate dehydrogenase levels in culture supernatants.[14]

The presence of persistently infected cells *in vivo* may ensure production of low levels of virus on a continual basis. Astrocytes could thus act as a reservoir for HIV and when stimulated with cytokines, lead to recurrent episodes of HIV production.

ROLE OF LYMPHOCYTE-ASTROCYTE CELL-TO-CELL CONTACT

Activated peripheral blood lymphocytes and CD4+ lymphoid cells readily adhere to astrocytes but not to microglia. Five to 15 lymphocytes of either subpopulation may adhere to an astrocyte, although in some instances the lymphocytes may completely obscure the astrocyte.[15] This interaction is mediated by cell adhesion molecules, and the phenomenon has been used to infect astrocytes in culture where HIV-infected lymphoblastic cells were cocultivated with astrocytes.[11,13,14] We have determined that 4-5 times more astrocytes can be infected by cell-to-cell contact than by free virus alone. One possibility is that the differences in the two systems represent the differences in the amount of inoculum present since the lymphoblasts continuously produce virus or it may be due to factors such as direct transmission of virus via cell fusion or due to activating factors produced by lymphoid cells.

Cell-to-cell contact is an important mechanism for viral transmission for those viruses that are cell membrane-associated. This method allows viral transmission to occur in the presence of neutralizing antibodies. Since astrocytes extend foot processes into the capillaries, viral transmission may occur from lymphocytes to astrocytes. This may serve as a route for viral entry into the brain.

GP120 BINDING SITE ON ASTROCYTES

Even though lymphotropic strains of HIV seem to preferentially infect astrocytes, we have been unable to detect CD4 on the surface of astrocytes by flow cytometry and immunocytochemistry. We have further been unable to block the binding of ^{125}I-gp120 to astrocytes with soluble CD4 or antibodies to CD4,[16] suggesting that an alternative binding site must be present on these cells. Gal C has been reported to be another receptor for HIV on neuroblastoma cells;[17] however, this molecule has not been detected on astrocytes either,[17] and antisera to Gal C does not block gp120 binding to the astrocyte cell membrane (Fig. 3).

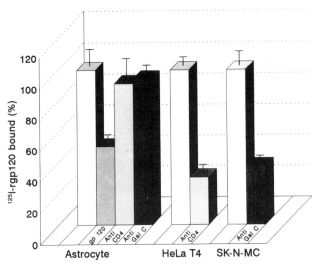

Figure 3. gp120 binding to astrocytes; 4 x 10⁴ cells were incubated with 1 nM ^{125}I-gp120 and competed with either 100 nM unlabeled gp120, monoclonal antibody to CD4a (4 µg/ml) or polyclonal antisera to Gal C (1:40). 50.4% ± 3.9% inhibition was seen with unlabeled gp120; no significant inhibition was seen with antibody to CD4 or Gal C. HeLa T4 cells and SK-N-MC cells were used as positive controls for CD4 and Gal C, respectively. All values represent mean ± SEM from two experiments, each done in triplicate.

Kinetic studies of ^{125}I-gp120 binding on human fetal astrocytes suggest that there is a single binding site on these cells. gp120 binds to astrocytes with a lower affinity than that for CD4 or Gal C (Table 1). Immunoprecipitation studies following surface labeling of astrocytes with ^{125}I, show that gp120 binds to a single molecule 260 kDa in size.[16] Whether this gp120 binding site is also the receptor for HIV remains to be determined.

Table 1. Receptors for gp120.

Cell Type	Biochemical Characteristics	Dissociation Constant (Kd)
Lymphocyte	glycoprotein (58 kDa)	$2\text{-}5 \times 10^{-9}$ M
SK-M-NC	lipid	11.6×10^{-9} M
Astrocyte	protein (260 kDa)	26×10^{-9} M

FUTURE DIRECTIONS

It seems to be well established that primary astrocytes can be infected with HIV *in vivo* and *in vitro*. Astrocytes are an interesting cell type to study since the mechanisms of viral entry and the virus-host relationships are different from those of lymphocytes and macrophages. Further studies on the mechanism of HIV infection in these cells and the life cycle of the virus will not only provide important information on the pathogenesis of HIV encephalopathy but will also provide new approaches to study other CD4 negative cells that may be infected with HIV.

A number of fundamental questions on the interaction of HIV and astrocytes remain unresolved. How does HIV enter astrocytes? Can gp120 binding protein serve as a receptor for HIV? Further biochemical and molecular characterization of this molecule will be necessary. What are the viral determinants for this interaction? What role do cell adhesion molecules play in viral entry by cell-to-cell contact, and which adhesion molecules are important in this interaction? Does infection of astrocytes lead to impairment of function of these cells? Which functions are affected and what is the mechanism? How do astrocytes regulate HIV genome expression? Why do different strains of HIV differ in their ability to infect and become expressed in astrocytes? Some of these questions can be best addressed by isolation of astrotropic strains of HIV. Clearly, much has been learned since HIV was first identified in the brain in 1986; yet many basic questions must be addressed. We hope this chapter has shed light on these elementary questions and will provide a conceptual model to incorporate the forthcoming answers.

ACKNOWLEDGMENTS

The authors would like to thank Eugene Major for helpful comments. This work was supported in part by grants from the Medical Research Council and National Health and Research Development Program (NHRDP) of Canada. A.N. is a NHRDP scholar and M.M. is a recipient of a graduate assistantship from the Manitoba Health Research Council.

REFERENCES

1. C. Cheng-Mayer, J.T. Rutka, M.L. Rosenblum, et al. Human immunodeficiency virus can productively infect cultured human glial cells. *Proc. Natl. Acad. Sci. USA* 84:3526 (1987).
2. C. Christofonis, L. Papadaki, Q. Sattentau, R.Ferns, and R. Tedder. HIV replicates in human brain cells. *AIDS* 1:229 (1987).
3. F. Gyorkey, J.K. Melnick, and P. Gyorkey. HIV in brain biopsies of patients with AIDS and progressive encephalopathy. *J. Infect.Dis.* 155:870 (1987).
4. L.G. Epstein, L.R. Sharer, V. V. Joshi, et al. Progressive encephalopathy in children with AIDS. *Ann. Neurol.* 17:488 (1985).
5. G.J. Nuovo. Personal communication (1993).
6. Y. Saito, L.R. Sharer, L.G. Epstein, et al. Overexpression of *nef* as a marker for restricted HIV-1 infection of astrocytes in postmortem pediatric central nervous system tissues. *Neurology* 44:474 (1994).
7. C. Tornatore, K. Myers, W.D. Atwood, and E.O. Major. HIV-1 infection of subcortical astrocytes in the pediatric central nervous system, *in*: "Pediatric AIDS: Clinical Pathology and Basic Science Perspectives," W. Lyman, ed., N.Y. Academy of Sciences, New York (in press).
8. C. Tornatore, R. Chandra, J.R. Berger, and E.O. Major. HIV-1 infection of subcortical astrocytes in the pediatric central nervous system *Neurology* 44:481 (1994).
9. O. Bagasra, and R. Pomerantz. Application of *in situ* PCR in the detection of HIV in brain specimens, *in*: "PCR Neuroscience," G. Shankar, ed., Academic Press Inc., New York (in press).
10. S. Murphy. "Astrocytes, Pharmacology, and Function," Academic Press Inc.,New York (1993).
11. R. Brack-Werner, A. Kleinschmidt, A. Ludvigsen, et al. Infection of brain cells with HIV: Restricted virus production in chronically infected glial cell lines. *AIDS* 6:273 (1992).
12. M. Tardieu, C. Hery, S. Peudenier, O. Boespflug, and L. Montagnier. Human immunodeficiency virus type 1 infected monocytic cells can destroy human neural cells after cell-to-cell adhesion. *Ann. Neurol.* 32:11 (1992).
13. C. Tornatore, A. Nath, K. Amemiya, and E.O. Major. Persistent human immunodeficiency virus infection type 1 in human fetal glial cells reactivated by T-cell factors or by the cytokines, tumor necrosis factor alpha and interleukin-1 beta. *J.Virol.* 65:6094 (1991).
14. A. Nath, V. Hartloper, M. Furer, and K.R. Fowke. Infection of human fetal glial cells with HIV: Viral tropism and the role of cell-to-cell contact in viral transmission. (Submitted).
15. M. Furer, V. Hartloper, J. Wilkins, and A. Nath. Lymphocyte emperipolesis in human fetal glial cells. *Cell Adhesion Commun.* (in press).
16. M. Ma, A. Nath, and J. Gieger. Characterization of a novel binding site for HIV-1 envelope protein gp120 on human fetal astrocytes. (Submitted)
17. J. Harouse, C. Kunsch, H.T. Hartle, et al. CD4 independent infection of human neural cells by human immunodeficiency virus type 1. *J. Virol.* 63:257 (1989).
18. F. Gonzalez-Scarano. Personal communication.

MODEL CELL CULTURES FROM ADULT BRAIN AND GLIOMA CELL LINES

MOLECULAR INTERACTION OF HIV-1 IN GLIOMA CELLS

Volker Erfle,[1] Andrea Kleinschmidt,[1] Markus Neumann,[1]
Alexandra Ludvigsen,[1] Barbara K. Felber,[2] George N. Pavlakis,[2],
Birgit Kohleisen,[1] and Ruth Brack-Werner[1]

[1]Institut für Molekulare Virologie, GSF-Forschungszentrum für
Umwelt und Gesundheit, GmbH
Ingolstaedterlandstrasse 1
D-85764 Neuherberg, Germany
[2]Basic Research Program
National Cancer Institute-Frederick Cancer Research and
Development Center
Frederick, Maryland 21702-1201 USA

INTRODUCTION

Analysis of brain specimens of HIV-1-infected individuals by immuno-chemistry as well as *in situ* hybridization indicate that the major cell types expressing HIV-1 antigens and nucleic acids in the central nervous system (CNS) are of macrophage origin and include microglia, macrophages and derivative multinucleated cells.[1,2] However, HIV-1 expression has been described in other cell types, including capillary endothelial cells, astrocytes, and oligodendrocytes.[3-7] Productive HIV-1 infection in brains of patients with AIDS-encephalitis is in many cases not abundant and often not in keeping with the severity of the disease.[8] On the other hand, high levels of HIV-1 DNA have been detected in brain tissue by Southern blot analysis[9,10] as well as the polymerase chain reaction (PCR) method.[11-13] Quantitative estimates of viral DNA in HIV-encephalitis autopsy samples indicate DNA levels comparable to or exceeding those in lymphoid tissues.[10,12] This suggests the presence of a latently infected virus reservoir in the brain. An indication that HIV-1 can directly infect cells of the nervous system came from *in vitro* infection studies of cultured human astrocytoma and neuroblastoma cells with HIV-1.[14-19] In addition, primary human brain cells expressing glial fibrillary acidic protein (GFAP) have also been found to be infected with HIV-1 *in vitro*.[20-22] *In vitro* infection of human glioma cells with HIV-1 differs markedly from infection of susceptible T-cell lines or peripheral blood mononuclear cells (PBMCs) by: (a) absence of virus-induced cytopathic effects in target cells; (b) lack of requirement for the presence of the CD4 cell surface receptor; and (c) the prevalence of a nonproductive infection phenotype.

The difficulties inherent in studying infection and disease development in the human brain necessitated development of *in vitro* systems for HIV-1 infection of cells of the CNS. To date, the molecular mechanisms governing HIV infection and expression in brain cells have been difficult to address because of the lack of stable continuous culture systems. To fulfill a basic requirement for such studies, we have established persistently HIV-1-infected glioma cell lines.

Technical Advances in AIDS Research in the Human Nervous System
Edited by E.O. Major and J.A. Levy, Plenum Press, New York, 1995

125

Establishment of Chronically HIV-1-Infected Human Glioma Cell Lines

The human cell line 85HG-66 was established from a primary brain tumor histologically defined as astrocytoma.[23] Infection with HIV-1 was achieved by cocultivation of 85HG-66 cells with T-lymphoma cells (KE37/1) productively infected with HIV-IIIB. Expression of HIV-1 antigen following exposure of cells to virus was monitored at a single-cell level by direct immunoperoxidase staining (IPS). Cocultivation of glioma cell lines with HIV-1-producing T-lymphoma cells led to about 1-6% of glioma cells becoming positive for the HIV-1 antigen. The HIV-1 antigen-positive cells disappeared after consecutive passages, indicating restricted spread of virus in the culture as well as a growth disadvantage of the HIV-1-infected cells. Therefore, glioma cells were cloned three times by limiting dilution shortly after HIV-1 infection, leading to clonal HIV antigen-expressing glioma cells isolates. In most glioma cell clones, the percentage of cells staining positive for HIV antigen ranged from 5 to 100% (see Figure 1).

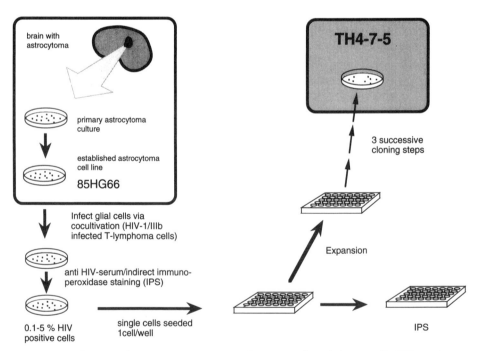

Figure 1. Strategy for establishing chronically HIV-1-infected glioma cells (TH4-7-5).

The nature of HIV antigen expression in persistently infected glioma cells was studied in more detail for cell line TH4-7-5, a representative clonal isolate of the third cloning generation consisting of 100% HIV antigen-expressing cells. Use of a panel of monoclonal and polyclonal antibodies for IPS revealed expression of gag (p24, p17, p15), env (gp160 and gp41), and pol (p66/51) antigens. Antibodies against viral nonstructural proteins Nef, Tat, Vif and Rev also yielded positive results. Western blot analysis using whole-cell extracts confirmed low-level intracellular expression of gag and env structural proteins.[24] Intracellular p24 antigen expression in TH4-7-5 cells was determined by p24 antigen capture ELISA. TH4-7-5 cells yielded only low p24 antigen levels, being <3% of p24 antigen levels in HIV-producer cells KE37/1-IIIB (T-lymphoma cells). The reproducibly high intensity of staining obtained with antibodies against Nef in IPS was also reflected by Western blot analysis. Whole-cell extracts from TH4-7-5 cells displayed strong reactivity for the 27 kD Nef protein, comparable in intensity with that of p24 antigen in H9-IIIB cells (human T-lymphoma cell line).

HIV-1 Production Is Restricted in Chronically Infected Glioma Cells

Culture supernatants from chronically infected glioma cell lines were examined for reverse transcriptase activity, p24, and for the ability to induce syncytia formation in C8166 indicator cell lines[25] to assess production of infectious HIV-1 progeny. All glioma cell lines yielded distinctly lower levels of reverse transcriptase activity, and p24 than productively HIV-1-infected T-lymphoma cells (KE37/1-IIIB), and for most HIV-infected glioma cell lines, reverse transcriptase activity did not exceed background levels. Incubation of HIV-susceptible C8166 target cells with culture supernatant led to induction of HIV antigen-positive syncytia in those target cells. However, the syncytia-inducing capacity of culture supernatant from chronically infected glioma cell lines was about three orders of magnitude below that of the HIV-producing KE37/1-IIIB. Infectious virus could not be transmitted by culture fluids from the TH4-7-5 cells to HIV-1-susceptible T-lymphoma (KE37/1) or fibroblast (LC5) cells or to primary macrophages. These results indicate that virus production in chronically infected glioma cells is restricted.

Virus rescue experiments were performed by cocultivation of TH4-7-5 cells with HIV-1 susceptible cells (KE37/1 T-lymphoma cells and peripheral blood-derived monocyte-macrophages). Cocultivation of TH4-7-5 cells with these target cells led to syncytia formation and virus recovery in both target cell types.[26] However, virus infection of target cells was first detected 13 and 19 days after cocultivation suggesting low-level virus production by TH4-7-5 cells. Following cocultivation, culture supernatant from the target cells contained infectious virus transmittable to uninfected KE37/1 cells as to be expected for T-lymphoma cells productively infected with HIV-IIIB.

Molecular Characterization of Restricted HIV-1 Expression in Chronically Infected Glioma Cells

The presence of a full-length HIV-1 proviral DNA in TH4-7-5 cells was demonstrated by repeated Southern blot hybridization of genomic DNA with various HIV-1 probes. Distinct fragment patterns were obtained after digestion with restriction enzymes and hybridization with a DNA probe encompassing a nearly full-length HIV-IIIB-related proviral genome (BH10). The restriction fragment patterns obtained demonstrated the presence of a single provirus integration site and allowed establishment of a restriction enzyme map of the TH4-7-5 virus. The TH4-7-5 provirus genome was amplified by PCR in four overlapping fragments, which were subcloned and sequenced. The nucleotide sequence of the TH4-7-5 provirus is closely related to the replication-competent molecular clone HXB2 indicating the presence of a functional proviral genome.[27] The *nef* sequence of TH4-7-5 provirus codes for serine at position 2 instead of the glycine conserved as a myristoylation site in *nef* sequences of HIV-1, HIV-2, and SIV.[28,29]

Low-level intracellular expression of major viral proteins and low-level production of infectious particles suggests that production of virus in TH4-7-5 cells is repressed at the transcriptional or translational level. Thus, regulation of HIV-LTR activity or an influence on posttranscriptional or translational mechanisms in persistently infected glioma cells may contribute to restricted virus production. To investigate this concept, first the chloramphenicol acetyltransferase (CAT) reporter gene activity of an HIV-LTR-CAT construct was compared to the activity of the corresponding deleted HIV-LTR construct containing only HIV-LTR sequences between positions -155 and +80 (HIV-1 strain BRU). The deleted construct showed an average 15-fold higher activity than the undeleted construct in TH4-7-5 cells, indicating that HIV-LTR activity of the full-length construct is suppressed by sequences not contained in the deleted construct. This negative regulatory effect was about 5-10 times higher in TH4-7-5 cells than in the other cell lines. The same tendency was observed in the presence of exogenous Tat. These results indicate that prominent negative regulation of HIV-LTR activity is specific for the chronically infected glioma cell line TH4-7-5 and may influence virus expression. The negative effect may be mediated by specific host cell factors induced in HIV-1-infected glioma cells which modulate HIV-LTR activity. These may interact directly or indirectly with sequences contained in the undeleted HIV-LTR-CAT construct and may involve a region of the HIV-LTR, termed the negative regulatory element (NRE). This region modulates HIV-LTR activity and has been shown to bind both known inducible transcriptional activators of cellular genes[30,31] as well as potential transcriptional repressors.[32,33]

To test the expression of HIV-1 mRNAs on a quantitative basis in chronically HIV-1-infected glioma cells (TH4-7-5), a quantitative RNA polymerase chain reaction (PCR) technique was developed which allows identification and evaluation of all HIV-1 mRNA species produced by HIV-1. This method was used to compare HIV-1 mRNA expression patterns in chronically infected glioma cells with HIV-1 producer fibroblasts. Both cell lines expressed the same mRNA species, indicating similar splicing of HIV-1 in glioma cells as in HIV-1 producer fibroblasts. However, there were major quantitative differences in mRNA expression patterns between both cell lines. Levels of Rev-dependent transcripts were generally much lower in the glioma cells with a restricted HIV-1 production than in the HIV-1 producer fibroblasts, which suggests perturbed function of the Rev/RRE regulatory axis in the glioma cells (Figure 2).

The chronically HIV-1-infected TH4-7-5 glioma cells were treated with cytokines and mitogens to study to what extent virus production can be increased. Induction of viral production was determined by measuring p24 antigen in culture supernatants. Stimulation of cells with phorbol ester, sodium butyrate and tumor necrosis factor-α (TNF-α) induced a modest 2-4-fold increase of viral protein in the glioma cells. Interferon-γ treatment of the cells inhibited HIV expression. Determination of infectivity of released virus particles was performed by measuring syncytia-inducing capacity in C8166 cells. The 2-3-fold p24 induction correlated with an average 10-fold increase in infectivity. No synergistic effects were observed by treating with combinations of the stimulatory agents (see Table 1). Much higher induction levels are reported for hematopoietic cell lines latently infected with HIV-1 (U1, ACH-2), ranging from 5-20-fold for phorbol esters and TNF-α.[34,35] In these cell lines, these compounds act by stimulating HIV-1 LTR activity. Lack of a substantial increase of HIV-1 expression in the glioma cells by these compounds indicates a possible involvement of posttranscriptional regulatory events in restricted virus production.

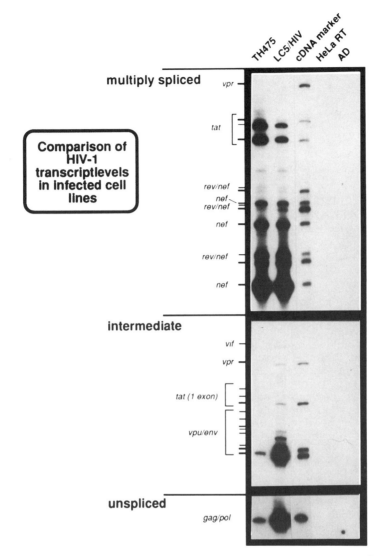

Comparison of HIV-1 transcriptlevels in infected cell lines

multiply spliced
- vpr
- tat
- rev/nef
- nef
- rev/nef
- nef
- rev/nef
- nef

intermediate
- vif
- vpr
- tat (1 exon)
- vpu/env

unspliced
- gag/pol

Figure 2. Semiquantitative reverse transcriptase-polymerase chain reaction (RT-PCR) was used to identify HIV-1 specific transcripts in total RNA from chronically HIV-1-infected glioma cells (TH4-7-5) and HIV-1 producer fibroblasts (LC5/HIV). RNA was reverse transcribed and subjected to PCR using one radiolabeled primer, whose binding site is common to all existing HIV-1 transcripts. After 20 cycles, the products were separated under denaturing conditions on polyacrylamide gels. Comparison with amplification products from previously cloned cDNAs used as template ("cDNA marker") allows quantitative estimation as well as exact functional definition of each band detected in this assay. Approximately 100 times lower levels of REV-dependent intermediate and unspliced transcripts are detected in the glioma cells whereas all members of the small class are produced at approximately the same levels in both cell lines.

Table 1. Induction of HIV-1 expression in chronically HIV-1-infected glioma cells (TH4-7-5) by various cytokines and mitogens. Relative levels of p24 in the cell culture supernatant in percent of mock-treated control.

	TH4-7-5 glioma cells	LC5/HIV fibroblast
Control (culture medium)	100	100
TPA	270	300
TNF-α	250	215
Sodium butyrate	250	450
TPA + TNF-α	120	300
TPA + sodium butyrate	150	115
TNF-α + sodium butyrate	65	380
TPA + TNF-α + sodium butyrate	180	300
Interferon-γ	70	75

Conclusions and Perspectives

The consistent observation that productive expression of HIV-1 is detected nearly exclusively in macrophage-derived cells in the CNS has led to the hypothesis that these cells are transporters of virus into the brain as well as being effectors of pathogenic mechanisms leading to the neurologic disorders associated with HIV infection. Thus, several virus gene products have been shown to possess neurotoxic potential. The gp120 surface glycoprotein[36,37] as well as the Tat[38] and the Rev proteins[39] contain peptide sequences that are neurotoxic when applied to neuronal cells *in vitro*. In addition to these viral compounds, HIV-1-infected cells are capable of releasing substances detrimental to CNS cells. HIV-infected macrophages secrete cytokines that are cytotoxic for neuronal and glial cells.[40] These *in vitro* results were extended to a more physiological system by treating brain aggregates with supernatants from HIV-infected macrophages. This treatment produced histochemical, ultrastructural, and functional abnormalities in the aggregates not observed with the supernatants of uninfected or LPS-activated macrophages or HIV-infected T-cells.[41]

However, the amount of HIV-1-expressing microglial nodules often does not correlate with the severity of the clinical signs. Large-scale neuronal cell destruction is uncommon in the AIDS-related cognitive motor complex,[42] and cytotoxic infections of neurons, astrocytes, and oligodendrocytes are not observed.[41] This suggests that indirect effects of HIV-1 infection rather than direct cytolysis by HIV-1 are responsible for the observed impairment of the CNS of AIDS patients. Furthermore, the infection of the brain takes place within the first weeks after the infection of the individual, as has also been shown in SIV-infected macaques,[43] and that virus expression cannot be detected until later stages of the disease. As already noted, the functional impairment induced by HIV-1 infection of the brain usually exceeds the observed physical damage, suggesting an important role for mechanisms based on noncytotoxic functional impairment of neural cells.

The observation of a restricted infection of glioma cells in culture as described here provides the basis for a somewhat different scenario of the HIV-1 infection and pathogenesis in the CNS. This would imply, after the early entry of the brain either by infected lymphocytes or via endothelial cells, that astroglial cells become infected and constitute the major long-term virus reservoir with a restricted virus expression phenotype. Because of the predicted low levels of structural proteins expressed by these infected cells, they would escape detection by immunohistochemical analysis with antibodies against p24, gp120 and gp41 which have been used classically in assessing HIV-1-infected cells in the

CNS. The use of Nef antibodies or oligonucleotides typical for Nef transcripts has now provided evidence that astroglial cells may be infected by HIV-1[44] and that these cells express HIV-1 Nef. Our finding that Nef is capable of inducing reversible alterations in the ion flux of neuronal cells provides clues to one potential mechanism for functional impairment of the CNS by HIV.[45] Sequence similarities with scorpion neuroactive peptides are also found in other viral proteins, including poliovirus VP2 and rhinovirus 14 VP2, although Nef is the only viral protein tested for electrophysiological activity so far. Rabies virus G protein bears a peptide similar to another neurotoxin, the cobra toxin.[46] Thus, the mode of neuronal impairment employed by scorpion and snake neurotoxins seems to be mimicked by several viruses and it is remarkable that two of these are also neurotropic (polio and rabies).

In the context of the above scenario, the appearance of the HIV-1-expressing multinucleated giant cells becomes a late event, assuming that macrophages from the peripheral blood pass the blood-brain barrier in later stages of the disease and become infected in the CNS through contact with infected astroglial cells. This event now may lead to a second phase of the HIV-1 infection in the brain which is characterized by processes leading to cytotoxicity and neuronal loss. Although it remains elusive why and how HIV induces neurologic abnormalities in AIDS patients, there is now evidence for several direct and indirect pathways, all of which may contribute to the observed neuropathology. Elucidation of the processes leading to HIV-associated neuro-pathy requires complementation of the *in vitro* studies of brain cells with suitable analyses of HIV-infected brains, especially at the early stages of CNS disease.

REFERENCES

1. A. Fauci, S. Koenig, H.E. Gendelman, et al. Detection of AIDS virus in macrophages in brain tissue from AIDS patients with encephalopathy. *Science* 233:1089 (1986).
2. R. Vazeux, N. Brousse, A. Jarry, et al. AIDS subacute encephalitis. *Am. J. Pathol.* 126:403 (1987).
3. L.G. Epstein, L.R. Sharer, E.-S. Cho, et al. HTLV-III/LAV-like retrovirus particles in the brains of patients with AIDS encephalopathy. *AIDS Res.* 1: 447 (1984-85).
4. F. Gyorkey, J.L. Melnick, and P. Gyorkey. Human immunodeficiency virus in brain biopsies of patients with AIDS and progressive encephalopathy. *J. Infect. Dis.* 15:870 (1987).
5. J.A. Levy, L.A. Evans, C. Cheng-Mayer, et al. Biologic and molecular properties of the AIDS-associated retrovirus that affect antiviral therapy. *Ann. Inst. Pasteur Virol.* 138:101 (1987).
6. T. Pumarola-Sune, B.A. Navia, C. Cordon-Cardo, et al. HIV antigen in the brains of patients with the AIDS dementia complex. *Ann. Neurol.* 21:490 (1987).
7. C.A. Wiley, R.D. Schrier, J.A. Nelson, et al. Cellular localization of human immunodeficiency virus infection within the brains of acquired immune deficiency syndrome patients. *Proc. Natl. Acad. Sci. USA* 83:7089 (1986).
8. R.W. Price, B. Brew, J. Sidtis, et al. The brain in AIDS: central nervous system HIV-1 infection and dementia complex. *Science* 239:586 (1988).
9. M.S. Saag, B.H. Hahn, J. Gibbons, et al. Extensive variation of human immunodeficiency virus type-1 *in vitro*. *Nature* 334:440 (1988).
10. G.M. Shaw, B.H. Hahn, S.K. Arya, et al. Molecular characterization of human T-cell leukemia (lymphotropic) virus type III in the acquired immune deficiency syndrome. *Science* 226:1165 (1984).
11. J. Bell, and L. Ratner. Specificity of polymerase chain amplification reactions for the human immunodeficiency virus type I DNA sequences. *AIDS Res. Hum. Retrovirus* 5:87 (1989).

12. S. Pang, Y. Koyanagi, S. Miles, et al. High levels of unintegrated HIV-1 DNA in brain tissue of AIDS dementia patients. *Nature* 343:85 (1990).
13. V.A. Varma, S. Hunter, R. Tickman, et al. Acute fatal HIV encephalitis with negative serologic assays for antibody and antigen: diagnosis by polymerase chain reaction. *N. Engl.J. Med.* 320:1494 (1989).
14. C. Cheng-Mayer, J.T.Rutka, M.L. Rosenblum, et al. Human immunodeficiency virus can productively infect cultured human glial cells. *Proc. Natl. Acad. Sci. USA* 84:3526 (1987).
15. F. Chiodi, S. Fuerstenberg, M Gidlund, et al. Infection of brain-derived cells with the immunodeficiency virus. *J. Virol.* 62:151 (1987).
16. P.R. Clapham, J.N. Weber, D. Whitby, et al. Soluble CD4 blocks the infectivity of diverse strains of HIV and SIV for T cells and monocytes but not for brain and muscle cells. *Nature* 337:368 (1989).
17. S. Dewhurst, K. Sakai, J. Bresser, et al. Persistent productive infection of human glial cells by human immunodeficiency virus (HIV) and by infectious molecular clones of HIV. *J.Virol.* 61:3774 (1987).
18. X.L. Li, T. Moudgil, H.V.Vinters, et al. CD-4 independent, productive infection of a neuronal cell line by human immunodeficiency virus type 1. *J. Virol.* 64:1383 (1990).
19. P. Shapshak, N.C.J. Sun, L. Resnick, et al. HIV-1 propagates in human neuroblastoma cells. *J. AIDS* 4:228 (1991).
20. G. Christofinia, L. Papadaki, Q. Sattentau, et al. HIV replicates in cultured human brain cells. *AIDS* 1:229 (1987).
21. C. Kunsch, and B.Wigdahl. Transient expression of human immunodeficiency virus type 1 genome results in a nonproductive infection in human fetal dorsal root ganglia glial cells. *Virology* 173:715 (1989).
22. P. Rytik, V.F. Eremin, Z.B. Kvacheva, et al. Susceptibility of primary human glial fibrillary acidic protein-positive brain cells to human immunodeficiency virus infection *in vitro*: Anti-HIV activity of memantine. *AIDS Res. Hum. Retrovirus* 7:89 (1991).
23. D. Stavrou, E. Keiditsch, F. Schmidberger, et al. Monoclonal antibodies against human astrocytomas and their reactivity pattern. *J. Neurol. Sci.* 80:205 (1987).
24. R. Brack-Werner, A. Kleinschimdt, A. Ludvigsen, et al. Infection of human brain cells by HIV-1: Restricted virus production in chronically infected human glial cell lines. *AIDS* 6:273-285.
25. S.Z. Salahuddin, P.D. Markham, F. Wong-Staal, et al. Restricted expression of human T-cell leukemia-lymphoma virus (HTLV) in transformed human umbilical cord blood lymphocytes. *Virology* 129:51 (1983).
26. V. Erfle, P. Stoeckbauer, A. Kleinschmidt, et al. Target cells for HIV in the central nervous system: macrophages or glial cells? *Res. Virol.* 142:139 (1991).
27. G.M. Shaw, B.H. Hahn, S.K. Arya, et al. Molecular characterization of human T-cell leukemia (lymphotropic) virus type III in the acquired immune deficiency syndrome. *Science* 226:1165 (1984).
28. B. Guy, Rivière, K. Dott, et al. Mutational analysis of the HIV nef protein. *Virology* 176:413 (1990).
29. K.P. Samuel, A. Seth, A. Konopka, et al. The 3'-orf protein of human immunodeficiency virus shows structural homology with the phosphorylation domain of human interleukin-2 receptor and the ATP-binding site of the protein kinase family. *FEBS Lett.* 218:81 (1987).
30. R. Franza, Jr., F.J. Rauscher, III, S.F. Josephs, et al. The fos complex and fos-related antigens recognize sequence elements that contain AP-1 binding sites. *Science* 239:1150 (1988).
31. J.-P. Shaw, P.J. Utz, D.B. Durand, et al. Identification of a putative regulator of early T cell activation genes. *Science* 241:202 (1988).
32. K. Orchard, N. Perkins, C. Chapman, et al. A novel T-cell protein which recognizes a palindromic sequence in the negative regulatory element of the human immunodeficiency virus long terminal repeat. *J. Virol.* 64:3234 (1990).
33. M.R. Smith, and W.C. Greene. The same 50 kDa cellular protein binds to the

negative regulatory elements of the interleukin 2 receptor alpha-chain gene and the human immunodeficiency virus type 1 long terminal repeat. *Proc. Natl. Acad. Sci. USA* 86:8526 (1989).

34. T.M. Folks, J. Justement, A. Kinter, C.A.Dinarello, A. Fauci, and J.H. Kehrl. Cytokine-induced expression of HIV-1 in a chronically infected promonocyte cell line. *Science* 238:800 (1987).

35. G. Poli, A. Kinter, J.S. Justement, et al. Tumor necrosis factor alpha functions in an autocrine manner in the induction of human immunodeficiency virus expression. *Proc. Natl. Acad. Sci. USA* 87:782 (1990).

36. D.E. Brenneman, G.L. Westbrook, S.P. Fitsgerald, et al. Neuronal cell killing by the envelope protein of HIV and its prevention by vasoactive intestinal peptide. *Nature* 335:639 (1988).

37. M.R. Lee, D.D. Ho, and M.E. Gurney. Functional interaction and partial homology between human immunodeficiency virus and neuroleukin. *Science* 237:1047 (1987),

38. J.-M. Sabatier, E.Vives, K. Mabrouk, et al. Evidence for neurotoxic activity of Tat human immunodeficiency virus type 1. *J. Virol.* 65:961 (1991).

39. K. Mabrouk, K. Vanrietschoten, E. Vives, et al. Lethal neurotoxicity in mice of the basic domains of HIV and SIV Rev proteins - study of these regions by circular dichroism. *FEBS Lett.* 289:13 (1991).

40. D. Giulian, K. Vaca, and C.A. Noonan. Secretion of neurotoxins by mononuclear phagocytes infected with HIV-1. *Science* 250:1593 (1990).

41. L. Pulliam, B.G. Herndier, N.M. Tang, et al. Human immunodeficiency virus-infected macrophages produce soluble factors that cause histological and neurochemical alterations in cultured human brains. *J.Clin. Invest.* 87:503 (1991).

42. M. Maj. Organic mental disorders in HIV-1 infection. *AIDS* 4:831 (1990).

43. L.R. Sharer, J. Michaels, M. Muerphy-Coreb, et al. Serial pathogenesis study of SIV brain infection. *J. Med. Primatol.* 20:211 (1991).

44. B. Kohleisen, K. Gaedigk-Nitschko, T. Werner, et al. Biological properties of Nef and its pathogenic potential in HIV-1-related central nervous system dysfunction. *AIFO* 5:175 (1993).

45. T. Werner, S. Ferroni, T. Saermark, et al. HIV-1 Nef protein exhibits structural and functional similarity to scorpion peptides interacting with K+ channels. *AIDS* 5:1301 (1991).

46. R.F. Garry, J.J. Kort, F. Koch-Nolte, et al. Similarities of viral proteins to toxins that interact with monovalent cation channels. *AIDS* 5:1381 (1991).

TRANSCRIPTION OF HUMAN IMMUNODEFICIENCY VIRUS PROMOTER IN CNS-DERIVED CELLS: EFFECT OF TAT ON EXPRESSION OF VIRAL AND CELLULAR GENES

Kamel Khalili, J. Paul Taylor, Crystina Cupp, Michael Zeira, and Shohreh Amini

Molecular Neurovirology Section
Jefferson Institute of Molecular Medicine
Thomas Jefferson University
Philadelphia, Pennsylvania 19107

HIV AND NEUROLOGIC DISEASE

Approximately 60% of patients with AIDS have neurologic symptoms, the so-called AIDS-related subacute encephalopathy, and more than 80% are found to have neuropathologic abnormalities at autopsy.[1,2] The most common neurologic problems include: toxoplasmosis, cryptococcosis, primary lymphoma of the central nervous system (CNS), and subacute encephalitis or AIDS encephalopathy.[3-8] Histologic analysis of CNS tissues from AIDS patients shows enlargement of oligodendrocytes and formation of multinucleated giant cells.[9-17] The detection of HIV DNA in the brain and recovery of infectious virus particles from cerebrospinal fluid and brain tissue of patients with AIDS have suggested that HIV-1 may be directly responsible for some of the neurologic deficits found in these patients.[18-22] The presence of CD4, the high-affinity receptor for HIV-1 in human brain tissue and in certain glioma cell lines, has been reported.[23,24] Furthermore, HIV-1 has been shown to infect glial cells *in vitro* and has been detected in oligodendrocytes and astroglial cells *in vivo*.[18,23,25-28] Together, these observations indicate that HIV-1 is not only lymphotropic but also neurotropic. However, the exact mechanisms involved in the neuropathogenesis of HIV-1 and AIDS dementia complex remain unclear. A simple model would envisage the direct infection of neurons and glia by neurotropic HIV-1 that results in indirect or direct cytotoxicity mediated by cytotoxic T cells. Alternatively, infection of monocytic macrophages with HIV-1 may lead to the release of a diffusible inflammatory component(s) that destroys neighboring neural cells, and/or results in the release of cytokines which are toxic to neural cells. Moreover, other neurotropic viruses, JCV and cytomegalovirus (CMV) may act as cofactors in the pathogenesis of AIDS-related neurologic disorders.

HIV-1: Genomic Structure and Control of the Life Cycle

In addition to the long terminal repeats (LTRs) and the gag, pol, and env genes, HIV has several genes that contribute to a system of genetic regulation far more complex than most retroviruses. These genes are termed virion

Technical Advances in AIDS Research in the Human Nervous System
Edited by E.O. Major and J.A. Levy, Plenum Press, New York, 1995

135

infectivity factor (vif), viral protein R (VPr), transactivator (Tat), regulator of expression of virion proteins (rev), viral protein u (VPu), and negative factor (nef). The gag and pol proteins are found in the core of viral particles, whereas env glycoproteins are within the lipid bilayer coat of the mature virion. A major 53 kD precursor polypeptide, the gag gene product, is cleaved during morphogenesis of the virion by the HIV-derived protease and produces a number of smaller peptides ranging from 25 kD to 7 kD in size. The pol polyprotein is also cleaved and produces protease, DNA-dependent RNA polymerase and endonuclease (integrase). The env gene encodes a precursor glycoprotein, gp160, which is subsequently cleaved to produce gp120 and gp41 (for review see ref. 29). The two major regulatory proteins, Tat and rev, are essential for viral replication.[30,31] The structure of the HIV regulatory sequence, LTR consists of a 543-bp U3 region, a 98-bp R region, and an 85-bp U5 region, similar to those of other known retroviruses.[30,31] Within the U3 and R regions, there are multiple cis-acting elements which are involved in HIV gene expression. Among these elements are the TATA box at position -27 with respect to the transcription start site, GC-rich sequences from -48 to -77, and an enhancer element located between nucleotides -82 to -105. It appears that the TATA box, as in other eukaryotic promoters, plays a role in the positioning of the transcription initiation site and contributes to the level of promoter efficiency.

Cellular factors interacting with this sequence may be universal components of RNA polymerase II initiation complexes. The GC-rich sequence binds to transcription factor SP1,[32] which has been purified and appears to potentiate transcription of any GC-containing promoter. The enhancer, which contains two 11-bp imperfect direct repeats (GGGGACTTTCC), increases transcription of the HIV-1 promoter irrespective of its position and orientation.[33,34] This sequence is analogous to the inducible transcription factor NF-kB binding site first identified in the light chain of the immunoglobulin enhancer region. *In vitro* DNA binding studies have indicated that, in fact, the HIV-1 11-bp imperfect repeats bind to NF-kB.[33, 34]

The lytic cycle of HIV-1 begins with the synthesis of a 2-kb RNA which encodes the two regulatory proteins Tat and rev, and nef. The shift from early to late phase results in the cytoplasmic appearance of unspliced 9-kb and singly spliced 4-kb viral mRNAs that produce the viral structural proteins, including gag, pol, and env. Tat increases the rate of transcription from the HIV-LTR, whereas rev is a posttranscriptional regulator that mediates the shift from early to late phase of the viral lytic cycle primarily by expediting the nuclear export of incompletely spliced and unspliced mRNAs.[31] However, a recent study shows that rev activity is also a function of the efficiency of splicing because the presence of efficient splice sites precludes rev responsiveness. The precise mechanism responsible for the shift from early to late phase during the lytic cycle is unknown.

Regulation of HIV-1 Gene Transcription

The transcriptional control sequences of HIV-1 are located in the U3 and R regions of the viral LTR within 450 bp of the sequence. Using a number of approaches, including transient transfection experiments with the LTR promoting transcription of reporter genes, *in vitro* transcription experiments, and employing mutant viruses, several positive and negative cis-acting transcriptional elements within the LTR have been identified. These cis-acting transcriptional elements are the targets for the binding of cellular transcription factors such as TF$_{IID}$, SP1, NF-kB, AP1, etc. Among these elements, NF-kB plays a significant role in the activation of the LTR by a variety of stimuli, including viral proteins, mitogens and several cytokines.[35] The transcription factor, NF-kB, belongs to a family of c-Rel-related proteins that are differentially expressed in a cell-type-specific manner.[35] In many cell types, including T-lymphocytes and HeLa cells, NF-kB was found only in an inducible form in the cytoplasm, whereas in B-lymphocytes, NF-kB DNA binding activity was present in the nucleus.[35]

In addition to the cellular proteins that control viral gene transcription, Tat, the HIV-1-encoded transacting protein, modulates expression of the viral promoter. Tat is an 86-amino acid protein produced from the multiply spliced transcripts during the early stages of the replicative cycle.[31] Mutational analysis has characterized multiple essential domains of the Tat protein, including a highly conserved basic domain that serves as a nuclear localizing signal and mediates nucleic acid binding, a cysteine-rich domain that mediates metal-linked dimer formation *in vitro*, and an acidic domain that is important in activation.[36] The Tat protein produced early during infection causes a remarkable increase in steady-state levels of LTR-directed transcripts.[31] It has been suggested that enhanced expression is due predominantly to increased transcriptional initiation and increased elongation, although there are reports that Tat may also influence translation of the transacting responsive (TAR) element-containing transcripts.[37-39] The positive feedback loop provided by Tat increases the expression of all viral genes, including Tat itself, and enables the virus to produce high levels of viral transcripts in a short time.

There has been substantial investigation into the mechanism of Tat transactivation of the HIV-1 LTR, with a focus on the interaction of the Tat protein with the target sequence TAR present just 3' to the start site of transcription.[40-44] TAR RNA, present in the leader of all HIV-1 transcripts, forms a stable stem-loop structure which can bind Tat and cellular factors *in vitro*.[45] Substantial evidence suggests that a specific interaction of Tat protein with TAR RNA is involved in mediating transactivation. Detailed mutagenesis experiments have characterized the TAR sequence and structural features required for Tat responsiveness in transient transfection assays; these correlate with the feature required for protein binding *in vitro*.

Recently, a model was proposed to explain the enhanced rate of transcription mediated by the Tat-TAR interaction.[33] According to this model, the TAR sequence in nascent HIV-1 transcripts, while still in the vicinity of the promoter, assumes a specific stable secondary structure that is bound by Tat and a 65 kD cellular protein.[45] From this position, Tat and cellular TAR-binding proteins can influence the events occurring at the promoter region. Thus, the TAR element would only serve as a localization signal that functions to localize the association of Tat, cellular TAR-binding proteins, and upstream transcription factors in the nucleus.

Whereas HIV-1 predominantly infects CD4+ cells both *in vivo* and *in vitro*, its ability to replicate is not limited to these cells, suggesting that viral tropism is restricted, at least in part, by infectivity mediated by the CD4 receptor, and not by the subsequent events, i.e., transcription, translation, etc. However, regulation of HIV-1 gene expression in a variety of CD4+ cells may differ depending on the cell type. Our results described below indicate that under identical conditions, the HIV-1 LTR promoter is more active in glial cells than any other cells, including human T-lymphocytes and H9 cells. More importantly, our studies indicate that Tat has the capacity to increase LTR activity in the absence of the TAR element in glial cells. This activity is glial cell-specific and not detected in nonglial cells so far examined. Finally, we demonstrated that a TAR-proviral construct replicates exclusively in glial and not in nonglial, H9 cells.

TAR-Independent Activation of HIV-1 LTR by Tat in Glial Cells

To evaluate the transcriptional activity of the HIV-1 LTR in CNS-derived cells, a plasmid expressing chloramphenicol acetyltransferase (CAT) under the direction of the HIV-1 LTR, was cointroduced with a Tat expression plasmid into the astrocytic glial cell lines, U87-MG and U138-MG (both derived from human glioblastoma cells), C6 (derived from rat glioblastoma cells), and several nonglial cell lines. The presence of Tat results in induction of LTR-directed transcription similar to that obtained in cell lines of non-CNS origin, i.e., H9, HeLa, and COS (Fig. 1A-F). To examine the dependence of Tat activity on the TAR element, the LTR-CAT construct was modified so that sequences encoding TAR were deleted.

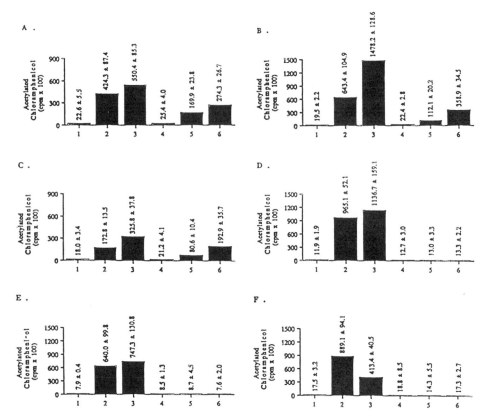

Figure 1. Activation of HIV-1 LTR by Tat in various cell lines. Either the wild type HIV-1 LTR-CAT construct (lanes 1-3) or TAR-deleted construct (lanes 4-6) were introduced alone (lanes 1 and 4) or together with 1 μg (lanes 2 and 5) or 5 μg (lanes 3 and 6) of a recombinant expressing Tat in U87-MG (A); U138-MG (B); C6 (C); H9 (D); HeLa (E); COS (F).

The TAR-deleted LTR was created by restriction digest to remove nucleotides downstream of +24 relative to the transcription start site (ΔTAR constructs). Previous studies have demonstrated that removal of the TAR sequence from the LTR abolishes Tat responsiveness in cells of nonglial origin. Indeed, we observe that Tat is unable to activate expression of the TAR-deleted LTR in either a lymphoid cell line (H9) or nonlymphoid cell lines (COS and HeLa) (Fig. 1D-1F). However, in the glial-derived cell lines, significant transactivation is still detected (Fig 1A-C).

To define the sequences responsible for TAR-independent activation of LTR by Tat in glial cells, a series of PCR-generated deletion mutants were constructed. These constructs were designed to allow sequential examination of small segments of the LTR within the region spanning -117 to -65 as well as sequences downstream of the transcription start site. Each of these segments has been previously implicated as a cis-element involved in transcription regulation (Fig. 2). Transient transfection results demonstrated that removal of sequences downstream of the cap site (construct p117/3) or upstream of the NF-kB binding domain (construct p105/3) does not influence TAR-independent Tat responsiveness (Fig. 2). Removal of one NF-kB binding site (construct p91/3) reduces Tat transactivation, while removal of both NF-kB binding sites (construct p80/3) eliminates Tat responsiveness. These results suggest that TAR-independent Tat transactivation in glial cells requires the kB domain.

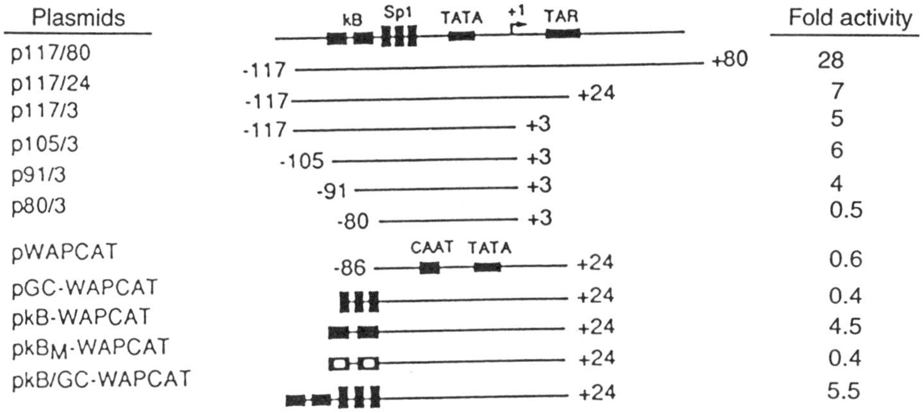

Plasmids	kB Sp1 TATA +1 TAR		Fold activity
p117/80	-117 ——————————————— +80		28
p117/24	-117 ———————————— +24		7
p117/3	-117 ——————————— +3		5
p105/3	-105 ——————————— +3		6
p91/3	-91 ———————————— +3		4
p80/3	-80 ——————————— +3		0.5
pWAPCAT	CAAT TATA -86 ———————— +24		0.6
pGC-WAPCAT	——————————— +24		0.4
pkB-WAPCAT	——————————— +24		4.5
pkB_M-WAPCAT	——————————— +24		0.4
pkB/GC-WAPCAT	——————————— +24		5.5

Figure 2. Deletion and hybrid-promoter analysis. Fold transactivation by Tat was determined by transient transfection analysis of U87-MG with the indicated CAT construct and a plasmid expressing Tat.

To confirm that the HIV-1 enhancer (NF-kB binding domain) can mediate TAR-independent Tat-responsiveness in glial cells, this sequence was examined in an heterologous background. A number of hybrid promoters were constructed by introducing the kB, mutant kB, and Sp1 domains of HIV-1 to the upstream region of an heterologous promoter from mouse whey acidic protein (WAP) (Fig. 2). Transient transfection assay of these constructs demonstrated that the presence of the kB domain is sufficient to confer TAR-independent Tat responsiveness in glial cells (Fig. 2). Mutant kB, on the other hand, shows no response to Tat activation. Transcription directed by the kB-containing WAP promoter is enhanced approximately 4-fold by Tat. This level of induction is similar to that observed for the TAR-deleted HIV-1-LTR promoter. The presence of the Sp1 domain has no influence on Tat responsiveness in the absence of the kB domain, but seems to contribute to a slightly greater Tat responsiveness when both the kB and Sp1 domains are present.

Identification of the kB domain as the element responsible for TAR-independent transactivation in the CNS prompted analysis of kB-binding activity of astrocytic cells. Utilizing electrophoretic mobility shift analysis, interesting differences were observed between glial-derived kB-binding activity and the prototypical NF-kB of T lymphocytic cells. The prototypic NF-kB induced by PMA in Jurkat T cells appears as two complexes that have been previously designated B1 and B2. The α complex of U87-MG astrocytic cells co-migrates with the B1 complex of Jurkat T cells (Fig. 3). Perhaps it should be noted that the B1 complex of Jurkat T cells consists of proteins of 105, 75, 86, and 50-55 kD, believed to represent p105 (a precursor of p50), p65, c-Rel, and p50, respectively. The B2 complex of Jurkat T cells, thought to represent a homo-dimer of p50, does not appear in astrocytic extracts demonstrating further heterogeneity in kB-binding factors in U87-MG astrocytic and Jurkat T cells. The β complex of U87-MG astrocytic cells migrates very slowly in the native gel, suggestive of a very large complex (Fig. 3). A similarly large complex which migrates more slowly than NF-kB, coincidentally termed BETA, was previously observed in astrocytes and neurons, and has also been found in mouse and human fetal brain nuclear extracts (unpublished observation). No complex of comparable migration is seen in Jurkat T cells, implying that astrocytic cells contain additional, or perhaps, novel kB-binding factors.

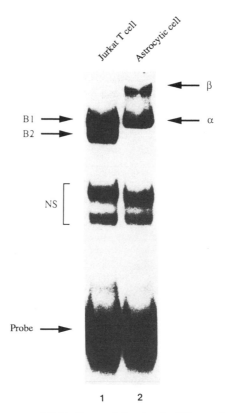

Figure 3. Astrocytic cells express kB-binding activity that is different from the NF-kB of Jurkat T cells. Electrophoretic mobility shift assay demonstrating kB-binding activity (α and β) of unstimulated U87-MG cells and Jurkat T cells stimulated for 20 hours with PMA before nuclear extract preparation.

To obtain further information regarding kB activity in glial cells, nuclear extracts from U87-MG cells treated with PMA for 1, 3, 6, 12, and 20 hours were used in a gel mobility shift assay. Results in Figure 4A illustrate that the activity of complex α comigrating with the NF-kB complex of T cells (as shown in Fig. 3) peaked at 1 to 3 hours after PMA treatment and diminished at 6-20 hours. Complex β, which was observed in glial but not T cell extracts, revealed the highest activity 20 hours after treatment. Note that formation of the β complex at 0-12 hours was detected at all times, suggesting a constitutive expression of this protein in glial cells. To examine the biologic significance of this finding with respect to HIV-1 gene expression, cell-free HeLa transcription extract was programmed with linearized HIV-1 LTR template in the absence or presence of 1 μg of PMA-treated glial nuclear extracts. Results in Figure 4B demonstrate that increased transcription of the LTR in HeLa cell extracts supplemented with nuclear extracts from 1-, 3-, and 20-hour PMA-treated glial cells. The concurrent enhancement of NF-kB activity in binding studies, and transcriptional activity of the LTR in mixing experiments suggest that both α and β complexes may increase the activity of the viral promoter in the nonglial extract.

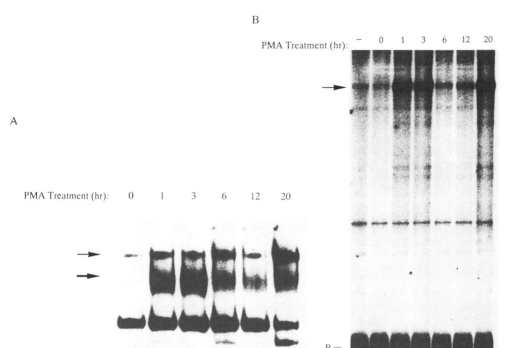

Figure 4. Biological activity of glial-derived kB binding protein. A. Gel mobility shift analysis of nuclear extracts derived from PMA-treated glial cells with the kB sequence. Nuclear extracts prepared from U87-MG cells treated with PMA for different periods of time were incubated with the kB probe. Lane 1, unstimulated U87-MG cells; lanes 2 to 7, U87-MG cells stimulated with 50 mg/ml of PMA for 0, 1, 3, 6, 12, and 20 hours. B. *In vitro* transcription of HIV-1 LTR promoter in the absence (lane 1) and presence of glial extracts treated with PMA (lane 2). Transcription reactions were performed in a final volume of 15 µl. The concentrations of ATP, CTP, and GTP were adjusted to a final value of 0.5 mM and the [32P] UTP to 10 mM. In order to minimize the basal activity of the promoter, 0.01 µg of the template DNA was used. The transcription cocktail was incubated at 30°C for 60 minutes. The arrow indicates the position of the run-off transcript, and "R" shows a reference band that remains constant upon treatment.

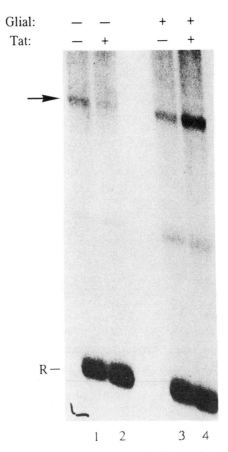

Glial: —   —   +   +

Tat: —   +   —   +

→

R —

1   2   3   4

Figure 5. TAR-independent activation of HIV-1 transcription by Tat *in vitro* requires astrocytic nuclear factors. *In vitro* transcription of template 117/3 in the presence of 0.5 µg of nuclear extract prepared from U87-MG cells is demonstrated. The arrow indicates run-off transcription of 279 nt and "R" shows a nonspecific reference band used as a control for loading. In this study, 0.5 µg/µl of highly purified Tat (kindly provided by Dr. S.A. Khan, Wistar Institute) was added to the reaction mixture. For use, Tat was dissolved in 20 mM Hepes-KOH (pH 7.9), 20% glycerol (v/v), 100 mM KCl, 0.2 mM EDTA, and 1 mM DTT.

To evaluate the transcriptional activity of the HIV-1 ΔTAR by Tat in the presence and absence of kB-binding proteins from glial cells, HIV-1 LTR template DNA carrying a deletion within the TAR sequence (-117 to +3) was incubated with HeLa extract according to the procedure described above. As shown in Figure 5, supplementation of HeLa transcription extract with nuclear factors from unstimulated astrocytic U87-MG cells does not influence transactivation of the template DNA (compare lanes 1 and 3). However, the presence of nuclear factors from unstimulated astrocytes supports activation of transcription by Tat approximately 4.5- to 5.0-fold (Fig. 5, compare lanes 3 and 4), demonstrating TAR-independent activation *in vitro*. Supplementation of the HeLa extract with equal amounts (0.5 µg per reaction) of nuclear extracts prepared from unstimulated Jurkat T lymphocytes did not permit Tat activation of the TAR-deleted template (Taylor et al., unpublished data).

Recognition of a novel kB complex in astrocytic cells that is capable of interaction with Tat implies that a CNS-specific DNA-binding factor was responsible for mediating TAR-independent transactivation. Understanding the molecular mechanism of this induction awaits cloning of the cDNAs from glial cells that encode the participant proteins and examination of the activities in highly purified *in vitro* systems.

Effect of Tat Protein on Cellular Gene Expression

In addition to its role in regulating HIV-1 transcription, Tat appears to play additional roles in the pathogenesis of AIDS. This probably reflects the recently recognized ability of Tat to influence the expression of select cellular genes.[46-48] Functional interaction between Tat and cellular transcription factors, such as those interacting with glial-derived kB, may be involved in initiating a cascade of altered cellular gene expression that contributes directly to disease. Consistent with this model, Tat has been directly implicated in the development of immunodeficiency as evidenced by its ability to specifically inhibit antigen-induced lymphocyte proliferation.[49] However, the effect seems to be indirect and may utilize cytokines, such as tumor growth factor beta 1 (TGFβ-1).[49] The increased levels of TGFβ-1 observed within the brains of HIV-1-infected individuals compared to the brains of noninfected individuals[50] suggests that HIV-1 infection directly or indirectly alters expression of TGFβ-1 and perhaps other regulatory proteins in the CNS. Therefore, we have designed a series of experiments to examine the effect of the HIV-1 Tat on the expression of the TGFβ-1 gene in human glial cell lines.

Toward this end, transient transfection assays were performed using TGFβ-1 promoter constructs driving the CAT reporter gene. Upon cotransfection with the Tat expressor plasmid, the TGFβ-1 promoter dose-dependently responded to Tat activation. This positive response to Tat transactivation was correlated with an increased steady-state CAT RNA level observed in an S1 nuclease protection assay.[51] Due to existing evidence that the Tat protein released from HIV-1-infected cells could exert a physiologic effect on surrounding uninfected cells through transcellular transactivation, we sought to study the effect of exogenously added Tat protein on the expression of the TGFβ-1 gene. The astrocytic glial cells were transfected with the TGFβ-1 promoter construct, and subsequently synthetic Tat protein was loaded on the cells. Interestingly, increased expression of TGFβ-1 promoter activity was evident indicating that these cells can internalize the Tat protein and, as a result, alter cellular gene expression (Fig. 6). Using deletion mutants in cotransfection studies allowed us to identify a region located between nucleotides -453 to -323 as a potential target for Tat-induced activation of the TGFβ-1 promoter.[51]

To examine the biologic significance of the transfection assay results, we investigated the ability of the Tat protein produced upon transfection of whole virus in primary human glial cells to stimulate expression of the endogenous TGFβ-1 gene. In this respect, the plasmid PNL4-3, a recombinant HIV-1 isolate clone,[52] was introduced into primary astrocytic glial cells, and after 48 hours, expression of TGFβ-1 was evaluated by Northern blot analysis. Results shown in Figure 7 indicate elevated levels of TGFβ-1 RNA in cells transfected with provirus HIV-1 DNA. The level of GAPDH transcript served as a control for RNA integrity and concentration. The significance of Tat transactivation of TGFβ-1 is several-fold: (a) TGF-β1 may function in a paracrine fashion resulting in the alteration of the expression of other cytokines and other responsive cellular genes such as those encoding matrix-associated proteins;[48] (b) TGF-β1 can act as a chemotactic agent for infected monocyte recruitment in the brain; and (c) TGF-β1, by up-regulating expression of other opportunistic latent viruses such as JCV in glial cells, results in induction of encephalopathy in the brains of AIDS patients. The exact mechanism by which Tat increases expression of TGF-β1 gene expression remains unclear. Experiments are in progress to identify glial-derived transregulatory factors that in combination with Tat result in alteration of TGF-β1 gene expression in the HIV-1-infected brain.

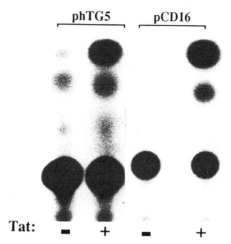

Figure 6. Addition of HIV-1 Tat protein to culture media of U87-MG cells transfected with TGFβ-1 or the HIV-1 LTR promoter constructs. U87-MG astrocytic glial cells were transfected with 5.0 µg phTG5 (left) or 0.2 µg of the HIV-1 LTR construct pCD16 (right). Twenty-four hours post-transfection, cells were washed twice with DMEM supplemented with 10% Serum Plus (J.R.H. Biosciences), then treated with 1 ml of the same media containing 25 µM chloroquine and synthetic Tat protein: 20.0 µg for plates transfected with phTG5 and 0.8 µg for plates transfected with pCD16. Cells were harvested 48 hours later and CAT assay was performed.[53] (Left) Promoter activity of phTG5 shows more than a 3-fold induction when HIV-1 Tat protein is present in the culture medium. (Right) Promoter activity of the HIV-1 LTR-CAT construct, pCD16 is induced nearly 80-fold when HIV-1 Tat is present in the culture medium.

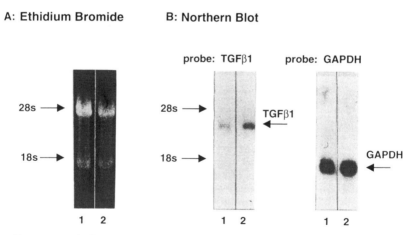

Figure 7. Expression of TGFβ-1 mRNA in transfected primary human fetal glial cells. 15 µg of pNL4-3 plasmid (lane 2) or nonspecific salmon sperm DNA (lane 1) were transfected into 5x10[5] primary human fetal glial cells by the calcium-phosphate precipitation procedure.[54] Total RNA was prepared by the hot phenol method,[55] and 15 µg of total RNA were electrophoresed in a 1.2% formaldehyde/agarose gel. The RNAs were transferred to Hybond-N nylon membrane (Amersham) and hybridized to |α32P| dCTP-labeled probes. Northern blot hybridizations were performed as described previously.[56] A. Ethidium bromide-stained formaldehyde/agarose gel demonstrating the integrity of the total RNAs. B. Nylon membrane probed with 1.0 kb fragment of a TGFβ-1 cDNA. C. Same nylon membrane reprobed with a 1.3-kb fragment of a GAPDH cDNA as a control for RNA loading.

Effect of Tat Protein on Expression of the Human Papovavirus, JCV, in Glial Cells

Progressive multifocal leukoencephalopathy (PML) is a rare human disease characterized by progressive demyelinating lesions in the brain secondary to viral infection and impaired cellular immunity.[57] JC virus, a ubiquitous human polyoma virus which replicates exclusively in glial cells, is the causative agent of this disease.[58] Although 70-80% of the adult population is seropositive

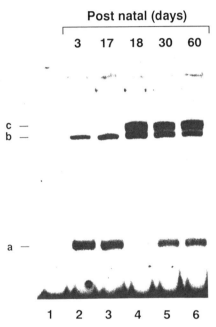

Figure 8. Interaction of upTAR with proteins from brain extracts. Binding activity of the upTAR probe to nuclear extracts derived from 2- to 3-day (lane 1), 7-day (lane 2), 18-day (lane 3), 30-day (lane 4), and adult (>60 day) (lane 5) mice was examined by band-shift assay. The positions of the a, b, and c complexes are shown on the left.

for JCV, the incidence of PML is very low. The cofactors responsible for activation of latent JCV and induction of PML are unknown, but this disease almost always occurs within the context of chronic immunosuppression. The incidence of PML among AIDS patients is approximately 4%, which is significantly higher than the incidence among individuals who are immunosuppressed by other diseases.[59] The surprisingly higher incidence of PML in AIDS patients than in other immunosuppressive disorders has suggested that the presence of HIV-1 in the brain may directly contribute to the pathogenesis of this disease.

Recently, we demonstrated that the HIV-1-encoded transregulatory protein, Tat, is a potent activator of JCV gene expression.[60] Tat greatly increases the rate of transcription from the JCV late promoter by a mechanism that is independent from and synergistic with the transactivation caused by the JCV regulatory protein, T-antigen.[61] The regulatory region of JCV contains two 98-bp tandem repeats that control cell-specific expression of viral early and late genes in glial cells. Of particular interest is the presence of a region with substantial sequence homology to the critical region of the HIV-1 TAR in the leader of the JCV late transcript.

Results from site-directed mutagenesis within the JCV TAR homologous sequence revealed that critical nucleotides required for the function of HIV-1 TAR that are conserved in the JCV TAR homolog play an important role in Tat activation of the JCV promoter.[62] In addition, *in vivo* competition experiments suggested that shared regulatory components mediate Tat activation of the JCV late and HIV LTR promoters. It should be emphasized that the JCV-derived TAR sequence behaves in the same way as HIV-1 TAR in response to two distinct Tat mutants, one of which has no ability to bind to HIV-1 TAR and the other which lacks transcriptional activity on the responsive promoter. These observations suggest that the TAR homolog of the JCV late promoter is responsive to HIV-1 Tat induction and thus may participate in the overall activation of the JCV promoter mediated by this transactivation.

In a separate set of experiments using deletion mutation analysis, a secondary region located upstream of the JCV late RNA start site, termed upstream target (upTAR) that positively responds to that activation in glial cells was identified. This region enriched in GA/GC confers Tat responsiveness to a heterologous promoter preferentially in glial cell lines. Using a gel mobility shift assay, we have demonstrated that at least three major complexes from glial cells, designated a, b, and c, interact with the upTAR sequences. An attractive possibility is the idea that the distribution of proteins participating in complex c are developmentally regulated during brain ontogeny (Fig. 8). Perhaps it should be mentioned that complex c was more abundant in glial cells than nonglial cells. These results suggest that complex c has a role in inducing transcriptional activity of the JCV late promoter by Tat. Experiments are underway to molecularly clone the gene encoding the protein associated with complex c in order to investigate the biological activity of these proteins in concert with the Tat protein in activating the JCV late promoter.

CONCLUSIONS

The observations presented in this chapter support the proposition that differential utilization of Tat proteins probably regulated by cellular factors, influences expression of HIV-1 and the heterologous promoters for host and other viruses. The presence of such cellular factors, or their level of activity, could be influenced by cell type or environmental stimuli. Perhaps Tat functions by directly or indirectly stabilizing the interaction of cellular transcription factors such as NF-kB, GC/GA-rich binding proteins, etc., to upstream promoter elements. Alternatively, Tat could play some role in regulating the activity of a promoter-bound transcription factor. The fact that in glial cells Tat activates HIV-1, JCV, and TGFβ-1 promoters independently of the TAR element may have implications for antiviral therapies that are aimed at Tat function or Tat/TAR interaction. The identity of cellular factors responsible for the TAR-independent regulation of eukaryotic promoters in glial cells and their mechanism of action are essential to understand the molecular pathogenesis of HIV-1-induced neurologic disorders in AIDS patients.

REFERENCES

1. R. Lechtenberg, and J.H. Sher. "AIDS in the Nervous System," Churchill Livingstone, New York.
2. B.A. Navia, E.S. Cho, C.K. Petito, and R.W. Price. The AIDS dementia complex: II. Neuropathology. *Ann. Neurol.* 19:525 (1986).
3. L.G. Epstein, L.R. Sharer, V.V. Joshi, M.M. Fojas, and M.R. Koenigsberger. Progressive encephalopathy in children with acquired immune deficiency syndrome. *Ann. Neurol.* 17:488 (1985).
4. J.L. Ho, P. Poldre, and D. McEniry. Acquired immunodeficiency syndrome with progressive multifocal leukoencephalopathy and monoclonal B-cell proliferation. *Ann. Intern. Med.* 100:693 (1984).
5. B.A. Navia, and R.W. Price. The acquired immunodeficiency syndrome dementia complex as the presenting or sole manifestation of human immunodeficiency virus infection. *Arch. Neurol.* 44:65 (1987).
6. R.W. Price, B.J. Brew, and M.K. Rosenblum. The AIDS dementia complex and HIV-1 brain infection: a pathologic model of virus-immune interaction. Research Publications: Association for Research in Nervous and Mental Disease 68:269 (1990).
7. R.W. Price, B. Brew, J. Sidtis, et al. The brain in AIDS: central nervous system HIV-1 infection and AIDS dementia complex. *Science* 239:586 (1988).
8. M.K.Rosenblum. Infection of the central nervous system by the human immunodeficiency virus type I. *Pathol. Ann.* 25:117 (1990).
9. J. Bedri, W. Weinstein, P. DiGregorio, and M.A. Verity. Progressive multifocal leukoencephalopathy in acquired immune deficiency syndrome. *N. Engl. J. Med.* 309:492 (1983).
10. J.R. Berger, L. Moskowitz, M. Fischer, and R.E. Kelly. The neurological complications of AIDS, frequently the initial manifestation. *Neurology* 34:134 (1984).
11. L.W. Blum, R.A. Chambers, R.J. Schwartzman, and L. Streletz. Progressive multifocal leukoencephalopathy in acquired immune deficiency syndrome. *Arch. Neurol.* 42:137 (1985).
12. B.R. Brook, and D.L. Walker. Progressive multifocal leukoencephalopathy. *Neurol. Clin.* 2:299 (1984).
13. J.D. England, Y. Hsu, P. Garen, J. Goust, and P. Biggs. Progressive multifocal leukoencephalopathy with the acquired immune deficiency syndrome. *South,. Med. J.* 77:1041 (1984).
14. L.B. Krupp, H. Lipton, M. Swerdlow, N. Leeds, and J. Liena. Progressive multifocal leukoencephalopathy: clinical and radiographic features. *Ann. Neurol.* 17:344 (1985).
15. J.R. Miller, R. Barrett, C. Britton, et al. Progressive multifocal leukoencephalopathy in a male homosexual with T-cell immune deficiency. *N. Engl. J. Med.* 307:1436 (1982).
16. W.D. Snider, D.M. Simpson, S. Neilson, et al. Neurological complications of acquired immune deficiency syndrome: analysis of 50 patients. *Ann. Neurol.* 14:403 (1983).
17. J.D. Speelman, J. ter Schegget, G. Bots, J. Stam, and B. Verbeeten. Progressive multifocal leukoencephalopathy in a case of acquired immune deficiency syndrome. *Clin. Neurol. Neurosurg.* 87:27 (1985).
18. F. Gyorkey, J.L. Melnick, and P.Gyorkey. Human immunodeficiency virus in brain biopsies of patients with AIDS and progressive encephalopathy. *J. Infect. Dis.* 155:870 (1987).
19. D.D. Ho, T.R. Rota, R.T. Schooley, et al. Isolation of HTLV-III from cerebrospinal fluid and tissues of patients with neurologic syndromes related to the acquired immunodeficiency syndrome. *N.Engl. J. Med.* 313:1493 (1985).
20. S. Koenig, H.E. Gendelman, J.M. Orenstein, et al. Detection of AIDS virus in macrophages in brain tissue from AIDS patients with encephalopathy. *Science* 233:1089 (1986).
21. J.A. Levy, J. Shimabukuro, H. Hollander, J. Mills, and L. Kaminsky.

Isolation of AIDS-associated retroviruses from cerebrospinal fluid and brain of patients with neurological symptoms. *Lancet* 2:586 (1985).

22. S. Pang, Y. Koyanagi, S. Miles, et al. High levels of unintegrated HIV-1 DNA in brain tissue of AIDS dementia patients. *Nature* 343:85 (1990).

23. S. Dewhurst, K. Sakai, J. Bresser, et al. Persistent productive infection of human glial cells by human immunodeficiency virus (HIV) and by infectious molecular clones of HIV. *J. Virol.* 61:3774 (1987).

24. C. Tornatore, A. Nath, K. Amemiya, and E.O. Major. Persistent human immunodeficiency virus type 1 infection in human fetal glial cells reactivated by T-cell factor(s) or by the cytokines tumor necrosis factor alpha and interleukin-1 beta. *J. Virol.* 65:6094 (1991).

25. J. Michaels, L.R. Sharer, and L.G. Epstein. Human immunodeficiency virus type 1 (HIV-1) infection of the nervous system: a review. *Immunodeficiency Rev.* 1:71 (1988).

26. R.H. Rhodes, J.M. Ward, D.L. Walker, and A.A. Ross. Progressive multifocal leukoencephalopathy and retroviral encephalitis in acquired immunodeficiency syndrome. *Arch. Path. Lab. Med.* 112:1207 (1988).

27. J.M. Ward, T.J. O'Leary, G.B. Baskin, et al. Immunohistochemical localization of human and simian immunodeficiency viral antigens in fixed tissue sections. *Am. J. Path.* 127:199 (1987).

28. C.A. Wiley, R.D. Schrier, J.A. Nelson, P.W. Lampert, and M.B. Oldstone. Cellular localization of human immunodeficiency virus infection within the brains of acquired immune deficiency syndrome patients. *Proc. Natl. Acad. Sci.* 83:7089 (1986).

29. M.B. Peterlin, and P. Luciw. Molecular biology of AIDS. *AIDS* 2:S29 (1988).

30. B.R. Cullen. The HIV-1 Tat protein: an RNA sequence-specific processivity factor? *Cell* 63:655 (1990).

31. B.R. Cullen, and W.C. Greene. Regulatory pathways governing HIV-1 replication. *Cell* 58:423 (1989).

32. K.A. Jones, J.T. Kadonga, P.A. Luciw, and R. Tijan. Activation of the AIDS retrovirus promoter by the cellular transcription factor, Sp1. *Science* 232:755 (1986).

33. K. Kawakami, C. Scheidereit, and R.G. Roeder. Identification and purification of a human immunoglobulin-enhancer-binding protein (NF-kappa B) that activates transcription from a human immunodeficiency virus type 1 promoter *in vitro*. *Proc. Natl. Acad. Sci. USA* 85:4700 (1988).

34. G. Nabel, and D. Baltimore. An inducible transcription factor activates expression of human immunodeficiency virus in T-cells. *Nature* 326:711 (1987).

35. P.A. Bauerle. The inducible transcription activator NFkB: regulation by distinct protein subunits. *Biochim. Biophys. Acta* 1072:63 (1991).

36. J. Rappaport, S.-J. Lee, K. Khalili, and F. Wong-Staal. The acidic amino-terminal region of the HIV-1 Tat protein constitutes an essential activating domain,. *New Biol.* 1:101 (1989).

37. M.B. Feinberg, D. Baltimore, and A.D. Frankel. The role of Tat in the human immunodeficiency virus life cycle indicates a primary effect on transcriptional elongation. *Proc. Natl. Acad. Sci. USA* 88:4045 (1991).

38. M.F. Laspia, A.P. Rice, and M.B. Mathews. Synergy between HIV-1 Tat and adenovirus E1A is principally due to stabilization of transcriptional elongation. *Genes Dev.* 4:2397 (1990).

39. M.F. Laspia, A.P. Rice, and M.B. Mathews. HIV-1 Tat protein increases transcriptional initiation and stabilizes elongation. *Cell* 59:283 (1989).

40. S. Calnan, S. Biancalani, D. Hudson, and A.D. Frankel. Analysis of arginine-rich peptides from the HIV Tat protein reveals unusual features of RNA-protein recognition. *Genes Dev.* 5:201 (1991).

41. B.J. Calnan, B.Tidor, S. Biancalana, D. Hudson, and A.D. Frankel. Arginine-mediated RNA recognition: the ariginine fork. *Science* 252:1167 (1991).

42. S. Feng, and E.C. Holland. HIV-1 Tat transactivation requires the loop sequence within TAR. *Nature* 334:165 (1988).

43. J.A. Garcia, D. Harrich, E. Soultanakis, et al. Human immunodeficiency

virus type 1 LTR TATA and TAR region sequences required for transcriptional regulation. *EMBO J.* 8:765 (1989).

44. C.A. Rosen, J.G. Sodrowski, and W.A. Haseltine. The location of cis-activating regulatory sequences in the human T cell lymphotropic virus type III (HIV-III/LAV) long terminal repeat. *Cell* 41:813 (1985).

45. R. Marciniak. Identification and characterization of a HeLa nuclear protein that specifically binds to the trans-activation-response (TAR) element of human immunodeficiency virus. *Proc. Natl. Acad. Sci. USA* 87:3624 (1990).

46. L. Buonaguro, G. Barillari, H.K. Chang, et al. Effect of the human immunodeficiency virus type 1 tat protein on the expression of inflammatory cytokines. *J. Virol.* 66:7159 (1992).

47. K.J. Sastry, R.H.R. Reddy, R. Pandita, K. Totpal, and B.B. Aggarwal. HIV-1 tat gene induces tumor necrosis factor-β (lymphotoxin) in a human B-lymphoblastoid cell line. *J. Cell Chem.* 265:20091 (1990).

48. J.P Taylor, C. Cupp, A.Diaz, et al. Activation of expression of genes coding for extracellular matrix proteins in tat-producing glioblastoma cells. *Proc. Natl. Acad.Sci. USA* 89:9617 (1992).

49. R.P. Viscidi, K. Mayur, H.M. Lederman, and A.D. Frankel. Inhibition of antigen-induced lymphocyte proliferation by Tat protein from HIV-1. *Science* 246:1606 (1989).

50. S.M. Wahl, J.B.Allen, N. McCartney-Francis, et al. Macrophage- and astrocyte-derived transforming growth factor β as a mediator of central nervous system dysfunction in acquired immunodeficiency syndrome. *J. Exp. Med.* 173:981 (1991).

51. C. Cupp, J.P. Taylor, K. Khalili, and S. Amini. Evidence of stimulation of the transforming growth factor β-1 promoter by HIV-1 Tat in cells derived from CNS. *Oncogene* 8:2231 (1993).

52. A. Adachi, H. Gendelman, S. Koenig, et al. Production of acquired immunodeficiency syndrome-associated retrovirus in human and nonhuman cells transfected with an infectious molecular clone. *J. Virol.* 59:284 (1986).

53. C.M. Gorman, L.F. Moffat, and B.H., Howard. Recombinant genomes which express chloramphenicol acetyl transferase in mammalian cells. *Mol. Cell. Biol.* 2:1044 (1982).

54. F.L.Graham, and A.J. van der Eb. A new technique for the assay of infectivity of human adenovirus 5 DNA. *Virology* 52:456 (1973).

55. C. Queen, and D. Baltimore. Immunoglobulin gene transcription is activated by downstream sequence elements. *Cell* 33:586 (1988).

56. F. Ausubel, R. Brent, R.E. Kingston, et al. "Current Protocols in Molecular Biology," John Wiley & Sons, Inc., New York (1989).

57. E.O. Major, K. Amemiya, C.S. Tornatore, S.A. Houff, and J.R. Berger. Pathogenesis and molecular biology of progressive multifocal leukoencephalopathy, the JC virus-induced demyelinating disease of the human brain. *Clin. Microbiol. Rev.* 5:49 (1992).

58. G.M. ZuRhein. Polyoma-like virions in a human demyelinating disease. *Acta Neuropathol. (Berl.)* 8:57 (1967).

59. C.A. Wiley, M. Grafe, C. Kennedy, and J.A. Nelson. Human immunodeficiency virus (HIV) and JC virus in acquired immune deficiency syndrome (AIDS) patients with progressive multifocal leukoencephalopathy. *Acta Neuropathol.* 76:338 (1988).

60. H. Tada, J. Rappaport, M. Lashgari, et al. Transactivation of the JC virus late promoter by the Tat protein of type 1 human immunodeficiency virus in glial cells. *Proc. Natl. Acad. Sci. USA* 87:3479 (1990).

61. M. Chowdhury, J.P. Taylor, H. Tada, et al. Regulation of the human neurotropic virus promoter by JCV-T antigen and HIV-1 Tat protein. *Oncogene* 5:1737 (1970).

62. M. Chowdhury, J.P. Taylor, C.-F. Chang, J. Rappaport, and K. Khalili. Evidence that a sequence similar to TAR is important for induction of the JC virus late promoter by human immunodeficiency virus type 1 Tat. *J. Virol.* 66:7355 (1992).

TUMOR NECROSIS FACTOR ALPHA DERIVED FROM HUMAN MICROGLIA ENHANCES HIV-1 REPLICATION AND IS TOXIC FOR RAT OLIGODENDROCYTES IN VITRO

Susan G. Wilt,[1] Jia Min Zhou,[1] Steve Wesselingh,[2]
Conrad V. Kufta,[3] and Monique Dubois-Dalcq[1]

[1]Laboratory of Viral and Molecular Pathogenesis
[3]Surgical Neurology Branch
National Institute of Neurological Disorders and Stroke
National Institutes of Health
Bethesda, Maryland 20892

[2]Department of Microbiology and Infectious Diseases
Flinders Medical Center
Adelaide, Australia

SUMMARY

In the brain of HIV-1-infected patients, some microglial cells are infected while many others are activated and express tumor necrosis factor alpha (TNF-α).[1] The abundance of TNF-α message in these brains correlates with the severity of clinical dementia.[2] To investigate the role of TNF-α in HIV-1 infection of the brain, we purified human microglial cells from adult brain and studied whether HIV-1 replication is influenced by neutralizing TNF-α antibodies and whether microglia secrete cytotoxic factor(s) for rat oligodendrocytes. In microglia cultures infected with HIV-1 JrFl, a neurotropic strain,[3] addition of TNF-α antibodies (TNF AB) to the medium delayed p24 expression and syncytium formation for several days, suggesting that microglia-derived TNF-α enhances viral replication. Conditioned medium (CM) of microglia cultures or live microglia were then added to rat oligodendrocytes (RO), and survival was assayed using staining with MTT, a vital dye detecting mitochondrial activity. Addition of CM from human microglia caused up to 30% RO death. A similar ratio of RO death was observed with maximal doses of recombinant human TNF-α (rhTNF) and the CM cytotoxic effect for RO was neutralized by TNF AB. These studies demonstrate a direct involvement of TNF-α derived from activated human microglia in oligodendrocyte damage and death *in vitro*. Thus, TNF-α specific inhibitors could possibly slow down viral replication and attenuate cytotoxicity for oligodendrocytes in HIV-1 encephalopathy.

Technical Advances in AIDS Research in the Human Nervous System
Edited by E.O. Major and J.A. Levy, Plenum Press, New York, 1995

INTRODUCTION

The most common neurologic complication of AIDS is the AIDS cognitive motor complex (also called AIDS dementia complex or ADC) which is characterized by cognitive, behavioral, and motor dysfunction (reviewed in refs. 4, 5). It has been classified as a 'subcortical dementia' because such cognitive dysfunction is also found in other degenerative diseases of the central nervous system (CNS) such as Huntington's and Parkinson's diseases.[4] In HIV-1-infected patients, inhibition of viral replication by zidovudine (AZT) significantly reduces the frequency of ADC. Brain atrophy and white matter abnormalities can be detected in ADC patients using computed tomographic (CT) scanning and magnetic resonance imaging (MRI). In addition, diffuse white matter pallor, reactive astrogliosis, and neuronal loss have been found at autopsy.[4,6]

The HIV-1-infected brain often harbors scattered microglial cells and/or macrophages expressing HIV-1 message and proteins; these cells are frequently located in the subcortical white matter, basal ganglia, and brainstem.[7] Intriguingly, these microglial cells are often found in association with areas of demyelination and vacuolation, especially in the AIDS-associated myelopathy.[8] Giant cells, probably resulting from the fusion of infected microglia or macrophages, as well as microglial nodules are also common features associated with dementia.[4,6] Neurons and oligodendrocytes appear to very rarely express either viral messages or proteins although infected microglial cells are seen in their vicinity.[7] Since cells of the monocyte/macrophage (MM) lineage, such as microglia, are the major population of productively HIV-1-infected cells in the adult brain, alteration of other cell types (namely, oligodendroglia, astrocytes and neurons) may result from microglia dysfunction. To understand the mechanism of the neuropathogenesis of AIDS dementia and the origin of the demyelinating lesions seen in some AIDS patients, we are using *in vitro* models in which human microglia are purified and then cocultured with rat oligodendrocytes.

PRIMARY CULTURES OF HUMAN BRAIN AS AN *IN VITRO* MODEL TO STUDY HIV-1 INFECTION OF THE CNS

Primary glial cell cultures established from adult human brain provide a suitable *in vitro* system to explore the mechanisms of HIV-1 neuropathogenesis. Tissue obtained from temporal lobe biopsies in patients with intractable epilepsy can be dissociated and cultured, yielding mature differentiated glial types, but not neurons.[5,9] Use of a Percoll gradient allows isolation of viable glial cells, with minimal contamination of meningeal or fibroblastic cells (modified from ref. 10; Dulbecco's modified Eagle's medium supplemented with 10% fetal calf serum was substituted for PBS in all but the Percoll centrifugation). Mixed glial cell cultures containing 50-70% microglial cells and 20-40% astrocytes have been used in experiments investigating entry and replication of HIV-1 in different CNS cells.[9] In addition, microglial cells can be purified[10] to homogeneity (>95% positive for the low-density lipoprotein receptor) and maintained for weeks *in vitro* when treated with growth factors enhancing survival of cells of the MM lineage[9] (Fig. 1).

Total RNA isolated from microglia cultures was analyzed by reverse transcription with polymerase chain reaction amplification (RT-PCR) using sets of specific primers to detect message for TNF-α, interleukin (IL)-1, IL-6, transforming growth factor-beta (TGF-β) and leukemia inhibitory factor (LIF).[11] Cultured human microglia expressed mRNAs for TNF-α, IL-1 and IL-6, but not TGF-β or LIF (data not shown).[12] Furthermore, TNF-α protein was detected in microglial cell extracts by Western and immunoprecipitation analysis, and in microglia culture supernatants by ELISA.[12] These initial studies demonstrated that human brain-derived microglia are activated *in vitro* and synthesize TNF-α.

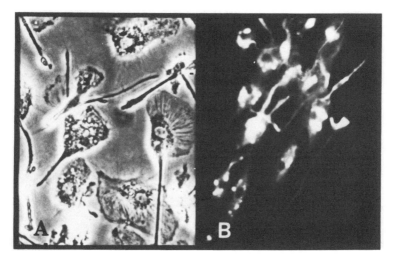

Figure 1. Micrograph of purified microglial cells in phase contrast (A) and after immunostaining for the low-density lipoprotein receptor (B). Magnification: 125X (A) and 135X (B).

Autocrine and/or Paracrine Enhancement of HIV-1 Replication by Microglia-Derived TNF-α

Human brain-derived microglia can be productively infected by MM tropic HIV-1 strains, such as Jr-Fl, which enters the cells through the CD4 receptor.[3,13,14] No evidence of productive or latent infection was observed in mature human astrocytes or oligodendrocytes *in vitro*.[14] The majority of primary isolates derived from the blood and cerebrospinal fluid (CSF) of patients at all stages of AIDS also have the ability to productively infect human brain microglia *in vitro*.[15]

Since microglial cells appear to be largely derived from bone marrow precursors and are members of the MM lineage, they may share with MM similar mechanisms of cytokine regulation. In MM, TNF-α triggers up-regulation of HIV-1 expression through activation of the transcription factor NF-kB.[16] Since microglia produce TNF-α *in vitro*, the role of TNF-α in regulating HIV-1 Jr-FL expression in microglial cells was examined in both mixed glial cultures and purified microglial cultures. We predicted that neutralizing TNF-α antibodies (AB) would inhibit the binding of TNF-α, secreted into the medium, to microglial TNF-α receptors. We therefore tested whether such antibodies added either prior to, concurrently or after viral adsorption, and continuously thereafter for 3 weeks, could have an effect on viral replication. Viral production was assayed by the release of HIV-1 p24 core antigen into the supernatant. In all experimental conditions with TNF-α AB, p24 antigen release was found to be delayed for 7-10 days compared to untreated HIV-1-infected dishes (Fig. 2).

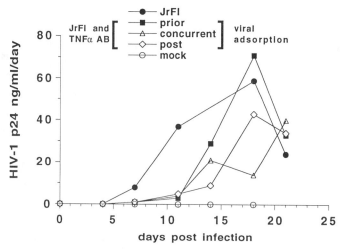

Figure 2. Infection of purified microglia cultures with the HIV-1 neurotropic strain JR-Fl in the presence or absence of TNF-α antibodies (neutralizing 10,000 U/ml rhTNF-α). HIV-1 p24 antigen production is inhibited for the first 11 days in the presence of TNF-α AB added to the medium prior to, concurrently, or after viral inoculation and replenished every 3 days for 3 weeks. Viral inoculum was 6 ng p24/35 mm dish containing about 80,000 microglial cells; adsorption was for 6 hours in DMEM with 5% GCT and 1% FBS at 37°C as previously described.[13] Production of p24 antigen in the supernatant (collected from triplicate dishes every 3-4 days) was followed for 21 days postinfection.

Moreover, syncytium formation characteristic of progressive HIV-1 infection was significantly reduced in the presence of TNF-α AB for a similar period of time (Fig. 3, panel D; compare with B and C). Addition of control antibody to CD14, a protein present on microglial cell surfaces, did not affect syncytium formation by Jr-FL (Fig. 3, panel C). The expression of HIV-1 p17 *gag* protein, as analyzed by immunofluorescence, was also found to be much decreased in TNF-α AB-treated cultures during the first 2 weeks. However, production of HIV-1 proteins and the number of syncytia increased during the third week postinfection, suggesting that anti-TNF-α AB interfere with the early events of TNF-α on viral replication rather than viral entry but that this block is overcome by the virus with time. In subsequent experiments described elsewhere[12] where microglia cultures were inoculated with different amounts of virus and treated with different TNF-α inhibitors, viral production was consistently inhibited for the first 10-13 days post-infection. The most potent inhibition was observed with pentoxifylline (PTX), an inhibitor of TNF-α message and protein synthesis,[17] as p24 production and syncytium formation (Fig. 3, panel E) were virtually abolished for 21 days post viral inoculation.[12]

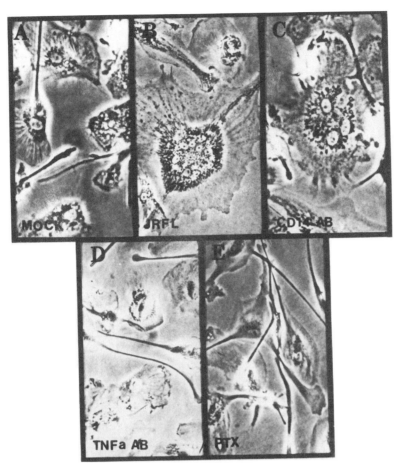

Figure 3. Syncytium formation in cultures of purified microglia infected with HIV-1 Jr-Fl in the presence and absence of TNF-α inhibitors. Cultures were infected as described in Fig. 2 and photographed at 9 days post-infection in phase microscopy. In (A), uninfected microglia. In (B), typical multinucleated cells are detected in HIV-1 Jr-Fl-infected cultures without any antibodies and in the presence of CD14 AB (C), while no multinucleated cells are seen in infected microglia cultures treated with neutralizing TNF AB (D) or PTX at 30 µg/ml (E). Magnification 125X.

Cytotoxicity of Microglia-Derived TNF-α for Rat Oligodendroglia

It has been proposed that production of toxic factors, such as nitric oxide (NO), quinolinic acid, IL-1 or TNF-α by microglia may damage other glial cell types in HIV-1 encephalitis.[4] In brain tissue from patients with ADC, a high proportion of microglia, infected or not, appeared activated and expressed increased levels of TNF-α message; moreover, this increase in TNF-α transcripts in ADC brain tissue has been directly correlated with severity of dementia.[1,2]

TNF-α has been shown to have direct cytotoxicity for primary rat oligodendrocytes in culture.[18-21] To determine whether TNF-α produced by microglia can mediate killing of oligodendrocytes, we used a cytotoxicity assay based upon 3-[4,5-dimethylthiazol-2-yl]-2,5-diphenyltetrazolium bromide (MTT) staining of live cells[22] and a rat oligodendrocyte (RO) cell line, the CG4,[23] as the target. Such an RO cell line can be expanded for more than 40 passages in neuroblastoma-conditioned medium, while retaining the ability to differentiate into mature oligodendrocytes, developing highly arborized processes and expressing galactocerebroside and myelin proteins when fed with defined medium without growth factors.[23] The effects of recombinant human TNF-α (rhTNF) on differentiated CG4 (RO) morphology and survival was compared to those of human microglia-conditioned medium (CM) and of addition of live human microglial cells.

We first analyzed the effects of rhTNF (Genzyme Corp., Boston, MA) on the survival of RO after 24 or 72 hours using the MTT assay (Figs. 4 and 5). A total of 5-6 random fields in each of triplicate wells per condition were photographed after MTT staining. Photographs of representative fields used for quantitation are shown in Figure 4. The ratio of dead (unstained or with less than 3 spots of mitochondrial staining) to total cells in each condition was counted blindly on the photographs and evaluated statistically by analysis of variance using the Scheffe's S test for significance level (SuperANOVA, Abacus Concepts Inc., Berkeley, CA).

When a range of 200-1,600 U/ml of rhTNF-α (0.14 - 2.4 nM) was applied to RO for 24 hours, a dose-dependent cytotoxicity was observed with a maximum of 35% dead RO as described in previous studies (Fig. 5).[18,19] In addition to cell death, a fraction of RO lost their highly arborized processes, while many surviving cells stained poorly with MTT, compared with control RO cultures, suggesting a decreased mitochondrial activity (Fig. 4, panel B). The observed cytotoxicity and morphological changes were entirely blocked by addition of TNF AB to the medium (Fig. 5, hatched bars and Fig. 4, panel C). Thus, rhTNF may directly induce killing of RO, presumably following binding to TNF-α surface receptor. Even in the absence of cell death, the mere disruption of oligodendrocyte processes due to TNF-α exposure could cause demyelination *in vivo*. These studies confirm that human TNF-α can directly damage RO.

The levels of TNF-α in the brain parenchyma during manifestation of AIDS dementia are not known. Measurements of TNF-α in the CSF indicate elevated levels, ranging from 50-100 pg/ml in AIDS patients, compared to less than 10 pg/ml observed in normal patients.[24,25] Therefore, we tested the effect of lower TNF-α concentrations (5-160 U/ml or 0.25 -8.0 ng/ml [0.006 - 0.2 nM]) for longer exposure times (72 hours). Again, approximately 25% RO were lost after addition of 160 U/ml rhTNF while others showed process disruption and this effect was fully neutralized by TNF AB (Fig. 5). The implication of these observations is that chronic exposure to moderately elevated TNF-α levels *in vivo* may contribute to oligodendrocyte damage and/or death of a significant number of oligodendrocytes. It is also possible that local concentrations of TNF-α released by or bound to microglia in close proximity to oligodendrocytes may approach, even briefly, the concentrations used *in vitro*.

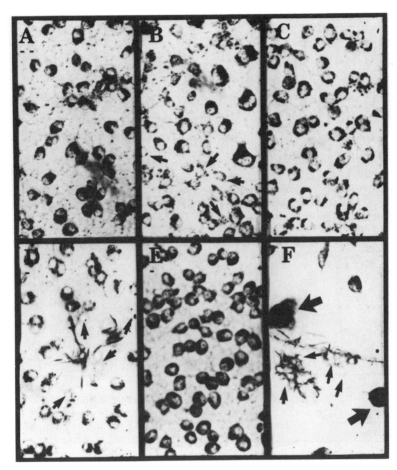

Figure 4. Brightfield photomicrographs of CG4 cultures treated with rhTNF, microglia CM, or live microglial cells in the presence or absence of neutralizing antibody for 24 hours and stained with MTT. Shown are representative photographs of random fields which were counted blindly to quantitate the cytotoxicity. Control cultures showing strong cytoplasmic staining in most cells (A); in cultures treated with 400 U/ml rhTNF (B) or microglia CM (arrows in D), unstained or weakly stained cells are seen at arrows. In contrast, in the presence of TNF AB and either 400 U of TNF-α/ml (C) or CM (E), cells are strongly stained as controls (A). In cocultures with 2x10⁴ microglia (large arrows on F) per 10⁴ RO, many fewer CG4 cells are seen, and those remaining are weakly stained and in clusters (F, small arrows). Magnification in 125X.

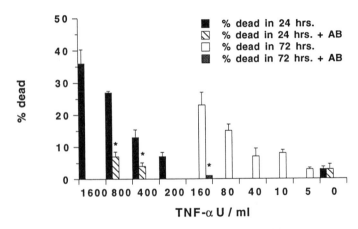

Figure 5. Cytotoxicity of recombinant human TNF-α for CF4 rat oligodendrocytes is dose-dependent. CG4 cells were plated in 24-well dishes (10,000 cells/well), differentiated as described,[22] and treated with increasing concentrations of rhTNF (0-1,600 U/ml for 24 hours or 0-160 U/ml for 72 hours). Parallel triplicate wells were treated with neutralizing TNF AB in some of the conditions. The cultures were stained with MTT,[21] and assayed as described in Fig. 4. The mean of 2 experiments (6 wells/condition) is presented with the standard error indicated. Asterisks indicate p = <0.01 determined by analysis of variance, Scheffe's S test at the 0.01 confidence level. The 24-hour dose response was repeated 5 times.

We then examined the cytotoxic effects, in the presence or absence of TNF-α inhibitors, of human microglia CM and live microglia on rat oligodendrocytes (RO) using a similar assay (Fig. 6). Addition of CM from microglia cultures caused a 25% cytotoxicity for RO, which was neutralized by TNF AB. The morphological changes and decreased MTT staining in the presence of CM were reversed in great part by addition of TNF AB (Fig. 4, panels D and E). Treatment of microglia cultures with lipopolysaccharide (LPS) prior to CM collection slightly increased the cytotoxicity for RO to over 30% cell death. Again, the cytotoxic effect in CM from LPS-treated microglia was largely neutralized by TNF AB, suggesting that the major toxin produced by microglia is TNF-α. Supporting this interpretation is the significant reduction (p = 0.005) in cytotoxicity when CM collected from microglia cultures was treated for 24 hours with PTX (Fig. 6). [Since the CM was collected 6 hours after withdrawal of PTX from the serum-free medium, the microglia may have resumed TNF-α production and secretion, accounting for the slight cytotoxic effect (15%) for RO observed with this CM.] Finally, when live human microglia were added to RO (at a ratio ranging from 0.5 to 2 microglial cells to 1 RO), RO death of up to 35% of the cells was observed and found to be proportional to the number of microglial cells added (Fig. 6). The highest numbers of dead RO were often observed in contact with or near clusters of human microglia (Fig. 4, panel F). The bulk of this cytotoxic effect was neutralizable by TNF AB (Fig. 6).

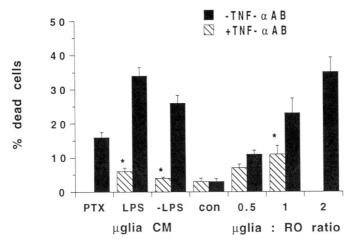

Figure 6. Microglial conditioned medium or live microglia is cytotoxic for differentiated CG4 cells. Cytotoxicity was quantitated as described in Figs. 4 and 5. Purified microglial cultures were first maintained in 5% giant cell supernatant and 5% fetal calf serum DMEM with or without either lipopolysaccharide (LPS) or PTX for 24 hours, then washed and refed with serum-free DMEM to collect conditioned medium (CM) after 6 hours. CM was centrifuged for 15 minutes at 2,000 rpm at 10°C, and stored at -70°C until use. CM was diluted 1:1 with 2X differentiation medium[22] and added to CG4 cultures for 24 hours. In experiments shown on the right, purified human microglial cells were added to differentiated RO at a ratio of microglia to RO of 0.5, 1 and 2. Cocultures were incubated in CG4 differentiation medium for 24 hours just as were control cultures. The graph shows the mean of 2 experiments (6 wells per condition) with bars corresponding to standard error or the mean. Asterisks indicate p<0.001 determined by analysis of variance, Scheffe's S test at the 0.01 confidence level.

These experiments have now been extended to human oligodendrocytes (HO).[12] Such cells can indeed be purified from adult human brain,[10] regenerate their processes *in vitro* in the presence of specific growth factors, and express differentiation markers such as galactocerebroside.[26] As no human oligodendrocyte cell line with differentiation capability has been described, one is entirely dependent upon available clinical specimens to perform such studies. The effects of rhTNF (500 to 2,000 U/ml) on the network of processes formed by purified HO (>98% positive for galactocerebroside) are shown in Fig. 7. HO demonstrated a dramatic retraction of arborized processes after 24 hours of TNF-α treatment as recently described.[27] Also noted was a decrease in the number of HO attached to the dish after exposure to TNF-α, presumably because HO death caused the cells to detach. These results differ from those of McLarnon et al.[27] probably because of differences in culture conditions and cytotoxicity assays. Since TNF-α produced by activated human microglia may adversely affect human oligodendrocyte function and survival in AIDS brain, we have recently studied the effects of microglia CM and live microglia, in the presence and absence of TNF-α inhibitors, on HO survival and morphology and have confirmed the results described here with the RO cell line.[12]

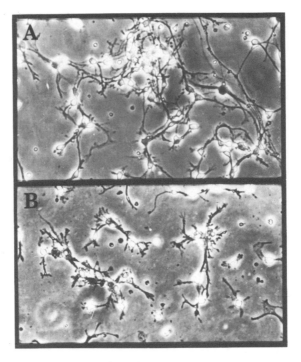

Figure 7. Phase contrast micrograph of purified human oligodendrocyte cultures grown for 12 days and exposed to 2,000 U/ml rhTNF-α for 24 hours (B). Oligodendrocytes often show retracted processes while, in the presence of neutralizing TNF AB, HO maintain their normal morphology (A). Magnification is 60X.

CONCLUSIONS

We have used *in vitro* systems derived from adult human brain as models to investigate cellular interactions occurring in HIV-1 infection of the CNS. In one model, human microglia were purified from adult human brain and infection with HIV-1 was studied in the presence of TNF AB. In the other model, human microglia or CM was added to RO to evaluate the role of microglia-derived TNF-α in oligodendrocyte alterations and death.

The results described suggest two independent roles for microglia-derived TNF-α in the neuropathogenesis of AIDS. First, an autocrine or paracrine enhancement of HIV-1 replication, especially during the early phase of microglial infection *in vitro*, may facilitate HIV-1 replication in the brain parenchyma. Slow replication of HIV-1 in infected but nonactivated microglia may occur until widespread activation of microglia is triggered by other factors, such as HIV-1 proteins, cytokines released by infiltrating leukocytes, or other neurologic injury. Overproduction of TNF-α could then enhance viral replication in the brain parenchyma by activating the NF-kB pathway[28] and possibly trigger progression to dementia.

Secondly, human microglia-derived TNF-α may be directly cytotoxic for oligodendrocytes as is observed with rhTNF. As activated microglia expressing TNF-α protein can be found in the white matter of ADC patients,[1] this cytokine may act *in vivo* in its membrane-bound form[20] and cause mild to severe dysfunction of the CNS myelin-forming cells. Future experiments in both rat and human cells should allow elucidation of the molecular events involved in TNF-α-mediated interactions between microglia and oligodendrocytes and should help design ways to interfere with the putative deleterious effects of this cytokine in ADC brain.

ACKNOWLEDGEMENTS

We thank J.C. Louis for providing the CG4 cell line, Ray Rusten for specimen dissection and excellent photographic work, G.D. Lange for invaluable assitance with statistical analysis, and Heather Patton for technical assistance with experiments. Additionally, we thank Claire Gibson for assistance with the manuscript.

REFERENCES

1. W.R. Tyor, J.C. Glass, J.W.Griffin, et al. Cytokine expression in the brain during AIDS. *Ann. Neurol.* 31:349 (1992).
2. S.L. Wesselingh, C. Power, J.D. Glass, et al. Intracerebral cytokine messenger RNA expression in acquired immunodeficiency syndrome dementia. *Ann. Neurol.* 33:576 (1993).
3. Y. Koyanagi, S. Miles, R.T. Mitsuyasu, et al. Dual infection of the central nervous system by AIDS viruses with distinct cellular tropisms. *Science* 236:819 (1987).
4. C. Spencer and R.W. Price. Human immunodeficiency virus and the central nervous system. *Annu. Rev. Microbiol.* 46:655 (1992).
5. M. Dubois-Dalcq, C. Jordan, W.B. Kelly, and B.A. Watkins. Understanding HIV-1 infection of the brain: a challenge for neurobiologists. *AIDS* 4 (suppl. 1):567 (1990).
6. J.D. Glass, S.L. Wesselingh, O.A. Selnes, and J.C. McArthur. Clinical-neuropathologic correlation in HIV-associated dementia. *Neurology* 43:2230 (1993).
7. R. Vazeux, M.C. Cumont, and L. Montagnier. HIV replication in the CNS of AIDS patients, *in*: "Modern Pathology of AIDS and Other Retroviral Infections," P. Racz, A.T. Haase, and J.C. Gluckman, eds., Karger, Basel (1990).
8. B. Weiser, N. Peress, D. LaNeve, et al. HIV-1 expression in the CNS correlates directly with the extent of disease. *Proc. Natl. Acad. Sci., USA* 87:3997 (1990).
9. B.A. Watkins, H.H. Dorn, W.B. Kelly, et al. Specific tropism of HIV-1 for microglial cells in primary human brain cultures. *Science* 249:549 (1990).
10. V.W. Yong and J.P. Antel. Culture of glial cells from human brain biopsies, *in*: "Protocol for Neural Cell Culture," S. Fedoroff and A. Richardson, eds., Humana Press (1992).
11. S.L. Wesselingh, N.M. Gough, J.J. Finlay-Jones, and P.J. McDonald. Detection of cytokine mRNA in astrocyte cultures using the polymerase chain reaction. *Lymphokine Res.* 9:177 (1990).
12. S.G. Wilt, E. Milward, J. Zhou, et al. HIV-1 replication in human microglia and killing of oligodendrocyte killing reduced by TNF alpha inhibitors. Submitted.

13. C.A. Jordan, B.A. Watkins, C. Kufta, and M. Dubois-Dalcq. Infection of brain microglial cells by HIV-1 is CD4 dependent. *J. Virol.* 65:736 (1991).
14. N.E. Sharpless, W.A. O'Brien, E. Verdin, et al. Human immunodeficiency virus type 1 tropism for brain microglial cells is determined by a region of the *env* glycoprotein that also controls macrophage tropism. *J. Virol.* 66:2588 (1992).
15. F.C. Chiodi, S.G. Wilt, M. O'Connor, and M. Dubois-Dalcq. Tropism for microglial cells is a common property of HIV-1 variants. Submitted.
16. G. Poli, A. Kinter, J.S. Justement, et al. Tumor necrosis factor alpha functions in an autocrine manner in the induction of human immuno-deficiency virus expression. *Proc. Natl. Acad. Sci. USA* 87:782 (1990).
17. C.C. Chao, H. Shuxian, K. Close, et al. Cytokine release from microglia: differential inhibition by pentoxifylline and dexamethasone. *J. Infect. Dis.* 166:847 (1992).
18. D.S. Robbins, D.S. Shirazi, B.E. Drysdale, et al. Production of cytotoxic factor for oligodendrocytes by stimulated astrocytes. *J. Immunol.* 139:2593 (1987).
19. K.W. Selmaj and C.S. Raine. Tumor necrosis factor mediates myelin and oligodendrocyte damage *in vitro*. *Ann. Neurol.* 23:339 (1988).
20. J.P. Zaijeck, M. Wing, N.J. Scolding, and D.A.S. Compston. Interactions between oligodendrocytes and microglia: A major role for complement and tumor necrosis factor in oligodendrocyte adherence and killing. *Brain* 115:1611 (1992).
21. J.C. Louis, E. Magal, S. Takayama, and S. Varon. CNTF protection of oligodendrocytes against natural tumor necrosis factor-α induced death. *Science* 259:689 (1993).
22. B.A. Barres, I.K. Hart, H.S.R. Coles, et al. Cell death and control of cell survival in the oligodendrocyte lineage. *Cell* 70:31 (1992).
23. J.C. Louis, E. Magal, D. Muir, M. Manthorpe, and S. Varon. CG4, a new bipotential glial cell line from rat brain, is capable of differentiating *in vitro* into either mature oligodendrocytes or type-2 astrocytes. *J. Neuro-sci. Res.* 31:193 (1992).
24. L.M.E. Grimaldi, G.V. Martino, D.M. Franciotta, et al. Elevated alpha-tumor necrosis factor levels in spinal fluid from HIV-1-infected patients with central nervous system involvement. *Ann. Neurol.* 29:21 (1991).
25. W.R. Tyor, J.D. Glass, N. Bauman, et al. Cytokine expression of macro-phages in HIV-1 associated vacuolar myelopathy. *Neurology* 43:1002 (1993).
26. N. Gogate, LK. Verma, J.M. Zhou, et al. Plasticity in the adult human oligodendrocyte lineage. *J. Neurosci.* (in press).
27. J.G. McLarnon, M. Michikawa, and S.U. Kim. Effects of tumor necrosis factor on inward potassium current and cell morphology in cultured human oligodendrocytes. *Glia* 9:120 (1993).
28. L. Osborn, S. Kunkel, and G.J. Nabel. Tumor necrosis factor-α and inter-leukin 1 stimulate the human immunodeficiency virus enhancer by activation of the nuclear factor kB. *Proc. Natl. Acad. Sci. USA* 86:2336 (1989).

NITRIC OXIDE MEDIATES A COMPONENT OF gp120 NEUROTOXICITY IN PRIMARY CORTICAL CULTURES

Valina L. Dawson,[1,2] and Ted M. Dawson[1,3]

[1]Department of Neurology and [2]Department of Physiology
[3]Department of Neuroscience
Johns Hopkins University School of Medicine
Baltimore, Maryland 21237

INTRODUCTION

A significant number of acquired immunodeficiency syndrome (AIDS) patients will suffer from multiple neurologic abnormalities including deficits in cognitive and motor functions.[1-3] Several studies have associated primary human immunodeficiency virus type 1 (HIV-1) with central nervous system (CNS) tissue damage in individuals without secondary or reactive opportunistic infections.[1,4,5] Tissue lesions of both white and grey matter have been reported;[1,4,6] however, productive HIV-1 infection has only been consistently described in brain macrophages and microglia,[7,8] and not in neurons, astrocytes or oligodendrocytes which constitute the major cell populations in the brain.[4,5] The exact pathogenesis of neurotoxicity in AIDS is unknown and in the absence of direct invasion of neurons by HIV-1 or opportunistic infection, other mechanisms have been examined. It is possible that viral products and cytokines initiate a complex network of cellular interactions that ultimately leads to neuronal cell death.[9-12] One viral protein that may contribute to neuronal cell death is the envelope glycoprotein, gp120. Both native and recombinant gp120 can increase intracellular calcium levels and injure rodent retinal ganglion cells, and hippocampal and cortical neurons *in vitro*.[13-15] Neurotoxicity may involve elevation of intracellular calcium levels through activation of the N-methyl-D-aspartate (NMDA) receptor subtype of glutamate receptors. The increase in intracellular calcium and the neurotoxicity of both retinal ganglion cells[16] and cortical neurons[14] is attenuated by NMDA receptor antagonists. Furthermore, gp120 neurotoxicity, *in vitro*, is entirely dependent upon the presence of extracellular glutamate.[14,16]

GLUTAMATE NEUROTOXICITY

Derangements in glutaminergic transmission have been implicated in a variety of neurodegenerative disorders, including Huntington's disease, Alzheimer's disease, amyotrophic lateral sclerosis, and epilepsy.[17,18] Additionally, excessive stimulation of glutamate receptors has been implicated in neuronal damage that follows cerebral infarction. Glutamate triggers the opening of cation-permeable channels. The entry of calcium through these channels, particularly the NMDA receptor/channel, into cells activates a number of calcium-dependent enzymes. Excess intracellular calcium mediates glutamate neuro-

Technical Advances in AIDS Research in the Human Nervous System
Edited by E.O. Major and J.A. Levy, Plenum Press, New York, 1995

163

toxicity through activation of calcium-dependent enzymes.[17,18] Recently, we provided evidence that activation of nitric oxide synthase (NOS) by entry of Ca^{2+} through these channels is involved in mediating components of glutamate neurotoxicity.[14,19] Activation of NOS results in formation of the soluble free radical gas, nitric oxide (NO).

NITRIC OXIDE AND NITRIC OXIDE SYNTHASE

NO, a newly identified messenger molecule, is an endogenous activator of soluble guanylyl cyclase (for review see refs.20-22). NO was first identified as endothelium-derived relaxing factor (EDRF) in which NO acts on adjacent smooth muscle cells to cause vasodilation via increases in cGMP levels.[21] Macrophages and other immune cells also produce NO which mediates their bactericidal and tumoricidal effects.[23,24] In the brain, NO mediates the actions of the excitatory neurotransmitter, glutamate, in stimulating cGMP formation while inhibitors of NO synthase (NOS) block the elevation of cGMP.[20,25,26] NO also modifies a critical cysteine in glyceraldehyde-3-phosphate dehydrogenase by adenosine diphosphate ribosylation,[27,28] or S-nitrosylation via NAD interactions.[29] NO also binds to many iron-sulfur-containing proteins.[30] Additionally, NO nitrosylates a variety of proteins,[31,32] and there may be other unidentified cellular targets. Immunocytochemical studies have localized NOS to selective neuronal populations in the brain as well as to neurons in the retina, adrenal medulla, intestine, and to nerve fibers in the posterior pituitary.[33,34] Inhibitors of NOS block the physiologic relaxation of the intestine induced by neurotransmitter stimulation, indicating that NO possesses some properties of a neurotransmitter.[22,24] Thus, NO seems to be a novel type of neuronal messenger in that unlike conventional neurotransmitters, it is not stored in synaptic vesicles and does not act on typical extracellular receptor proteins on synaptic membranes. NO is synthesized from the amino acid, L-arginine, by the enzyme NOS. Several different isoforms of the enzyme have been purified to homogeneity and molecularly cloned.[30,35] The neuronal and endothelial NOS enzymes are constitutive calcium/calmodulin-dependent enzymes which release NO for short periods in response to receptor activation. The NO released by these enzymes mediates several physiologic responses. Two isoforms of inducible NOS have been purified and molecularly cloned as well, and these include the macrophage NOS and the human inducible hepatic NOS.[36-39] These forms of NOS are induced after activation by a variety of cytokines and once expressed, synthesize NO for long periods of time. Macrophage NOS differs from the neuronal and endothelial enzymes in being calcium independent.[24] Its induction is inhibited by glucocorticoids. So far, the only clearly established role for macrophage NO is as a cytotoxic molecule for invading microorganisms and tumor cells. It is likely however, that the release of NO via this enzyme may have other biological consequences, such as vasodilation, pathologic tissue damage and septic shock.[21,24,30] From the molecular cloning and subsequent biochemical studies, the NOS enzymes have recognition sites for NADPH, flavin adenine mono- and dinucleotide, calmodulin, heme, and several phosphorylation sites.[35] All the NOS enzymes utilize tetrahydrobiopterin which is thought to stabilize the enzyme; these sites combine for very tight regulation and control of NO formation.[35]

The unique pattern of NOS localization corresponds with the histochemical stain, neuronal NADPH diaphorase, throughout the brain and periphery.[33,34] NADPH diaphorase is a histochemical activity in which tetrazolium dyes in the presence of NADPH, but not NADH, provide a dark blue formazan precipitant.[40] The small population of neurons which stain positive for NADPH diaphorase are uniquely resistant to degeneration in Huntington's disease, hypoxia or excitatory amino acid neurotoxicity.[41-44,46] By applying the NADPH diaphorase stain to human kidney cells transfected with the cDNA for NOS, we showed that the NADPH diaphorase staining reflects and is proportional to the amount of transfected cDNA. These findings and those of Hope et al.[45] established that NOS was responsible for NADPH diaphorase staining of neurons.

NITRIC OXIDE AND NEUROTOXICITY

Recently, Bredt and Synder[25] provided evidence that glutamate acting primarily via NMDA receptors, leads to the influx of calcium (Ca^{2+}) which subsequently binds calmodulin and activates NOS to form NO. Under conditions of excessive glutamate receptor stimulation, NO has been implicated in mediating components of NMDA toxicity. In primary rat cortical cultures, we showed that NMDA neurotoxicity was prevented by several L-arginine analogs which are inhibitors of NOS including nitro-L-arginine (N-Arg), L-arginine methyl ester, N-methylarginine, and N-iminoethylornithine. The potency of each analog in blocking neurotoxicity was proportional to its potency as a NOS inhibitor, with N-Arg being most potent. Addition of 10-fold excess L-arginine reverses the effects of the NOS inhibitors. Moreover, the reversal by arginine and arginine derivatives was closely related to their capacity to serve as precursors of NO. Removal of L-arginine from the media by treatment with the enzyme arginase or by using arginine-free tissue culture media prevented neurotoxicity. Hemoglobin which complexes NO and inactivates it was also neuroprotective.[14,19,46] We have also compared the effects of NOS inhibitors on neurotoxicity on primary cultures from cortex, hippocampus and striatum, and neurotoxicity elicited by glutamate, NMDA, quisqualate and kainate.[19,46] Glutamate and its three analogs produce substantial neurotoxicity in all three brain regions. In all brain regions, N-Arg provides the most protection against glutamate and NMDA neurotoxicity, with somewhat less protection against quisqualate and negligible protection in the cerebral cortex and hippocampus against kainate. In the caudate-putamen, N-Arg produces modest but statistically significant protection against kainate. In all brains regions versus all glutamate analogs, excess arginine reverses the effects of N-Arg.[19,46]

NOS can be regulated at sites other than the L-arginine catalytic site. Calmodulin is an essential cofactor and the calmodulin antagonists, calmidazolium and W-7, are potent inhibitors of NOS catalytic activity and are neuroprotective against NMDA neurotoxicity in primary neuronal cultures. The shuttling of electrons by the flavoprotein moieties is critical for the conversion of L-arginine to citrulline and NO. NOS can be inhibited by diphenyleneiodonium (DPI) which binds flavins critical to NOS activity. DPI potently inhibit NMDA toxicity with an ED_{50} of 30 nM.[46]

NO generated in culture by structurally unrelated NO donors such as sodium nitroprusside (SNP), S-nitroso-N-acetylpenacillamine (SNAP) and SIN-1 elicits neurotoxicity.[46,47] The shapes of the concentration response relationships of cell death for SNP and NMDA in cortical cultures are essentially the same with increases in neurotoxicity from 10% to more than 80%, over two orders of magnitude, suggesting the absence of cooperativity. The time course for development of SNP and NMDA neurotoxicity is identical, suggesting a similar mechanism and furthering the concept that NO mediates NMDA toxicity.[46] A well known cellular target for NO is the heme-containing enzyme, guanylyl cyclase. In cerebellar slices and also primary neuronal cultures, NMDA induces an increase in cGMP which is attenuated by NOS inhibitors.[19,25,46] Inhibition of guanylyl cyclase or addition of cell-permeable cGMP derivatives did not modulate either NMDA- or SNP-induced neurotoxicity, indicating that activation of guanylyl cyclase and elevation of intracellular cGMP plays some other physiologic role in neuronal tissue than mediating toxicity.[46,47]

NO can be formed by NOS in macrophages, endothelial cells, as well as in neurons expressing NOS. In the brain, microglia function as macrophages. To determine whether NOS neurons in culture are the source of neurotoxic NO, we took advantage of the differential sensitivity of NOS neurons and other neurons to various toxins.[44,48] While about 60% of the total neuronal population of cortical cultures are killed by 300 µM NMDA or 300 µM SNP, only about 10-35% of NOS neurons die with either treatment. In striking contrast, 20 µM quisqualate kills less than 20% of the total neuronal population but kills about 85-

95% of NOS neurons.[46] Neurotoxicity induced by 300 µM NMDA is attenuated 60-70% in cultures treated 24 hours earlier with 20 µM quisqualate, a concentration that destroys 85-95% of NOS neurons. In sister cultures exposed to 20 µM quisqualate, normal NMDA Ca^{2+} currents can still be measured. These experiments strongly implicate NOS neurons as the source of NO that mediates NMDA toxicity.[46] Additionally, immature neuronal cultures do not express NOS activity and are relatively resistant to NMDA-type neurotoxicity. For an NO component of NMDA toxicity to be observed, primary rat cortical cultures need to be grown for at least 19-21 days, at which time NOS is fully expressed.[46] Although young cultures are resistant to NMDA toxicity, they are sensitive to 200 µM SNP, and also elicit NMDA-induced Ca^{2+} currents.[46]

Many groups have shown that NO mediates a component of NMDA neurotoxicity in hippocampal[49-51] and striatal slices,[52] and a variety of culture systems.[19,46,47,53-58] Despite the established role of NO as mediating components of glutamate neurotoxicity in primary cultures, some investigators did not detect an involvement of NO in glutamate neurotoxicity.[59-61] Lipton and collaborators showed that NO may be neuroprotective or neurodestructive, depending upon its oxidative reductive status.[62] The NO free radical (NO•) is toxic whereas the nitronium form of NO (NO+) is neuroprotective. Both SIN-1 and SNP tend to release neurodestructive NO, whereas the NO releaser nitroglycerine releases neuroprotective NO. These results suggest that the oxidative state of the cell at the time NOS is activated may determine the physiologic activity of NO.

Although NO has been implicated in glutamate neurotoxicity, it may not by itself, be sufficient for neuronal injury, and it has been suggested that NO is toxic only in the presence of other factors.[46] It has been proposed that NO interacts with the superoxide anion to form peroxynitrite (ONOO-) which is an extremely reactive and toxic molecule. Peroxynitrite rapidly decomposes and can form the hydroxyl free radical and the nitrogen dioxide free radical, potent activators of lipid peroxidation.[26,63-66] Superoxide dismutase (SOD) scavenges the superoxide anion converting it to hydrogen peroxide which is subsequently converted into water by catalase or glutathione peroxidase. Recently, the superoxide anion has been implicated as mediating components of NMDA neurotoxicity in primary cerebellar granule cell cultures.[67] In transgenic mice overexpressing SOD, infarct volume in response to focal ischemia is reduced, and in primary neuronal cultures of these transgenic mice, NMDA neurotoxicity is attenuated.[68,69] Addition of exogenous SOD also reduces the NMDA and SNP neurotoxicity in primary cortical cultures.[46] Thus, both NO and superoxide anion appear to be involved in glutamate neurotoxicity.

gp120 AND NITRIC OXIDE NEUROTOXICITY

A component of gp120 neurotoxicity involves activation of the NMDA receptor.[13-16] In primary rat cortical cultures, gp120 neurotoxicity is abso-lutely dependent on extracellular glutamate with an ED_{50} of 18 µM glutamate. In the presence of glutamate, gp120 elicits neurotoxicity in a dose-dependent manner with significant neurotoxicity observed at a concentration as low as 100 fM gp120 and maximal neurotoxicity attained at 1 nM gp120. Antagonists for the NMDA and non-NMDA receptor subtypes of glutamate receptors, MK-801 and 6,7-dinitroquinoxaline-2,3-dione (DNQX) respectively, are neuroprotective against gp120 neurotoxicity. Both agents combined provide additional sparing of neurons from cell death (Fig. 1). These data correlate with previous studies in retinal ganglion cultures where NMDA antagonists were effective in blocking toxicity of gp120.[16] Calcium has been identified as an intracellular signaling molecule that initiates mechanisms leading to neuronal death.[17] L-type voltage-dependent Ca^{2+} channel antagonists such as nimodipine and nifedipine as well as calcium-free media diminish the neurotoxicity of gp120 in retinal ganglion cells.[15,16] In primary cortical cultures, we showed that both nifedipine and calcium-free media attenuate gp120 neurotoxicity (Fig. 1).

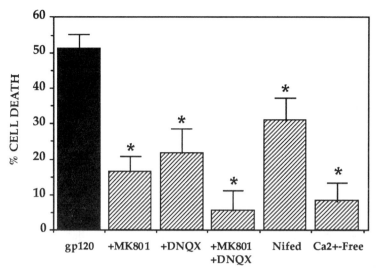

Figure 1. Attenuation of gp120 neurotoxicity. Primary cortical cultures were exposed to 100 pM gp120 + 25 μM glutamate in the presence or absence of 10 μM MK-801, 100 μM DNQX, 100 μM nifedipine, or in calcium-free media. Data are the means S.E.M. (n $\geq$ 8). Cell death was determined by 0.4% trypan blue exclusion by viable cells. Significance was determined by Student's t-test for independent means (*p $\leq$ 0.001).

Glutamate stimulation of NMDA receptors results in the formation of NO through activation of NOS through elevated intracellular calcium. NO mediates a component of glutamate neurotoxicity as NOS inhibitors and NO scavengers are neuroprotective.[19,46,55] Neurotoxicity in cortical cultures elicited by gp120 was examined to determine if there was an NO component. Depletion of L-arginine, the precursor of NO, from the media resulted in a 70% decrease in gp120 neurotoxicity (Fig. 2). Various classes of NOS inhibitors were also neuroprotective against gp120 neurotoxicity. Nitroarginine (N-Arg) which competes with L-arginine for the catalytic site on NOS attenuates gp120 neurotoxicity 70% and was reversible with 10-fold excess L-arginine (Fig. 2). Inhibiting NOS catalytic activity with the flavoprotein inhibitor, diphenyliodonium (DPI) produces 90% neuroprotection (Fig. 2). Reduced hemoglobin provided neuroprotection against gp120 neurotoxicity.[14]

One cellular target for NO that may be necessary for NO neurotoxicity is the superoxide anion. SOD scavenges the superoxide anion and the addition of SOD to the exposure solution results in significant neuroprotection against gp120 neurotoxicity (Fig. 2). Addition of both N-Arg and SOD results in nearly complete attenuation of gp120 neurotoxicity suggesting that both NO and superoxide anion contribute to gp120 neurotoxicity (Fig. 2).

Exposure of cortical neurons to gp120 results in increased cGMP levels which is inhibited by NOS inhibitors or reduced hemoglobin indicating that NO is formed in response to gp120 (Fig. 3). There are several possible cellular sources of NO in cortical cultures. Microglia, astrocytes and macrophages can be induced to express; in addition, these cells have been shown to be essential for gp120 neurotoxicity in retinal ganglion cultures.[70] Furthermore, constitutive NOS in both neurons and astrocytes could account for NO neurotoxicity. To determine the source of neurotoxic NO in primary cortical cultures exposed to gp120, NOS neurons were selectively removed from the culture well by prior

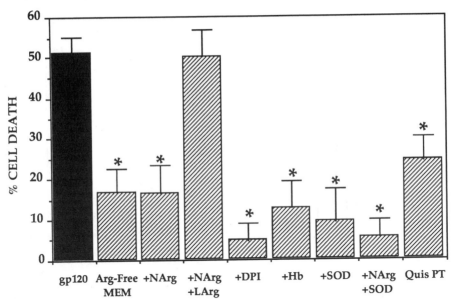

Figure 2. Attenuation of gp120 neurotoxicity. Primary cortical cultures were exposed to 100 pM gp120 + 25 μM glutamate in the presence or absence of 100 μM N-Arg, 100 μM N-Arg + 1 mM L-Arg, 500 nM DPI, 500 μM Hb, 100 units SOD, 100 μM N-Arg + 100 units SOD, or pretreated with 20 μM quisqualate. Data are the means ±S.E.M. (n≥8). Cell death was determined by 0.4% trypan blue exclusion by viable cells. Significance was determined by student's t-test for independent means (* p≤0.001). Abbreviations: DPI, diphenyleneiodonium; Hb, hemoglobin; L-Arg, L-arginine; N-Arg, nitroarginine; NMA, N-methylarginine; SOD, superoxide dismutase; Quis, quisqualate.

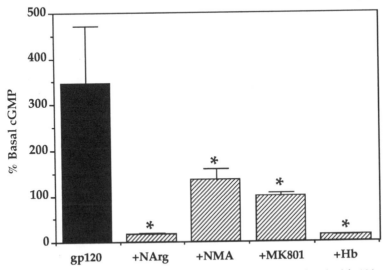

Figure 3. cGMP formation after primary cortical cultures were stimulated with 100 pM gp120 + 25 μM glutamate in the presence or absence of 100 μM N-Arg, 500 μM NMA, 10 μM MK-801 or 500 μM Hb. Data are the means S.E.M. (n≥6). Abbreviations: N-Arg, nitroarginine; NMA, N-methylarginine; Hb, hemoglobin.

exposure to 20 µM quisqualate.[46] Treating the cortical cultures with 20 µM quisqualate 24 hours prior to exposure of these cells to gp120 attenuated the gp120-induced neurotoxicity by 65%, suggesting that in this primary cortical culture system, neuronal NOS is the primary source of neurotoxic NO (Fig. 2). gp120 can induce NOS expression in human astrocyte cultures,[71] suggesting that both neuronal and astrocyte NOS may contribute to gp120 neurotoxicity.

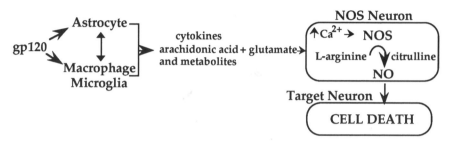

Figure 4. Proposed mechanism of gp120 neurotoxicity. The HIV-1 coat protein, gp120, is shed by the virus. gp120 interacts with macrophages/microglia and astrocytes to release cytokines, arachidonic acid and its metabolites, which may interact synergistically with endogenous glutamate to activate NMDA receptors. The increase in intracellular calcium stimulates NOS and excessive NO formation kills adjacent cells.

Although gp120 neurotoxicity is dependent on extracellular glutamate, NMDA receptors are not directly activated by gp120.[16] How does gp120 initiate glutamate excitotoxicity in neuronal cultures? Arachidonic acid metabolites and cytokines are produced by cell-to-cell interactions between HIV-infected macrophages and microglia,[11] and cultures exposed to gp120.[12] Arachidonic acid potentiates NMDA receptor currents by increasing the open-channel probability. It is conceivable that gp120 stimulates macrophages and microglia in neuronal cultures to release arachidonic acid, arachidonic acid metabolites and cytokines which act synergistically with endogenous extracellular glutamate to overactivate NMDA receptors resulting in neurotoxic NO production (Fig. 4). In some animal models of focal ischemia in which neuronal cell death is associated with the overstimulation of the NMDA receptor, administration of the NOS inhibitor, nitroarginine, can markedly reduce neuronal damage.[72] It is possible that NOS inhibitors may have a therapeutic value in the treatment of AIDS dementia.

REFERENCES

1. B.A. Navia, B.D. Jordan, R.W. Price. The AIDS dementia complex: I. Clinical features. *Ann. Neurol.* 119:517 (1986).
2. B.A. Navia, E-S. Cho, C.K. Petito, and R.W. Price. The AIDS dementia complex: II. Neuropathology. *Ann. Neurol.* 19:525 (1986).
3. R.W. Price, B. Brew, J. Sidtis, et al. The brain in AIDS: Central nervous system infection and AIDS dementia complex. *Science* 238:586 (1988).
4. C.A. Wiley, R.D. Schrier, J.A. Nelson, P.W. Lampert, and M.B.A. Oldstone. Cellular localization of human immunodeficiency virus infection within the brains of acquired immune deficiency syndrome patients. *Proc. Natl. Acad. Sci. USA* 83:7089 (1986).
5. J. Michaels, L.R. Sharer, and L.F. Epstein. Human immunodeficiency virus type-1 (HIV-1) infection of the nervous system: a review. *Immunodefic. Rev.* 1:71 (1988).
6. C.A. Wiley, E. Masliah, M. Morey, et al. Neocortical damage during HIV infection. *Ann. Neurol.* 29:651 (1991).
7. M.H. Stoler, T.A. Eskin, S. Benn, R.C. Angerer, and L.M. Angerer. Human T-cell lymphotrophic virus type III infection of the central nervous system - a preliminary *in situ* analysis. *J.A.M.A.* 256:2381 (1986).
8. J. Michaels, R.W. Price, and M. Rosenblum. Microglia in the glial cell encephalitis of AIDS: Proliferation, infection, and fusion. *Acta Neuropathol.* 76:373 (1988).
9. Guilian, D. E. Wendt, K. Vaca, and C.A. Noonan. The envelope glycoprotein of human immunodeficiency virus type-1 stimulates release of neurotoxins from monocytes. *Proc. Natl. Acad. Sci. USA* 90:2769 (1993).
10. D. Guilian, K. Vaca, and C.A. Noonan. Secretion of neurotoxins by mononuclear phagocytes infected with HIV-1. *Science.* 250:1593 (1990).
11. P. Genis, M. Jett, E.W. Bernton, et al. Cytokines and arachidonic acid metabolites produced during human immunodeficiency virus (HIV)-infected macrophage-astroglia interactions: Implications for the neuropathogenesis of HIV disease. *J. Exp. Med.* 176:1703 (1992).
12. L.M. Wahl, M.L. Corcoran, S.W. Pyle, et al. Human immunodeficiency virus glycoprotein (gp120) induction of monocyte arachidonic acid metabolites and interleukin 1. *Proc. Natl. Acad. Sci.* 86:621 (1989).
13. D.E. Brenneman, G.L. Westbrook, S.P. Fitzgerald, et al. Neuronal cell killing by the envelope protein of HIV and its prevention by vasoactive intestinal peptide. *Nature* 335:639 (1988).
14. V.L. Dawson, T.M. Dawson, G.R. Uhl, and S.H. Snyder. Human immunodeficiency virus-1 coat protein neurotoxicity mediated by nitric oxide in primary cortical cultures. *Proc. Natl. Acad. Sci. USA* 90:3256 (1993).
15. E.B. Dreyer, P.K. Kaiser, J.T. Offerman, and S.A. Lipton. HIV-1 coat protein neurotoxicity prevented by calcium channel antagonists. *Science* 248:364 (1990).
16. S.A. Lipton, N.J. Sucher, P.K. Kaise, and E.B. Dreyer. Synergistic effects of HIV coat protein and NMDA receptor-mediated neurotoxicity. *Neuron* 7:111 (1991).
17. D.W. Choi. Glutamate neurotoxicity and disease of the nervous system. *Neuron* 1:623 (1988).
18. B. Meldrum, and J. Garthwaite. Excitatory amino acid neurotoxicity and neurodegenerative disease. *Trends Pharmacol. Sci.* 11:379 (1990).
19. V.L. Dawson, T.MN. Dawson, E.D. London, D.S. Bredt, and S.H. Snyder. Nitric oxide mediates glutamate neurotoxicity in primary cortical culture. *Proc. Natl. Acad. Sci. USA* 88:6368 (1991).
20. J. Garthwaite. Glutamate, nitric oxide and cell-cell signaling in the nervous system. *Trends Neurol. Sci.* 14:60 (1991).
21. S. Moncada, R.M.J. Palmer, and E.A. Higgs. Nitric oxide: physiology, pathophysiology, and pharmacology. *Pharmacol. Rev.* 43:109 (1991).
22. S.H. Snyder. Nitric oxide: First in a new class of neurotransmitters? *Science* 257:494 (1992).

23. M.A. Marletta. Nitric oxide: biosynthesis and biological significance. *Trends Biol. Sci.* 14:488 (1989).
24. C. Nathan. Nitric oxide as a secretory product of mammalian cells. *FASEB J.* 6:3051 (1992).
25. D.S. Bredt, and S.H. Snyder. Nitric oxide mediate glutamate-linked enhancement of cGMP levels in the cerebellum. *Proc. Natl. Acad. Sci USA* 86:9030 (1989).
26. T.M. Dawson, V.L. Dawson, and S.H. Snyder. A novel neuronal messenger molecule in brain: the free radical, nitric oxide. *Ann. Neurol.* 32:297 (1992).
27. J. Zhang, and S.H. Snyder. Nitric oxide stimulates auto-ADP-ribosylation of glyceraldehyde-3-phosphate dehydrogenase in brain,. *Proc. Natl. Acad. Sci. USA* 89:9382 (1992).
28. S. Dimmeler, F. Lottspeich, and B. Brune. Nitric oxide causes ADP-ribosylation and inhibition of glyceraldehyde-3-phosphate dehydrogenase. *J. Biol. Chem.* 267:16771 (1992).
29. L.J. McDonald, and J. Moss. Stimulation by nitric oxide of an NAD linkage to glyceraldehyde-3-phosphate dehydrogenase. *Proc. Natl. Acad. Sci. USA* 90:6238 (1993).
30. C.J. Lowenstein, and S.H. Snyder. Nitric oxide, a novel biologic messenger. *Cell* 70:705 (1992).
31. J.S. Stamler, D.I. Simon, J.A. Osborne, et al. S-nitrosylation of proteins with nitric oxide: synthesis and characterization of biologically active compounds. *Proc. Natl. Acad. Sci. USA* 257:494 (1992).
32. J.S. Stamler, D.J. Singel, and J. Loscalzo. Biochemistry of nitric oxide and its redox-activated forms. *Science* 258:1898 (1992).
33. D.S. Bredt, C.E. Glatt, P.M. Hwang, et al. Nitric oxide synthase protein and mRNA are discretely localized in neuronal populations of the mammalian CNS together with NADPH diaphorase. *Neuron* 7:615 (1991).
34. T.M. Dawson, D.S. Bredt, M. Fotuhi, P.M. Hwang, and S.H. Snyder. Nitric oxide synthase and neuronal NADPH diaphorase are identical in brain and peripheral tissues. *Proc. Natl. Acad. Sci. USA* 88:7797 (1991).
35. M.A. Marletta. Nitric oxide synthase structure and mechanism. *J. Biol. Chem.* 268:12231 (1993).
36. D.A. Geller, C.J. Lowenstein, R.A. Shapiro, et al. Molecular cloning and expression of inducible nitric oxide synthase from human hepatocytes. *Proc. Natl. Acad. Sci. USA* 90:3491 (1993).
37. C.J. Lowenstein, C.S. Glatt, D.S. Bredt, and S.H. Snyder. Cloned and expressed macrophage nitric oxide synthase contrasts with brain enzyme. *Proc. Natl. Acad. Sci. USA* 89:6711 (1992).
38. C.R. Lyons, G.J. Orloff, and J.M. Cunningham. Molecular cloning and functional expression of an inducible nitric oxide synthase from a murine macrophage cell line. *J. Biol. Chem.* 267:6370 (1992).
39. Q-W. Xie, H.J. Cho, J. Calaycay, et al. Cloning and characterization of inducible nitric oxide synthase from mouse macrophages. *Science* 256:225 (1992).
40. E. Thomas, and A.G.E. Pearse. The solitary active cells. Histochemical demonstration of damage-resistant nerve cells with a TPN-diaphorase reaction. *Acta Neuropathol.* 3:238 (1964).
41. R.J. Ferrante, N.W. Kowall, M.F. Beal, et al. Selective sparing of a class of striatal neurons in Huntington's disease. *Science* 230:561 (1985).
42. Y. Uemura, N.W. Kowall, and M.F. Beal. Selective sparing of NADPH-diaphorase-somnatostatin-neuropeptide Y neurons in ischemic gerbil striatum. *Ann. Neurol.* 27:620 (1990).
43. M.F. Beal, N.W. Kowall, D.W. Ellison, et al. Replication of the neurochemical characteristics of Huntington's disease by quinolinic acid. *Nature* 321: 168 (1986).
44. J.-Y. Kohn, S. Peters, and D.W. Choi. Neurons containing NADPH-diaphorase are selectively resistant to quinolinate toxicity. *Science* 234:73 (1986).
45. B.T. Hope, G.J. Michael, K.M. Knigge, and S.R. Vincent. Neuronal NADPH

diaphorase is a nitric oxide synthase. *Proc. Natl. Acad. Sci. USA* 88:2811 (1991).

46. V.L. Dawson, T.M. Dawson, D.A. Bartley, G. Uhl, and S.H. Snyder. Mechanisms of nitric oxide mediated neurotoxicity in primary brain cultures. *J. Neurosci.* 13:2651 (1993).

47. H.S. Lustig, K.L. von Brauchitsch, J. Chan, and D.A. Greenberg. Ethanol and excitotoxicity in cultured cortical neurons: differential sensitivity of N-methyl-D-aspartate and sodium nitroprusside toxicity. *J. Neurochem.* 59:2193 (1992).

48. J.-Y. Koh, and D.W. Choi. Vulnerability of cultured cortical neurons to damage by excitotoxins: Differential susceptibility of neurons containing NADPH-diaphorase. *J. Neurosci.*, 8:2153 (1988).

49. Y. Izumi, A.M. Benz, D.B. Clifford, and C.F. Zormumski. Nitric oxide inhibitors attenuate N-methyl-D-aspartate excitotoxicity in rat hippocampal slices. *Neurosci. Lett.* 135:227 (1992).

50. S. Moncada, D. Lekieffre, N. Arvin, and B. Meldrum. Effect of NO synthase inhibition of NMDA- and ischaemia-induced hippocampal lesions. *NeuroReport* 3:530 (1992).

51. R.A. Wallis, K. Panizzon, C.G. Wasterlain. Inhibition of nitric oxide synthase protects against hypoxic neuronal injury. *NeuroReport* 3:645 (1992).

52. H. Kollegger, G.J. McBean, and K.F. Tipton. Reduction of striatal N-methyl-D-aspartate toxicity by inhibition of nitric oxide synthase. *Biochem. Pharmacol.* 45:260 (1993).

53. C. Cazevieille, A. Muller, F. Meynier, and C. Bonne. Superoxide and nitric oxide cooperation in hypoxia/reoxygenation-induced neuron injury. *Free Rad. Biol. Med.* 14:389 (1993).

54. M. Corasaniti, R.L. Tartaglia, G. Melino, G. Nistico, and A.Finazzi-Agro. Evidence that CHP100 neuroblastoma cell death induced by N-methyl-D-aspartate involves L-arginine-nitric oxide pathway activation. *Neurosci. Lett.* 147:221 (1992).

55. T.M. Dawson, J.P. Steiner, V.L. Dawson, et al. The immunosuppressant, FK506, enhances phosphorylation of nitric oxide synthase and protects against glutamate neurotoxicity. *Proc. Natl. Acad. Sci. USA* 90:9808 (1993).

56. D.W. Reif. Delayed production of nitric oxide contributes to NMDA-mediated neuronal damage. *NeuroReport* 4:566 (1993).

57. Y. Tamura, Y. Sato, A. Akaike, and H. Shiomi. Mechanisms of cholecystokinin-induced protection of cultured cortical neurons against N-methyl-D-aspartate receptor-mediated glutamate cytotoxicity. *Brain Res.* 592: 317-325.

58. X. Vige, A. Carreau, B. Scatton, and J. Nowicki. Antagonism by N^{G}-nitro-L-arginine of L-glutamate-induced neurotoxicity in cultured neonatal rat cortical neurons. Prolonged application enhances neuroprotective efficacy. *Neuroscience* 55:893 (1993).

59. C. Demerle-Pallardy, M.O. Lonchampt, P.E. Chabrier, and P. Braquet. Absence of implication of L-arginine/nitric oxide pathway on neuronal cell injury induced by L-glutamate or hypoxia. *Biochem. Biophys. Res. Commun.* 181:456 (1991).

60. P.J. Pauwels, and J.E. Leysen. Blockade of nitric oxide formation does not prevent glutamate-induced neurotoxicity in neuronal cultures from rat hippocampus. *Neurosci. Lett.* 143:27 (1992).

61. R.F. Regan, K.E. Renn, and S.S. Panter. NMDA neurotoxicity in murine cortical cell cultures is not attenuated by hemoglobin or inhibition of nitric oxide synthesis. *Neurosci. Lett.* 153:53 (1993).

62. S.A. Lipton, Y-B. Choi, Z-H. Pan, et al. A redox-based mechanism for the neuroprotective and neurodestructive effects of nitric oxide and related nitroso-compounds. *Nature* 364:626 (1993).

63. J.S. Beckman, T.W. Beckman, J. Chen. Apparent hydoxyl radical production by peroxynitrite: implications for endothelial injury from nitric oxide and superoxide. *Proc. Natl. Acad. Sci. USA* 87:1620 (1990).

64. J.S. Beckman. The double-edged role of nitric oxide in brain function and superoxide-mediated injury. *J. Dev. Physiol.* 15:53 (1991).
65. R. Radi, J.S. Beckman, K.M. Bush, and B.A. Freeman. Peroxynitrite-induced membrane lipid peroxidation: the cytotoxic potential of superoxide and nitric oxide. *Arch., Biochem. Biophys.* 288:481 (1991).
66. R. Radi, J.S. Beckman, K.M. Bush, B.A. Freeman. Peroxynitrite oxidation of sulfhydryls. The cytotoxic potential of superoxide and nitric oxide. *J. Biol. Chem.* 266:4244 (1991).
67. M. Lafon-Cazal, S. Pietri, M. Culcasi, and J. Bockaert. NMDA-dependent superoxide production and neurotoxicity. *Nature* 364:535 (1993).
68. P.H.Chan, L. Chu, S.F. Chen. Reduced neurotoxicity in transgenic mice overexpressing human copper-zinc-superoxide dismutase. *Stroke* 21:80 (1990).
69. H. Kinouchi, C.J. Epstein, and T. Mizui. Attenuation of focal cerebral ischemic injury in transgenic mice overexpressing CuZn superoxide dismutase. *Proc. Natl. Acad. Sci. USA* 88:11158 (1991).
70. S.A. Lipton. Requirement for macrophages in neuronal injury induced by HIV envelope protein gp120. *NeuroReport* 3:913 (1992).
71. V. Mollace, M. Colasanti, T. Persichini, et al. HIV gp120 glycoprotein stimulates the inducible isoform of NO synthase in human cultured astrocytoma cells. *Biochem. Biophys. Res. Comm.* 194:439 (1993).
72. J.P. Nowicki, D. Duval, H. Poignet, and B. Scatton. Nitric oxide mediates neuronal death after focal cerebral ischemia in the mouse. *Eur. J. Pharmacol.* 204:339 (1991).

NEUROTROPISM OF HIV-1 STRAINS

CONTRIBUTION OF V3 AND REVERSE TRANSCRIPTASE
SEQUENCE ANALYSIS TO UNDERSTANDING THE CONCEPT OF
HIV-1 NEUROTROPISM

Francesca Chiodi, Mariantonietta Di Stefano, and Farideh Sabri

Laboratory for Virology
Microbiology and Tumorbiology Center
Karolinska Institute
c/o SMI, Lundagatan 2
S-10521 Stockholm, Sweden

INTRODUCTION

Recovery of HIV-1 from brain tissue and the cerebrospinal fluid (CSF) of a large number of infected patients,[1,2] together with the neurologic clinical picture and brain histopathology,[3] have contributed to establishing the concept of HIV-1 neurotropism. The main target cells for HIV-1 infection within the brain are cells of the macrophage/microglia lineage.[4,5] It is likely that application of more sensitive methods to identify HIV-1-infected cells in the brain will add interesting findings in this context, as reviewed in this volume by Nuovo.[6] For now, however, one of the attributes needed to include HIV-1 among the "strict" neurotropic viruses, namely infection and replication of the virus in neural cells, is missing. One of the hypotheses formulated with regard to the pathogenesis of AIDS-related neurologic symptoms is that the infection of the brain should be carried out by HIV-1 variants with increased capacity to replicate in brain parenchyma, i.e., the neurotropic HIV-1 strains. This chapter focuses on the sequence variability and biologic properties of HIV-1 strains recovered from the brain and discusses whether these viral properties signify the existence of HIV-1 variants having special brain tropism.

NEUROTROPIC VARIANTS AMONG RETROVIRUSES

Retroviral infections in animals are often accompanied by the appearance of neurologic symptoms. In the case of lentiviruses, however, the brain is not the only target organ for virus infection and replication, and symptomatology is not confined to the nervous system. Caprine arthritis encephalitis virus induces leukoencephalomyelitis, arthritis, and interstitial pneumonia in goats.[7] Visna virus, an ovine lentivirus, causes slowly progressive disease of the central nervous system (CNS) and chronic progressive pneumonia.[8] The virus can be recovered from lung, brain, CSF, and peripheral mononuclear cells (PBMCs).[9] HIV-1 is also present in a large variety of body fluids, including blood, CSF, seminal and vaginal fluid, saliva, and milk.[10] Although neuropsychiatric symptoms, may in some patients, precede most other clinical signs of AIDS,[11] in the

Technical Advances in AIDS Research in the Human Nervous System
Edited by E.O. Major and J.A. Levy, Plenum Press, New York, 1995

majority of patients, neurologic clinical symptoms and signs follow, or occur in parallel with overt immunodeficiency.

The distinction between tropism for different organs is better defined in some variants of the animal oncovirus murine leukemia virus. The neuropathogenic variants PVC-211 murine leukemia virus (MuLV), Cas-Br-E MuLV and temperature-sensitive 1 (*ts*1) Moloney MuLV have been derived either by adaptation *in vivo*, or by *in vitro* selection. Little of the leukemogenic properties of the parental MuLV strains can be recovered in these viruses, and they infect predominantly neural cells and cause only neurologic symptoms. The molecular determinants for the pathogenicity of these viruses have been mapped within the 5' half of the coding region for the outer glycoprotein.[12-14] In the case of the *ts*1 mutant of Moloney MuLV, the neurovirulent properties of the virus have been linked to one Val-25-to-Ile substitution in the envelope precursor protein; this mutation, at the restrictive temperature, appears to affect the transport of the glycoprotein from the endoplasmic reticulum to the Golgi apparatus.[12] Identification of viral sequences that account for the neurotropic property may be easier in oncoviruses, which show less genetic variability than lentiviruses.

SPREAD OF THE VIRUS TO THE BRAIN COMPARTMENT IS A COMMON EARLY EVENT DURING HIV-1 INFECTION

Isolation of the virus from the CSF during acute infection and in the asymptomatic phase of the disease[1,2,15] indicates that HIV-1 spread to the nervous system occurs soon after the initial contact with the virus. The pathway(s) of invasion of the brain compartment is not known but it is reasonable to believe that the virus crosses the blood-brain barrier (BBB) through infected T-cells and macrophages. Symptomatic acute HIV-1 infection is often complicated by mild meningeal signs[16] which could contribute to the establishment of brain infection through increased permeability of the BBB. Studies aimed at characterizing the degree of HIV variability acquired during sexual transmission, indicated that a highly homogeneous virus population was present in the blood of the recipients within three months of seroconversion.[17] Hence, if HIV-1 reaches the brain early during infection, the virus genotype that enters the nervous system is likely to be similar to the virus population present, at that time point, in other body compartments. The virus might, however, be carried to the brain compartment through multiple infection events, distinguished in time and modality of spread.

What then would be the fate of the HIV-1 variants that reach the brain early in infection, and are they competent to infect the cells present there? Blood HIV-1 strains isolated early during infection from the majority of asymptomatic carriers and acutely infected individuals can replicate in primary blood macrophages.[18,19] In view of the fact that the major target cells for HIV-1 infection within the brain are microglia, which also belong to the macrophage lineage, the HIV-1 variants present at early stages of infection could possibly establish persistent infection in the brain parenchyma.

That this might indeed be the case is indicated by the current collaborative project with the National Institute of Neurological Disorders and Stroke, National Institutes of Health (Chiodi, in preparation). Previous work has shown that primary human brain cultures containing microglial cells can be infected *in vitro* with HIV-1 via the CD4 molecule.[20,21] To assess the possibility that tropism for microglial cells might be a common property of HIV-1 isolates, we selected viruses from the blood and CSF of patients with varying degrees of symptoms, including asymptomatic carriers, and passaged them in primary microglial cultures. Ten of the 13 isolates used in the study replicated to a high degree in microglial cells, comparable to what has been observed for the macrophage/microglia tropic Jr-F1 isolate.[22, 23] These results indicate that virus isolates present during the initial phase of HIV-1 infection can, indeed, establish infection of the brain tissue. Histopathologic changes and virus production within the brain are minor during the asymptomatic phase of the disease,[24] as opposed to the terminal stage of AIDS.[25] If infection of microglia occurs early *in vivo*, expression of the viral proteins in microglial cells may be controlled until overt immunodeficiency occurs by the same, or other, factors which determine latency in lymphocytes and macrophages in blood.[26]

GENETIC VARIATION AND BIOLOGIC PROPERTIES OF HIV-1 ISOLATES

The HIV-1 isolates consist of a complex mixture of genotypically distinguishable viruses. Intra- and interpatient genomic diversity of HIV-1 is a well-documented phenomenon,[27] and genetic variation over time in viruses isolated from the same individual has also been reported.[28] In the presence of this complexity of virus quasispecies, the identification of regions responsible for HIV-1 tropism and biologic properties appears to be an arduous task. Recombination between different HIV-1 genomes may further complicate this picture.[29] The efforts of many research teams have, however, contributed to our present knowledge of the variable region 3 (V3) of the outer glycoprotein, gp120, as important determinant of tropism, immunoprotective responses, and replicative capacity of HIV-1 isolates.

Comparison of several HIV-1 sequences has revealed the presence of five hypervariable regions in the gp120 outer glycoprotein;[30] these regions are interspaced by amino acid stretches with a higher degree of conservation. Conserved sequences and structural elements have been found in the approximately 35 amino acids forming the V3 domain of several HIV-1 isolates; the two cysteine residues at the boundary of this region allow the formation of a loop.[31] The V3 region serves as a major target for neutralizing antibodies.[32,33] The relatively conserved motif Gly-Pro-Gly-Arg (GPGR), present at the tip of the loop, is believed to play a role, yet unidentified, in viral fusion and penetration into target cells.[34]

Several studies, involving the exchange of envelope regions from viruses with well-defined T-cell or macrophage tropism have correlated those properties to amino acids sequences present within the V3 loop.[35-37] Mostly viral molecular clones and laboratory-adapted HIV-1 strains have been used in these studies and, therefore, it remains to be seen if this observation also applies to primary HIV-1 isolates. A correlation between the biological phenotype of HIV-1 isolates, the amino acid sequence of the V3 region, and the clinical course of infection has been demonstrated. In the asymptomatic stage of the disease, the viral isolates obtained from the blood show slow replicative capacity and do not form syncytia [non-syncytia inducing (NSI)] in primary cell cultures from the peripheral blood.[38,39] These variants persist throughout the AIDS phase in approximately one-half of the patients,[40] whereas variants with increased replicative capacity, broader cellular tropism, and syncytium-inducing (SI) ability arise in others. It has been proposed that the switch from NSI to SI variants is accompanied by specific size variations in V2 and amino acid changes in positions flanking the GPGR motif of V3, which in turn, result in higher net charge thereby modifying the secondary structure of this region.[41,42]

Conceivably, the V3 domain could play an important role in determining the neurotropic properties of HIV-1 isolates. The comparison of V3 sequences from blood and brain may therefore pinpoint differences in biologic properties of HIV-1 in the two compartments. Receptor molecules other than CD4, such as galactosyl ceramide,[43] have been suggested to mediate HIV-1 infection of brain cells. The finding that monoclonal antibodies to V3 block the interaction of galactosyl ceramide with the virus adsorption protein reinforces the importance of studying and analyzing V3 sequences even in this context (Gonzales-Scarano, personal communication).

SEQUENCE ANALYSIS OF THE V3 REGION AND THE REVERSE TRANSCRIPTASE OF PAIRED HIV-1 ISOLATES FROM CSF AND BLOOD

The presence of infectious virus in the CSF of both asymptomatic and AIDS patients offers the possibility of analyzing the molecular and biological characteristics of HIV-1 variants present in the brain compartment during the early phase of infection. We have selected paired isolates obtained from CSF and blood of five asymptomatic HIV-1 carriers and five AIDS patients for studies by nucleotide sequencing. Following PCR amplification and cloning, the V3 loop and flanking regions were sequenced.[44] Similar to Epstein and collaborators,[45] we were unable to identify amino acid positions that would allow the grouping of HIV-1 isolates according to tissue specificity. The paired isolates from blood and CSF clustered, without exception, according to the host of origin.

Intrapatient variation (blood versus CSF) in amino acid sequence of the V3 loop and flanking regions increased in the symptomatic group, as shown in Figure 1. The sequences of the V3 region were derived as follows. PBMCs infected with low-passage virus supernatant were used to prepare DNA for PCR and sequencing of the V3 region of gp120. The cells were washed twice in phosphate-buffered saline (PBS) and then lysed in 0.1 ml of PCR lysing buffer.[46]. The PCR was performed in a two-step reaction according to the method of Albert and Fenyö.[46] Four nucleotide primers derived from the HIV-1 env type B consensus sequences[47] were used to amplify V3 and flanking regions.[44] The amplified products consisted of 798 bp (nucleotides 315 to 1092). The PCR products were cloned[44] and nucleotide sequence determination was performed using the T7 sequence kit (Pharmacia, Uppsala, Sweden) by the dideoxynucleotide chain termination method.[48] Sequences of the amplified fragments were determined in two orientations with primers binding to env 716-735 and env 1071-1090. Four clones were sequenced for each of the isolates used to generate consensus nucleotide and amino acid sequences. The V3 sequence data have been deposited with the EMBL/Gen Bank Data Libraries under Accession Numbers Z23177-Z23188 and Z23190-Z23255. The V3 loop and its carboxy terminal flanking region showed the highest variation whereas the degree of variability in the amino terminus was similar throughout infection. It is tempting to speculate that distinct mechanisms of immunomodulation and/or adaptation within different body compartments may account for these variations. Some of our previous results pointed to the lack of neutralizing activity in the CSF of infected patients, whereas antibodies capable of neutralizing several HIV-1 isolates were found in the corresponding sera.[49]

That the intrapatient variations found within the V3 loop might not only be due to the inaccuracy of the HIV-1 reverse transcriptase during transcription of the virus genome, or Taq-polymerase during PCR amplification, is indicated by the following. Amino acid positions 10 and 24 of the loop have been shown to determine the virus biological phenotype.[41] These positions were found to be different in the blood versus the CSF isolates of three of the AIDS patients but in none of the asymptomatic carriers. Covariation, as opposed to independent mutation, of these paired sites, along with others within the V3 loop, has been shown to occur by using an information theoretical analysis.[50] Whatever the meaning of the V3 variations found between blood and CSF isolates, we determined that variants with substantial differences in V3 can still replicate in primary microglial cells, including HIV-1 isolates with SI properties.

The study by Korber and collaborators[50] also indicated that covariation of mutations does not occur when analyzing a large number of HIV-1 reverse transcriptase sequences. The pol region of HIV-1, which includes the gene coding for reverse transcriptase, is the most conserved region of the viral genome, with an estimated nucleotide change of 1.7×10^{-3} sites/year, approximately ten times less than what was observed for the variable regions in the viral envelope.[51] A number of mutations occur in the HIV-1 RT gene in patients undergoing therapy with 3'-azido-3'-deoxythymidine (AZT); the mutations, resulting in the amino acid substitution of Met[41] to Leu, Asp[67] to Asn, Lys[70] to Arg, Thr [215] to Phe or Tyr and Lys[219] to Gln render HIV-1 isolates less sensitive, or resistant to the

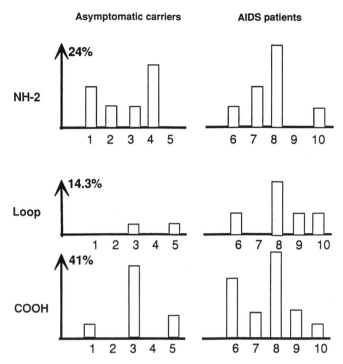

Figure 1. Percentage of amino acid variation (shown as vertical boxes) between blood and CSF HIV-1 isolates in the V3 loop and flanking regions (NH$_2$ and COOH termini). Isolates obtained from 5 asymptomatic HIV-1 carriers and 5 AIDS patients were included in the study. The percentage figures next to the vertical axis indicate the maximum intrapatient variation found within that region. The loop comprises 35 amino acids; 25 amino acids were sequenced in the NH$_2$ terminus and 17 in the COOH portion.

drug *in vitro*.[52,53] A study is in progress in our laboratory to understand whether CSF HIV-1 isolates of AIDS patients under AZT treatment become resistant to the drug and if HIV-1-resistant isolates from the brain are characterized by the same RT mutations present in resistant blood isolates (Di Stefano *et al.*, unpublished data).

Amino acids 20 to 250 of the RT gene of blood and CSF isolates from five patients, obtained before and up to 39 months after therapy, have been directly sequenced after PCR amplification of cultured material. The sequence analysis revealed that the amino acid substitution involved in AZT resistance can also be found in CSF isolates (Table 1). Interestingly, in two of the patients (No. 2 and 3), different patterns of mutations could be found in the HIV-1 from blood and brain compartments 27 and 29 months post-therapy, respectively. This finding agrees

Table 1. Reverse transcriptase mutations in paired blood and CSF isolates from AZT-treated patients.

Patient No.	Months of AZT	Blood Isolates 41 67 70 215 219					CSF Isolates 41 67 70 215 219				
1	0	W	W	W	W	W	W	W	W	W	W
	22	W	W	W	W	W	W	W	W	W	W
	35	W	W	W	W	W	W	W	W	W	W
2	0	W	W	W	W	W	W	W	W	W	W
	27	W	W	M	W	W	M	M	M	M	W
3	0	W	W	W	W	W	W	W	W	W	W
	29	W	W	M	M	W	W	W	M	W	W
	39	W	W	M	M	W	W	W	M	M	W
4	0	W	W	W	W	W	W	W	W	W	W
	13	M	W	W	M	M	M	W	W	M	W
5	0	W	W	W	W	W	W	W	W	W	W
	5	W	W	W	W	W	W	W	W	W	W
	29	W	M	M	M	M	W	M	M	M	M

W = wild type
M = mutated

with the results obtained from the V3 study, and shows that the HIV-1 population present in CSF at a certain timepoint can be different from the genotypes found in the blood. A dissimilarity in drug concentrations between the brain and blood tissues is likely to account for these differences. Moreover, the pattern of mutations found in the viruses isolated from the two patients may indeed indicate targeting to and replication in tissue-specific cell types. It has to be pointed out that the anabolic phosphorylation pathway of AZT, necessary to exert its anti-HIV activity, is different in activated lymphocytes or resting macrophages.[54]

The genetic distance of the RT proteins of paired blood and CSF isolates can add information about diversification and/or adaptation in the nervous tissue. Targets for neutralizing antibodies and markers for virus tropism have not been described to lie within these sequences and, therefore, variation may be ascribed to RT infidelity. An analysis of the HIV-1 RT amino acid sequences from blood and CSF over approximately 2.5-year period is shown in Figure 2 for two of the patients studied. When the positions directly involved in AZT resistance are excluded from the calculation, the percentage of amino acid variations between isolates obtained from the same compartment over time remains approximately the same (3.7% and 4.2% in patient No. 2, and 4.1% and 4.7% in patient No. 3). Variation was similar (3.7 to 4.2%; 27 months of observation) when comparing blood and CSF isolates over time in patient No. 2, whereas a slight increase of mutated positions was found in patient No. 3, from 3.7 to 6.4% in 29 months. The changes in the RT amino acid sequence within the two separate compartments, apart from the positions involved in AZT resistance, do not appear to follow a linear process.

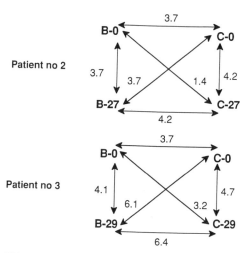

Figure 2. Amino acid differences (expressed in percentage) in the reverse transcriptase sequences of HIV-1 isolates obtained from the blood and CSF of two AIDS patients treated with AZT. B = blood; C = CSF; 0 = pretherapy; 27 and 29 months of AZT therapy. DNA from PBMC infected with the different isolates was used for PCR. The RT-PCR products were directly sequenced in an automated laser sequencer (Pharmacia Biotechnology, AB, Sweden) according to Wahlberg and collaborators.[55] The sequencing primers were RIT 136F (5'-FITC-GATGGA-GTTCATAACCCARCCAAA-3') and RIT227 (5'-FITC-AATCTGTTGACTCAFGATTGG-3')[56].

In conclusion, the sequence analysis of V3 and RT regions from parallel blood and CSF isolates suggests that the variations found in the V3 loop in the two compartments could arise upon distinct immunomodulation events or following tissue adaptation.

FUTURE DIRECTIONS

Culturing lentiviruses induces selection in the virus population present in the tissue.[57] The possibility that replication-competent HIV-1 variants may be selected against during this procedure must be taken into account. To further address the question whether HIV-1 in the brain undergoes a process of selection and adaptation, PCR-amplified envelope fragments from postmortem material will be sequenced. This study will include brain tissue from asymptomatic virus carriers, deceased for causes unrelated to HIV-1 infection, and from AIDS patients. This very valuable material has been obtained within the framework of the European Concerted Action for AIDS Neuropathology from Dr. F. Gray (Hospital Henry Mondor, Creteil, France).

The role of biologically active anti-HIV-1 antibodies in the spread and modulation of infection to and within the brain is a completely unexplored field. Simian immunodeficiency virus (SIV) infection of cynomolgus macaques represents a valuable model to study the pathogenesis of lentivirus infection in humans, including neurologic syndromes. Using combinatorial libraries,[58] we have generated macaque monoclonal Fab fragments[59] with neutralizing activity. Biologically active Fab (or corresponding whole immunoglobulin) will be used to study the role of neutralizing antibodies on virus variability in the brain.

CONCLUSIONS

A number of observations indicate that spread of the virus to the brain is common during HIV-1 infection. The recovery of infectious virus from the CSF of a large number of asymptomatics,[2] and the expression of HIV-1 proteins in cells of the macrophage/microglia lineage in the brain of the majority of autopsied patients,[25] suggest that neuroinvasiveness is a common property of HIV-1 isolates. HIV-1 macrophage-tropic variants can be found in the blood of the majority of asymptomatic virus carriers.[18] The major target cells for HIV-1 within the brain are microglial cells, which share origin and surface markers with monocyte/macrophage cells present in other tissues.[60,61] Viruses that reach the nervous system early during the infection should, therefore, be fully competent to initiate infection of the brain parenchyma.

Accordingly, if the term "neurotropic variants" is to be applied to the HIV-1 variants present early during infection, a proportion of the virus quasispecies found in all patients has these characteristics or, rather, its macrophage-tropic property allows establishment of the infection in the brain. Yet, very little is known about the functions and characteristics of microglia. It cannot be excluded that HIV-1 replication in these cells may be under the control of specific cellular factors unique to these cells. Cellular transcription factors that bind to the long terminal repeat (LTR) sequences of the virus genome have been shown to alter HIV-1 expression *in vitro*.[62] Several studies conducted *in vitro* have shown that cell lines of neural origin can be infected by HIV-1.[63-65] If additional cell types are infected in the brain via molecules other than CD4, a new virus population -- the real neurotropic strain -- may emerge which may then be adsorbed onto cellular receptors. Future efforts should be directed toward identifying the molecular determinants for the adaptation of HIV-1 variants in brain tissue.

Acknowledgements

This study was supported by grants from the Swedish Medical Research Council, Swedish Physicians Against AIDS, and the Swedish Society of Medicine. The authors would like to thank Dr. E.M. Fenyö for critical reading of the manuscript and the coauthors of the studies presented in this paper: Drs. M. Dubois-Dalcq, S. Wilt, L. Hagberg, G. Norkrans, A. Samuelsson, and B. Keys.

REFERENCES

1. J.A. Levy, J. Shimabukuro, H. Hollander, J. Mills, and L. Kaminsky. Isolation of AIDS-associated retroviruses from cerebrospinal fluid and brain of patients with neurological symptoms. *Lancet* ii:586 (1985).
2. F. Chiodi, B. Keys, J. Albert, L. Hagberg, J. Lundeberg, M. Uhlén, E.M. Fenyö, and G. Norkrans. Human immunodeficiency virus type 1 is present in the cerebrospinal fluid of a majority of infected individuals. *J. Clin. Microbiol.* 30:1768 (1992).
3. H. Budka, G. Costanzi, S. Cristina, A. Lechi, C. Parravicini, R. Trabattoni, and L. Vago. Brain pathology induced by infection with the human immunodeficiency virus (HIV). A histological, immunocytochemical, and electron microscopical study of 100 autopsy cases. *Acta Neuropathol.* 75:185 (1987).
4. C.A. Wiley, R.D. Schrier, J.A. Nelson, P.W. Lampert, and M.B.A. Oldstone. Cellular localization of the human immunodeficiency virus infection within the brains of acquired immunodeficiency syndrome patients. *Proc. Natl. Acad. Sci. USA* 83:7089 (1986).
5. S. Koenig, H.E. Gendelman, J.M. Orenstein, M.C. Dal Canto, G.H. Pezeshkpour, M. Yungbluth, F. Janotta, A. Aksamit, M.A. Martin, and A.S. Fauci. Detection of AIDS virus in macrophages in brain tissue from AIDS patients with encephalopathy. *Science* 233:1089 (1986).
6. G. Nuovo -- this volume.
7. L.C. Cork, W.J. Hadlow, J.R. Gorham, R.C. Piper, and T.B. Crawford. Pathology of viral leukoencephalomyelitis of goats. *Acta Neuropathol.* 29:281 (1974).
8. B. Sigurdsson, P.A. Palsson, and H. Grimson. Visna, a demyelinating transmissible disease of sheep. *J. Neuropathol. Exp. Neurol.* 16:389 (1957).
9. G. Petursson, N. Nathanson, G. Georgsson, H. Panitch, and P.A. Palsson. Pathogenesis of Visna. I. Sequential virologic, serologic and pathologic studies. *Lab. Invest.* 35:402 (1976).
10. J.A. Levy. Pathogenesis of human immunodeficiency virus infection. *Microbiol. Rev.* 57:183 (1993).
11. B.A. Navia, and R.W. Price. The acquired immunodeficiency dementia complex as the presenting or sole manifestation of human immunodeficiency virus infection. *Arch. Neurol.* 44:65 (1987).
12. P.F. Szurek, P.H. Yuen, J.K. Ball, and P.K.Y. Wong. A Val-25-to Ile substitution in the envelope precursor polyprotein, gPr80env, and neurovirulence of ts1, a mutant of Moloney murine leukemia virus TB. *J. Virol.* 64:467 (1990).
13. Y. Paquette, Z. Hanna, P. Savard, R. Brousseas, Y. Robitaille, and P. Jolicoeur. Retrovirus-induced murine motor neuron disease: mapping the determinant of spongiform degeneration within the envelope gene. *Proc. Natl. Acad. Sci. USA* 86:3896 (1989).
14. M. Masuda, P.M. Hoffman, S.K. Ruscetti. Viral determinants that control the neuropathogenicity of PVC-211 murine leukemia virus in vivo determine brain capillary endothelial cell tropism of the virus in vitro. *J. Virol.* 67:4580 (1993).
15. H. Hollander, and J.A. Levy. Neurologic abnormalities and recovery of human immunodeficiency virus from cerebrospinal fluid. *Ann. Intern. Med.* 106:692 (1987).
16. D.A. Cooper, J. Gold, P. Maclean, B. Donovan, R. Finlayson, T.G. Barnes, H.M. Michelmore, P. Brooke, and R. Penny. Acute AIDS retrovirus infection: definition of a clinical illness associated with seroconversion. *Lancet* i:537 (1985).
17. T.F.W. Wolfs, G. Zwart, M. Bakker, and J,. Goudsmit. HIV-1 genomic RNA diversification following sexual and parenteral virus transmission. *Virology* 189:103 (1992).
18. H. Schuitemaker, M. Koot, N.A. Kootstra, M.W. Dercksen, R.E.Y. de Goede, R.P. van Steenwijk, J.M.A. Lange, J.K.M. Eeftink-Schattenkerk, F. Miedema, and M. Tersemette. Biological phenotype of human immuno-

deficiency virus type 1 clones at different stages of infection: progression of disease is associated with a shift from monocytotropic to T-cell-tropic virus populations. *J. Virol.* 66:1354 (1992).

19. T. Zhu, H., Mo, N. Wang, D.S. Nam, Y. Cao, R.A. Koup, and D.D. Ho. Genotypic and phenotypic characterization of HIV-1 in patients with primary infection. *Science* 261:1179 (1993).

20. B.A. Watkins, H.H. Dorn, W.B. Kelly, R.C.Armstrong, B. Potts, F. Michael, C.V. Kufta, and M. Dubois-Dalcq. Specific tropism of HIV-1 for microglial cells in primary human brain cultures. *Science* 249:549 (1990).

21. C.A. Jordan, B.A. Watkins, C. Kufta, and M. Dubois-Dalcq. Infection of brain microglial cells by human immunodeficiency virus type 1 is CD4-dependent. *J. Virol.* 65:736 (1991).

22. Y. Koyanagi, S. Miles, R.T. Mitsuyasu, J.E. Merrill, H.V. Vinters, and I.S.Y. Chen. Dual infection of the central nervous system by AIDS viruses with distinct cellular tropism. *Science* 236:819 (1987).

23. N.E. Sharpless, W.A. O'Brien, E. Verdin, C.F. Kufta, I.S.Y. Chen, and M. Dubois-Dalcq. Human immunodeficiency virus type 1 tropism for brain microglial cells is determined by a region of the env glycoprotein that also controls macrophage tropism. *J. Virol.* 66:2588 (1992).

24. F. Gray, M.C. Lescs, C. Keohane, F. Paraire, B., Marc, M. Durigon, and R. Gheradi. Early brain changes in HIV infection. Neuropathological study of 11 HIV-seropositive, non-AIDS cases. *J. Neuropathol. Exp. Neurol.* 51:177 (1992).

25. H. Budka. Human immunodeficiency virus (HIV) envelope and core proteins in CNS tissues of patients with the acquired immune deficiency syndrome (AIDS). *Acta Neuropathol.* 79:611 (1990).

26. J. Embretson, M. Zupancic, J. Beneke, M. Till, S. Wolinsky, J.L.Ribas, A. Burke, and A.T. Haase. Analysis of human immunodeficiency virus-infected tissues by amplification and *in situ* hybridization reveals latent and permissive infections at single-cell resolution. *Proc. Natl. Acad. Sci. USA* 90:357 (1993).

27. J. Goudsmit, N.K.T. Back, and P.L. Nara. Genomic diversity and antigenic variation of HIV-1: links between pathogenesis, epidemiology and vaccine development. *FASEB J.* 5:2427 (1991).

28. B.H. Hahn, G.M. Shaw, M.E. Taylor, R.R. Redfield, P.D. Markham, S.Z. Salahuddin, F. Wong-Staal, R.C. Gallo, E.S. Parks, and W.P. Parks. Genetic variation in HTLV-III/LAV over time in patients with AIDS or at risk for AIDS. *Science* 232:1548 (1986).

29. W.-S. Hu, and H.M. Temin. Genetic consequences of packaging two RNA genomes in one retroviral particle: pseudodiploidy and high rate of genetic recombination. *Proc. Natl. Acad. Sci. USA* 87:1556 (1990).

30. B.R.Starcich, B.H. Hahn, G.M. Shaw, P.D. McNeely, S. Modrow, H. Wolf, E.S. Parks, W.P. Parks, S.F. Josephs, R.C. Gallo, and F. Wong-Staal. Identification and characterization of conserved and variable regions in the envelope gene of HTLV-III/LAV, the retrovirus of AIDS. *Cell* 45:637 (1986).

31. G.J. LaRosa, J.P.Davide, K. Weinhold, J.A. Waterbury, A.T. Profy, J.A. Lewis, A.J. Langlois, Dreesman G.R., R.N. Boswell, P. Shadduck, L.H. Holley, M. Karplus, D.P. Bolognesi, T.J. Matthews, E.A. Emini, and S.D. Putney. Conserved sequences and structural elements in the HIV-1 principal neutralizing determinant. *Science* 249:932 (1990).

32. T.J. Palker, M.E. Clark, A.J. Langlois, T.J. Matthews, K.J,. Weinhold, R.R. Randall, D.P. Bolognesi, and B.F. Haynes. Type-specific neutralization of the human immunodeficiency virus with antibodies to env-encoded synthetic peptides. *Proc. Natl. Acad. Sci. USA* 85:1932 (1988).

33. J.R. Rusche, K. Javaherian, C. McDanal, J. Pedtro, D. Lynn. R. Grimaila, A. Langlois, R.C. Gallo, L.O. Arthur, P.J. Fischinger, D.P. Bolognesi, S.D. Putney, and T.J. Matthews. Antibodies that inhibit fusion of human immunodeficiency virus-infected cells bind a 24-amino acid sequence of the viral envelope, gp120. *Proc. Natl. Acad. Sci. USA* 85:3198 (1988).

34. T. Hattori, A. Koito, K. Takatsuki, H. Kido, and N. Katanuma. Involvement

of tryptase-related cellular protease(s) in human immunodeficiency virus type 1 infection. *FEBS Lett.* 248:48 (1989).

35. B. Chesebro, J. Nishio, S. Perryman, A. Cann, W. O'Brien, I.S.Y. Chen, and K. Wehrly. Identification of human immunodeficiency virus envelope gene sequences influencing viral entry into CD4-positive HeLa cells, T-leukemia cells, and macrophages. *J. Virol.* 65:5782 (1991).

36. S.S. Hwang, T.J. Boyle, H.K. Lyerly, and B.R. Cullen. Identification of the envelope V3 loop as the primary determinant of cell tropism in HIV-1. *Science* 253:71 (1991).

37. P. Westervelt, D.B. Trowbridge, L.G. Epstein, B.M,.Blumberg, Y. Li, B.H. Hahn, G.M. Shaw, R.W. Price, and L. Ratner. Macrophage tropism determinants of human immunodeficiency virus type 1 in vivo. *J. Virol.* 66:2577 (1992).

38. E.M.Fenyö, M.L. Morfeldt, F.Chiodi, B. Lind, A. von Gegerfelt, J. Albert, E. Olausson, B. Asjö. Distinct replicative and cytopathic characteristics of human immunodeficiency virus isolates. *J. Virol.* 62:4414 (1988).

39. M. Tersmette, R.E. de Goede, B.J. Al, I.N. Winkel, R.A. Gruters, H.T. Cuypers, H.G. Huisman, and F. Miedema. Differential syncytium-inducing capacity of human immunodeficiency virus isolates: frequent detection of syncytium-inducing isolates in patients with acquired immunodeficiency syndrome (AIDS) and AIDS-related complex. *J. Virol.* 62:2026 (1988).

40. M. Tersmette, R.A. Gruters, F. de Wolf, R.E. de Goede, J.M. Lange, P.T. Schellekens, J. Goudsmit, H.G. Huisman, and F. Miedema. Evidence of a role of virulent human immunodeficiency virus (HIV) strains in the pathogenesis of acquired immunodeficiency syndrome obtained from studies on a panel of sequential HIV isolates. *J. Virol.* 63:2118, 1989.

41. R.A. Fouchier, M. Groenink, N.A. Kootstra, M. Tersmette, H.G. Huisman, F. Midema, and H. Schuitemaker. Phenotype-associated sequence variation in the third variable domain of the human immunodeficiency virus type 1 gp120 molecule. *J. Virol.* 66:3183 (1992).

42. M. Groenink, R.A.M. Fouchier, S. Broersen, C.H. Baker, M. Koot, A.B. van't Wout, H.G. Huisman, F. Miedema, M. Tersmette, and H. Schuitemaker. Relation of phenotype evolution of HIV-1 to envelope V2 configuration. *Science* 260:1513 (1993).

43. S. Bath, S.L. Spitalnid, F. Gonzales-Scarano, and D.H. Silberberg. Galactosyl ceramide or a derivative is an essential component of the neural receptor for human immunodeficiency virus type 1 envelope glycoprotein gp120. *Proc. Natl. Acad. Sci. USA* 88:7131 (1991).

44. B. Keys, J. Karis, N. Fadeel, A. Valentin, G. Norkrans, L. Hagberg, and F. Chiodi. V3 sequences of paired HIV-1 isolated from blood and cerebrospinal fluid cluster according to host and show variation related to the clinical stage of disease. *Virology* 196:475 (1993).

45. L.G. Epstein, C. Kuiken, B.M. Blumberg, S. Hartman, L.R. Sharer, M. Clement, and J. Goudsmit. HIV-1 V3 domain variation in brain and spleen of children with AIDS: tissue-specific evolution within host-determined quasispecies. *Virology* 180:583 (1990).

46. J. Albert and E.M. Fenyö. Simple, sensitive, and specific detection of human immunodeficiency virus type 1 in clinical specimens by polymerase chain reaction with nested primers. *J. Clin. Microbiol.* 28:1560 (1990).

47. G. Myers, B. Korber, J.A. Berzofsky, R.F. Smith, and G.N. Pavlakis. Human retroviruses and AIDS 1992. *Theoretical Biology and Biophysics*, Los Alamos (1992).

48. F. Sanger, S. Nicklen, and A.R. Coulson. DNA sequencing with chain-terminating inhibitors. *Proc. Natl. Acad. Sci. USA* 74:5463 (1988).

49. A. Von Gegerfelt, F. Chiodi, B. Keys, G. Norkrans, L. Hagberg, E.M.Fenyö, and K. Broliden. Lack of autologous neutralizing antibodies in the cerebrospinal fluid of HIV-1 infected individuals. *AIDS Res. Retroviruses* 8:1133 (1992).

50. B.T. M. Korber, R.M. Farber, D.H.Wolpert, and A.S. Lapedes. Covariation of

mutations in the V3 loop of human immunodeficiency virus type 1 envelope protein: an information theoretic analysis. *Proc. Natl. Acad Sci. USA* 90:7176 (1993).

51. W.-H. Li, M. Tanimura, and P.M. Sharp. Rates and dates of divergence between AIDS virus nucleotide sequences. *Mol. Biol. Evol.* 5:313 (1988).

52. B.A. Larder, and S.D. Kemp. Multiple mutations in HIV-1 reverse transcriptase confer high-level resistance to zidovudine (AZT). *Science* 246: 1155 (1989).

53. P. Kellam, C.A.B. Boucher, and B.A. Larder. Fifth mutation in human immunodeficiency virus type 1 reverse transcriptase contributes to the development of high-level resistance to zidovudine. *Proc. Natl. Acad. Sci. USA* 89:1934 (1992).

54. B. Kierdaszuk, and S. Eriksson. Selective inactivation of the deoxyadenosine phosphorylating activity of pure human deoxycytidine kinase stabilization of different forms of the enzyme by suubstrates and biological detergents. *Biochemistry* 29:4109 (1990).

55. J. Wahlberg, J. Albert, J. Lundeberg, S. Cox, B. Wahren, and M. Uhlen. Dynamic changes in HIV-1 quasispecies from azidothymidine (AZT)-treated patients. *FASEB J.* 6:2843 (1992).

56. J. Wahlberg, J. Fiore, J. Angarano, M,. Uhlen, and J. Albert. Apparent selection against transmission of AZT resistant HIV-1 variants. *J. Infect. Dis.*169:611 (1994).

57. S. Meyerhans, R. Cheynier, J. Albert, M. Seth, S. Kwok, J. Sninsky, L. Morfeldt-Månson,B. Asjö, and S. Wain-Hobson. Temporal fluctuations in HIV quasispecies in vivo are not reflected by sequential isolations. *Cell* 48:901 (1992).

58. C.F. Barbas III, A.S. Kang, R.A. Lerner, and S.J. Benkovic. Assembly of combinatorial antibody libraries on phage surfaces: the gene III site. *Proc. Natl. Acad. Sci. USA* 88:7978 (1991).

59. A. Samuelsson, F. Chiodi, E. Norny, and M.A. Persson. Macaque monoclonal Fab molecules derived from a combinatorial library are specific for the SIV envelope glycoprotein, *in:* "Vaccine 94," Cold Spring Harbor Laboratories, in press.

60. W.F. Hickey, and H. Kimura. Perivascular microglial cells of the CNS are bone marrow-derived and present antigen in vivo. *Science* 239:290 (1988).

61. V.H. Perry and S. Gordon. Macrophages and microglia in the nervous system. *Trends Neurosci.* 11:2273 (1988).

62. R.B. Gaynor. Intracellular factors influencing HIV replication, *in:* "Focus on HIV," H.C. Neu, J.A. Levy, R.A. Weiss, eds., Churchill Livingstone, London (1993).

63. C. Cheng-Mayer, J.T. Rutka, M.L. Rosenblum, T. McHugh, D.P. Stites, and J.A. Levy. Human immunodeficiency virus can productively infect cultured human glial cells. *Proc. natl. Acad. Sci. USA* 84:3526 (1987).

64. F. Chiodi, S. Fuerstenberg, M. Gidlund, B. Åsjö, E.M. Fenyö. Infection of brain-derived cells with the human immunodeficiency virus. *J. Virol.* 61:1244 (1987).

65. C. Tornatore, A. Nath, K. Amemiya, and E.O. Major. Persistent HIV-1 infection in human fetal glial cells reactivated by T cell factor(s) or cytokines, tumor necrosis factor-alpha and interleukin-1 beta. *J. Virol.* 65:6094 (1991).

SEQUENCE ANALYSIS OF NEUROINVASIVE AND BLOOD-DERIVED HIV-1 *NEF* GENES

Ruth Brack-Werner, Thomas Görblich, Thomas Werner,[1]
Francesca Chiodi,[2] Lutz Gürtler,[3] Josef Eberle,[3] Annemarie
Schön, and Volker Erfle

Institut für Molekulare Virologie, and
[1]Institut für Säugetiergenetik, GSF
D-85764 Oberschleissheim,
Neuherberg, Germany
[2]Department of Virology, Karolinska Institute
S-10521 Stockholm, Sweden
[3]Max von Pettenkofer Institute, University of Munich
D-880336 Munich, Germany

INTRODUCTION

Neurological disease associated with acquired immune deficiency syndrome (AIDS) relates to the presence of human immunodeficiency virus-1 (HIV-1) in the central nervous system (CNS). In support, HIV-1, like other lentiviruses, invades the CNS and can be readily isolated from cerebrospinal fluid (CSF) and brain of HIV-infected individuals. Several studies have identified large amounts of HIV-1 proviral DNA in the brain, indicating that the brain may constitute a reservoir for the virus.[1,2]

A question of considerable interest has been whether HIV-1 evolves separately in the CNS and peripheral blood, and whether different selection pressures govern formation of distinct quasispecies populations in each compartment. These selection pressures are expected to be reflected in the tissue-specific conservation of viral sequence motifs required for invasion and replication of HIV in each cellular compartment. Virus strains isolated from blood and CNS have been found to differ in their capacity to replicate in various cell types. This led to the concept that HIV-1 strains in CNS are predominantly macrophage-tropic, whereas those in blood are mainly T-lymphotropic, mirroring the predominant HIV-producing cell type of each compartment.

HIV entry into a cell is governed by interaction of viral envelope proteins with host-cell surface receptors. Therefore, the envelope gene is an important determinant of cellular tropism. Persistence of HIV in the CNS has been equated with its capacity to replicate in neural tissue, leading to the concept of "neurotropic" variants The envelope gene has thus been a target for investigating the genetic basis of neurotropism.[3-5] These studies indicate sequestration and separate evolution of HIV in blood and CNS within an HIV-infected individual. However, this conclusion still remains to be confirmed by independent sequence data derived for other regions of the HIV genome.

Technical Advances in AIDS Research in the Human Nervous System
Edited by E.O. Major and J.A. Levy, Plenum Press, New York, 1995

The *nef* Gene: A Potential Determinant for Viral Replication and Pathogenesis in Blood and CNS

Another possible determinant of virus replication in HIV-infected individuals is the *nef* gene. Within the viral genome, the *nef* gene is unique in that it overlaps with the HIV long-term repeat (LTR), containing several DNA binding sites for modulators of HIV LTR activity, as well as coding for a protein, which is expressed early in the virus' life cycle. *In vitro* studies have indicated many different functions of Nef protein, including suppression or enhancement of virus replication, down-regulation of cell surface CD4 expression, direct or indirect influence on HIV-LTR activity and involvement in signal transduction pathways (reviewed in refs. 6,7). In some cases, Nef has even been shown to be indispensable for HIV replication *in vitro*. Nef exhibits pleiotropic functions which may differ with respect to target cell, viral genetic context and localization in cellular compartments. However, experiments in simian immune virus (SIV)-infected rhesus macaques showed maintenance of high virus burden and immune dysfunction required presence of an intact *nef* gene.[8] Therefore, Nef seems to play a crucial role *in vivo* in viral replication and pathogenesis, at least for SIV.

There are several lines of evidence that Nef may also be involved in persistence and pathogenesis of HIV-1 in the CNS. Chronically HIV-1-infected nonproducer astrocytoma cell lines have been found to express much higher levels of Nef than stably HIV-1-infected T-lymphoma or fibroblasts.[9] In agreement with the generally nonproductive phenotype observed for HIV-1-infected glial cells (reviewed in ref. 10), viral structural proteins are expressed at only very low levels in these glial cell lines. This predominant expression of Nef protein may be indicative of a restricted infection phenotype in brain cells, in which virus replication has been arrested at an early stage of the viral life cycle. Detection of Nef *in vivo* has been complicated by the existence of cellular proteins which cross-react with antibodies against Nef,[11] the lack of unique *nef*-specific mRNA probes for *in situ* hybridization and the difficulties inherent in simultaneously detecting Nef and cell-specific markers for unambiguous identification of target cells. However, expression of Nef protein in astrocytes *in vivo* is suggested by several recent reports of immunohistochemical staining of brain sections from AIDS patients with anti-Nef antibodies.[7,12,13]

Sequence comparisons of HIV-1 LAI Nef and cellular proteins led to identification of a potential neuroactive domain shared by Nef and scorpion neuroactive peptides known to interact with potassium channels. Patch-clamp analysis revealed that peptides derived both from the neuroactive domain of Nef and from a representative scorpion neurotoxin reversibly increased the total voltage-dependent potassium current of chicken dorsal root ganglia without killing the cells.[14] This effect was shared by recombinant Nef protein. These results suggest that Nef is a potential neuropathogenic factor, affecting neuronal cell function in a manner similar to scorpion neurotoxins which are not cytotoxic.

For further investigation of the potential role of Nef *in vivo*, we analyzed *nef* gene sequences from brain tissue as well as from paired HIV-1 isolates from blood and CSF of the same patients. We compared *nef* gene sequences derived from CNS and blood to assess whether separate virus populations exist in each cellular compartment. In addition, the *nef* gene was analyzed for tissue-specific conservation, indicative of selection for neurotropic or lymphotropic Nef functions, respectively.

General Methodology

A schematic of the methodology involved is given in Fig. 1. Briefly, HIV-1 was isolated from CSF or blood of HIV-1-infected individuals by cocultivation of patient material with peripheral blood mononuclear cells (PBMCs). *Nef* genes were obtained from HIV isolates in PBMCs containing first-passage virus (C-isolates) or from multiple-passage virus propagated in H9 cells after isolation in PBMCs (G-isolates). Alternatively, virus sequences were amplified from high molecular weight DNA extracted from brains of deceased AIDS patients. Nef-

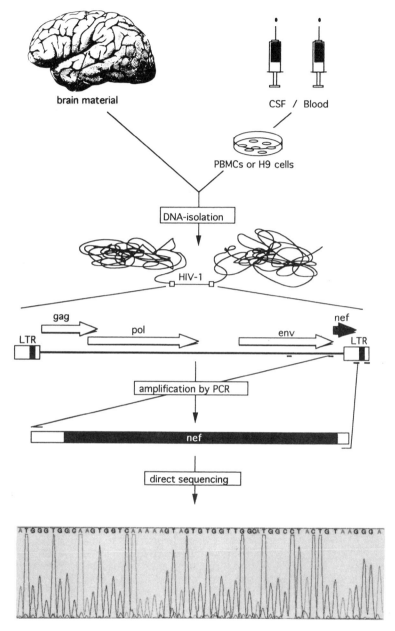

Figure 1. General methodology for analysis of *nef* gene sequences from patient material. HIV-1 was isolated from CSF or blood from HIV-infected individuals by cocultivation with PBMCs. *Nef* genes were either amplified directly from cell lysates of these PBMCs (first-passage virus: C-isolates) or from high molecular weight DNA isolated after further propagation of HIV-1 isolates in H9 cells (multiple-passage virus: G-isolates). For *ex vivo* analysis of *nef* genes from brain, high molecular weight DNA was isolated from various regions of the brain. *Nef* genes amplified by two-step PCR were directly sequenced by dideoxy chain termination method, using fluorescent labelled dideoxynucleotide triphosphates and Taq polymerase.

-containing polymerase chain reaction (PCR) amplification products were sequenced directly without additional cloning steps to obtain the sequence of the predominant virus variant in each sample.

Isolation of HIV-1 from CSF and Blood

HIV-1 isolates were obtained by short-term cocultivation of PBMCs (isolates G2B, G4B, C14B) or CSF (G1L, G3L, C11L, C15L, C17L) or brain (frontal lobe: G5H) from 7 patients with PHA-stimulated PBMCs from normal blood donors. Isolation procedures for C-isolates are described in more detail in Keys et al.[15] HIV-1 isolates G1L, G2B, G3L, G4B, and G5H were propagated further on H9 cells. Clinical features of the HIV-1 infected subjects are shown in Table 1.

Table 1. HIV Isolates

Sequence Code	Source of isolate	Patient	Clinical Condition	Years from sero-conversion
G1L	CSF	c	AIDS (pediatric);	2
G2B	Blood		neurologic symptoms	
G3L	CSF	h	AIDS (adult);	6
G4B	Blood		neurologic symptoms	
G5H	Brain	i	AIDS	unknown
C11L	CSF	b	CDC class II	2
C13L	CSF	g	CDC class II	unknown
C14B	Blood			
C15L	CSF	e	AIDS/CDC class IV	6
C17L	CSF	k	AIDS/CDC class IV	unknown

Ex vivo analysis of nef Genes in Brain Samples

For direct assessment of *nef* genes in CNS *in vivo*, high molecular weight genomic DNA was extracted from frozen brain tissue homogenized in liquid nitrogen.[16] Three brains were analyzed, two of which showed no neuropathologic evidence of productive HIV-1 infection and one with visible signs of HIV encephalopathy (Table 2). Since we have previously found evidence for nonhomogeneous distribution of HIV in brain, samples were taken from 11 different regions of each brain.

PCR Amplification of nef Genes

Primers for amplification of *nef* genes were designed to bind to conserved sequences flanking *nef* from the *env* gene and the LTR, resulting in a product of approximately 770 bp (positions 8281-9050 of HIV-1 LAI[17]). Conditions for PCR reactions were established with high molecular weight genomic DNA from chronically HIV-1-infected glial cells.[9] Under these conditions, *nef* PCR reaction products were obtained only with purified genomic DNA containing multiple-passage HIV-1 isolates propagated in H9 cells (G isolates). There was some heterogeneity with respect to the size of the amplification product, the isolate from brain (G5H), yielding a somewhat larger fragment than the other isolates.

Table 2. Brain Samples From HIV-1 Infected Patients

Sequence Code	Location in Brain	Patient	Neuropathology of CNS
8a 8d	midbrain medulla oblongata	d	HIV-encephalitis negative; lymphoma
10e	cerebellum	f	no morphological changes
11a 11d	medulla oblongata basal ganglia	a	HIV encephalopathy; un-specific nodules; vacuolar myelopathy

The amounts of amplification product varied from one isolate to the other, and the weakest product was obtained for G2B. This suggests variation in numbers of target sequences in the primary samples. For enhanced sensitivity, a two-step nested PCR amplification procedure was established. In the initial step, a 1.9 kb *env*/LTR region (positions 7389-178 of HIV-1 LAI[17]) was amplified, which was then used as target for amplification of the nef gene fragment in a second step. This procedure yielded high levels of *nef* fragment for G2B.

PCR amplification of *nef* genes from HIV-1 isolates

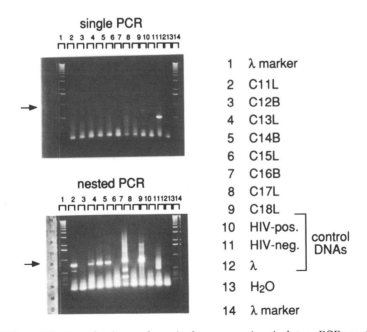

single PCR

1 2 3 4 5 6 7 8 9 10 11 12 13 14

nested PCR

1 2 3 4 5 6 7 8 9 10 11 12 13 14

1	λ marker
2	C11L
3	C12B
4	C13L
5	C14B
6	C15L
7	C16B
8	C17L
9	C18L
10	HIV-pos.
11	HIV-neg.
12	λ
13	H₂O
14	λ marker

control DNAs (lanes 9–12)

Figure 2. PCR amplification of *nef* genes from single-passage virus isolates. PCR reactions were carried out with cell lysates from PBMCs containing single-passage virus isolates (C-isolates) from blood (B) or CSF (L). High molecular weight control DNAs were obtained from chronically HIV-1 infected (HIV-positive) or uninfected (HIV-negative) glial cells or from phage λ. Location of *nef* amplification product is indicated by an arrow.

Nested PCR with whole-cell extracts from PBMCs yielded high-level amplification products for several first-passage virus isolates, although these were negative in single-step PCR (Fig. 2). More than one discrete PCR fragment ≤770 bp was obtained with samples C11L and C17L. Sequence analysis of the 300-bp product of C17L revealed a truncated *nef* gene, containing only the first 80 nucleotides. Interestingly, the sequence of the truncated product was identical with the sequence of the full-length *nef* gene determined for this sample.

One-step PCR with genomic DNA from various locations of three brains did not reveal *nef* amplification products. An example of nested PCR analysis of various samples from the same brain is shown in Figure 3. We found extensive variation in reactivities of high molecular weight DNA samples derived from different locations of a single brain in nested PCR. In summary, samples from midbrain (a) and medulla oblongata (d) of brain 8, cerebellum (e) of brain 10, and medulla oblongata (a) and basal ganglia (d) of brain 11 yielded amplification products in at least two independent PCR reactions. Positive results obtained from the pons of brain 8 and hippocampus and temporal cortex of brain 11 could not be reproduced in a second independent PCR reaction. Presence of virus in *nef*-positive samples has been confirmed by an independent PCR approach involving evaluation of results from multiple amplification reactions with primers targeted to the *gag* gene. Lack of consistent amplification of *nef* gene from these samples may reflect extremely low copy numbers of target molecules.

PCR amplification of *nef* genes from brain samples

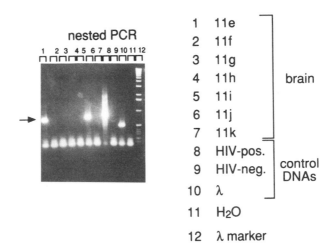

Figure 3. Heterogeneity of PCR amplification of HIV-1 *nef* genes for samples from different locations of brain from an AIDS patients. Nested PCR reactions for amplification of HIV-1 *nef* genes were carried out for samples from different regions of brain 11. For control DNAs, see legend to Figure 2. Location of *nef* amplification product is indicated by an arrow.

Analysis of *nef* Genes by Direct Sequence Analysis of PCR Products

Nef sequences were assessed by direct sequence analysis of amplified proviral DNA. The sequence information obtained in this manner reflects the consensus sequence of the predominant variant existing in the sample. This is a major advantage over isolation of molecular clones of the amplified product for sequence analysis. In this case, each clone represents only one amplified DNA molecule. Thus, numerous clones must be sequenced to determine the frequency with which each sequence is represented in the sample. In addition, sequences obtained from cloned PCR products may reflect errors made by the Taq polymerase, which has an error rate of approximately 1 in 9,000 nucleotides.[18] Since each misincorporation is generally contained in a small subgroup of amplified molecules (maximally 25%),[19] direct sequence analysis minimizes these errors. Finally, cloning in *E. coli* may represent an artificial level of selection, since not all sequences may be cloned and propagated with equal efficiency, and some may not be amenable to cloning in *E. coli*-based vector systems.

For direct sequence analysis, PCR amplification products were purified by spin dialysis. Multiple amplification products obtained for C17L were separated by high-pressure liquid chromatography[20] prior to sequence analysis. Sequence analysis was carried out by the method of dideoxy-mediated chain termination, using fluorescent labelled dideoxynucleotide triphosphates and Taq polymerase. Sequence reactions were analyzed on an Applied Biosystems Sequencer. Six primers were used for sequence analysis of each amplification product, largely covering both strands of the *nef* gene. Two independent *nef* amplification products were sequenced for each HIV-1 isolate. Both products yielded identical results.

Results from independent analysis of two amplification products from brain samples yielded ambiguous results for 1.1% (8d), 1.6% (11a, 11d), and 3.1% (8a) of the nucleotide positions. Therefore, a renewed sequence analysis of a third independent PCR product was carried out for 8a, 11a, and 11d. For each ambiguous position, the nucleotide determined in the third analysis agreed with one of the previously determined nucleotides. No new ambiguities were detected.

Direct sequence analysis of PCR products will only yield unambiguous results as long as the amplification product contains a major population of uniform molecules. This seemed to be the case of amplification of proviral DNA from samples containing HIV-1 isolated from patient material. However, the population of amplified molecules derived from brain was more heterogeneous. This indicates the coexistence of two or more major subpopulations in the brain samples which are amplified at similar frequencies.

Nef Genes from Patient Material Contain Open-Reading Frames of Variable Lengths

A total of 15 samples derived from 10 patients were analyzed. Each sample contained a *nef* gene with a full-length open-reading frame. Two samples yielded additional *nef* amplification products (see above). In a separate study analyzing 11 pediatric patients with AIDS, the *nef* reading frame was found to be open in 92% of *nef*-containing molecular clones derived from both brain and lymphocytic tissue.[21] Conservation of Nef protein coding capacity in HIV-1 from patient material argues for an important role for Nef function(s) *in vivo*. Whatever function this may be, it does not seem to be required for *in vitro* virus replication, since laboratory isolates exist in which the *nef* gene is disrupted by a termination codon (e.g., HXB2).[22]

The length of the *nef* gene sequences ranged from 615 (205 a.a.) to 648 (216 a.a.) nucleotides (Figure 4). Sequence alignment showed that heterogeneity in length was localized exclusively in the NH2-terminal region of the nef gene encompassing the first 80 amino acids. Size heterogeneity was especially pronounced in the region between amino acids 20 and 30, which in isolates G5H, C17L, 10e and C15L contained 4-10 amino acids in length (Figure 4).

HIV-1* isolate	Insertion region	length in aa ins.	length in aa nef gene	Source
BRVA	RRAE P A R E R M R R A E P R A E P	14	218	Brain
JRCSF	RRAE R A T D R V R Q T E P	10	216	CSF
JRFL	RRAE P A A D R V R R T E P	10	216	Brain
HIVSF162	KRAE P A E P	3	208	CSF
G5H	RRAE P R Q A E P R R A E P	10	216	CSF
C17L	RRIN P A A E R R T E P	8	216	CSF
10e	HRAE P T A E P	4	212	Brain
C15L	KRAE P Q A E P	4	211	CSF
C13L	ERA E P	-	205	CSF
G3L	RRA E P	-	205	CSF
G1L	RR E P	-	207	CSF
8a	RRA E P	-	207	CSF
8d	RRA E P	-	207	CSF
11a	RRT E P	-	207	CSF
11d	RRT E P	-	207	CSF
C14B	ERA E P	-	205	
G2B	RRT E P	-	205	
G4B	RRA E P	-	206	
HIVLAI, HIVNL43	RRA E P	-	206	
HIVOY1	KRAE L Q P P E P	5	211	
HIVSF2	RRAE P R A E P	4	210	
HIVCAM1	RRAE P R A E P	4	210	Blood
HIVHE120B1	QRAE P A A E P	4	208	
HIVHE128B1	RRA E P	-	207	
HIVHE139B1	RQAE P A E P	3	210	
HIVHE14BL	RRA E P	-	206	
HIVSF33	KRA E P	-	205	
HIVSWB84	KQA E P	-	205	
HIVHAN	KQAE P E P	2	200	
HIVD31	KRA E P	-	205	
HIVRF	KQA E P	-	208	

*Sequences of isolates in bold face were determined in this study.

Figure 4. Larger size of some HIV-1 *nef* genes from CNS can be attributed to sequence insertions at a distinct region. The insertion region comprises amino acids 19-37 in HIV-1 brain isolate HIV-1BR.[22] The lengths of the inserted sequence stretches and the corresponding *nef* genes are given in amino acids.

The longest insertions were observed for G5H and C17L, which had been derived from brain and CSF, respectively. Insertions 10-14 a.a. in length are contained in the HIV-1 isolates HIV-1$_{BR}$[23] and HIV-1JRFL and HIV-1 JRCSF.[24] HIV-1$_{BR}$ and HIV-1JRFL were both isolated from brain tissue of AIDS patients. HIV-1 JRCSF was obtained from the CSF of the same patient used for isolation of HIV-1JRFL. In HIV-1$_{BR}$, the inserted sequence contains a tandem duplication of a 10-amino acid sequence at positions 14-23. In G5H, a.a. 19 to 33 contain 3 almost perfect repeats of the motif RRAEP. No obvious duplications of downstream sequences are found in the inserts of JR isolates and C17L.

Shorter inserts (3-4 a.a.) are contained in the *nef* genes of isolates HIV-SF162 and C15L from CSF and proviral DNA amplified directly from brain material (sample 10e) (Figure 4). No inserted sequences were found in 3 HIV-1 isolates from CSF (C13L, G3L, G1L) and 4 amplified *nef* genes from brain tissue (8a, 8d; 11a, 11d). HIV-1 isolates from blood (n = 15) contain only short inserted sequences in this region (2-5 a.a.), if at all (Figure 4).

Only some *nef* genes from the CSF are distinguishable from blood-borne sequences by the presence of longer sequence inserts (10-14 a.a.). However, their exclusive detection so far in *nef* genes from the CNS suggests that appearance of such inserts may be a genetic indicator of CNS origin of a *nef* gene.

Nef Genes Cluster in a Patient-Specific Rather than A Tissue-Specific Manner

Variation between *nef* gene sequences was investigated by multiple alignments using Gene Works and Genalign programs (Intelligenetics). In addition, sequences of the V3 region of the *env* gene of the HIV-1 isolates in this study were analyzed for comparison. V3-env sequences of C-isolates were taken from

Keys et al.[15] V3-*env* sequences of G-isolates were obtained by direct sequencing of PCR amplification products obtained by two-step PCR.

Nucleotide sequence identities between *nef* genes from HIV-1 isolates and brain samples ranged from 78-99%, with an average identity of 87.3±4.7% (Table 3). Interpatient variability of *nef* gene sequences from the blood did not differ markedly from the CNS. However, paired HIV-1 isolates from blood and CSF of the same patients were highly similar (98±1.0%), as were samples from different regions of the same brain (97%). The sequences of the V3 region show higher variability than the *nef* genes (71.3±14.36%). Again, sequences from blood and CSF showed equivalent levels of similarity and the highest level of similarity was observed between paired HIV-1 isolates from blood and CSF of the same patients (99.3±0.58%). Thus, sequence analysis of two independent regions of the HIV-1 genome indicates a much higher degree of sequence conservation within a patient than within the same tissue from different patients.

Table 3. Percentage of nucleotide identifies in *nef* genes and *env*-V3 sequences.

| | n[b] | Pairwise Identities (%)[a] | |
		nef	V3
Average	105	87.3 ±4.7	71.3± 14.36 (n = 45)
Same Patient			
Blood/CSF	3	98±1.0	99.3±0.58
Brain/Brain	2	97	n.d.[c]
Total	5	87.6±0.9	n.d.[c]
Different Patients			
Blood	3	89±2.0	71±12.12
CNS:			
CSF	15	85.9± 5.3	73±12.13
CSF + brain isolate	21	84.9±5.0	68.8±13.9
Brain (direct)	8	89.6±1.8	n.d.[c]
Brain (direct) + brain isolate	13	86.9±4.0	n.d.[c]
Total	64	83.3±4.4	n.d.[c]

[a]Values given are mean values ± standard deviation.

[b]n = number of pairwise sequence alignments.

[c]n.d. = not done

This is also reflected by the dendrograms of the respective amino acid sequences of the *nef* genes and the *env*-V3 regions (Figures 5A, B). Again, clustering was observed for sequences derived from the same patients, including sequences derived from different regions of the same brain. Although this analysis included only three blood-derived isolates, patient-specific clustering of *nef* genes was also observed for an extended analysis including additional published blood-derived *nef* sequences (n = 11; 8 from Myers et al.[22]).

None of the *nef* gene sequences were identical, including any of the paired *nef* sequences in the five patient clusters. In contrast, identity of *env*-V3 sequences was observed for G1L and G2B (patient c) on nucleotide and amino acid levels. Since the *nef* gene is roughly three times the size of the *env*-V3 region, it may be more suitable for analysis of sequence diversity than the *env*-V3 region used in several studies.[5,25]

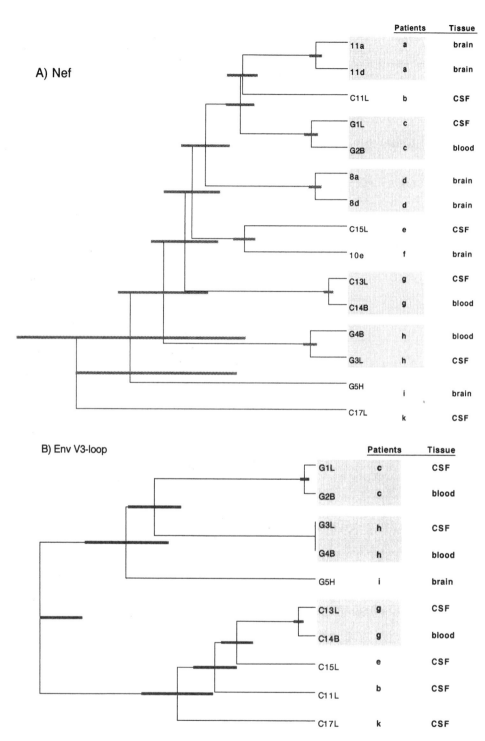

Figure 5. Patient-specific clustering of HIV-1 sequences from blood and CNS (amino acid sequences). (A) Dendrograms of the relationship of *nef* genes from HIV-1 isolates from CSF and blood and from *ex vivo* brain samples. (B) Cluster analysis of the corresponding *env*-V3 amino acid sequences determined for the HIV-1 isolates.

In this study, HIV-1 proviral sequences were obtained either directly from patient material (brain sequences), from single-passage (C-isolates) or from multiply passaged (G-isolates) virus. There was no clustering of *nef* gene sequences with respect to isolation method, suggesting that *in vitro* propagation of the virus did not result in selection of *nef* genes. Genetic diversity of *nef* sequences indicates the presence of a distinct HIV variant population (quasispecies) in each sample (n = 15). This suggests that HIV-1 evolves separately in the CSF and blood of the same individual. Steueler et al.[3] suggested separate evolution of HIV-1 in blood and CSF by analysis of the nucleotide sequence encoding gp41 transmembrane protein. In their study, 3 of 6 paired samples showed distinct sequence differences between blood and CSF.

Highly Conserved Sequence Features of *nef* Genes: Conservation of a Neurotoxin-Like Domain

Sequence conservation within the derived Nef protein sequences was investigated by calculation of amino acid identities as well as similarities assessed by Dayhoff mutation data matrix (PLOTSIMILARITY Program of UWGCG program package for sequence analysis) for each amino acid position. As expected from the analysis of nucleotide identities, the carboxy-terminal half of the *nef* gene was generally more highly conserved than the amino-terminal half (Figure 6). Several highly conserved sequence stretches correspond with regions previously reported to be of potential functional significance for Nef. These include the amino-terminal myristoylation signal[26] as well as potential phosphorylation sites[27] and a glycine-rich motif resembling the ATP binding site of *src*-like protein kinases (KEKGGLEG).[28]

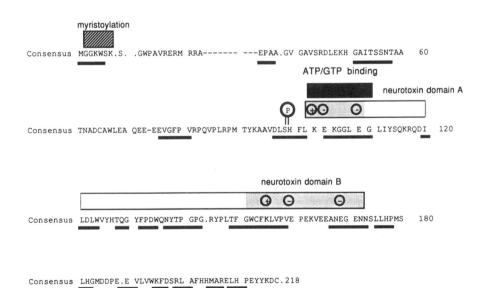

Figure 6. Conserved features of HIV-1 *nef* genes from patient material. The consensus sequence was derived from the 15 HIV-1 *nef* genes determined in this study. Conserved sequence features include the amino-terminal myristoylation signal,[26] the potential phosphorylation sites[27] (encircled P), a glycine-rich motif resembling the ATP binding site of *src*-like protein kinases (KEKGGLEG),[28] and the two-peptide neurotoxin domain.[14] Conserved locations of charged amino acid residues within the neurotoxin domain are indicated by encircled + or -. Horizontal bars underline positions of amino acids identical in at least 14 of the 15 *nef* genes analyzed.

In addition, the putative neuroactive domain of Nef[14] was found to be highly conserved. In this domain, sequence features shared with neuroactive peptides from scorpions are distributed to two peptides (a.a. 102-109, encompassing the putative ATP/GTP binding site, and a.a. 162-170) separated by a 42-amino acid spacer region. The conserved sequence pattern identified only HIV Nef proteins and several scorpion neuroactive peptides in the Swiss Prot 14 data base ($p = 0.5 \times 10^{-7}$). The putative neuroactive domain contains a conserved pattern of charged amino acids distributed to both peptides. In scorpion neurotoxins, these are in close spatial contact, forming a loop. Thus, this region of Nef may be involved in formation of a "neurotoxin loop", stabilized by electrostatic interaction between charged amino acid residues in both peptides. An additional conserved feature between scorpion neurotoxins and Nef is a WCY/FKL-motif (a.a. 152-156). In agreement with the "neurotoxin loop" model, this motif was shown to be located at the surface of scorpion neurotoxins molecules by crystallography.

The high-level conservation of the sequence features of the neurotoxin loop in *nef* genes independent of tissue origin indicates that significance of this region for function(s) of Nef *in vivo* goes beyond the CNS. Although the nature of these function(s) is still unclear, the influence of Nef on total potassium current in chicken dorsal root ganglia suggests interaction of Nef with membrane proteins. Such interactions may be crucial for virus spread or pathogenesis *in vivo*, where, opposite to *in vitro* conditions, the virus needs to replicate in a network of multiple cell types.

HIV-1 Isolates from Blood and CNS Cannot be Distinguished by Their Replicative Capacities

A previous study of 10 paired isolates from blood and CSF indicated that the majority of HIV-1 isolates were able to replicate in macrophage cultures and could not be grouped according to their replicative capacities.[15] This study included the C-isolates analyzed here.

Growth properties of G-isolates were assessed in T-lymphoma cell lines (HUT-78, C8166), a monocytic cell line (U937) and in an astrocytoma cell line (85HG66), previously shown to be infectible with HIV-1.[9] Cells were infected with equal amounts of cell-free infectious virus (100 $TCID_{50}$) and infection of target cells assessed by PCR amplification of HIV proviral sequences. Virus replication in target cells was analyzed by syncytia including capacity and levels of p24 antigen and reverse transcriptase activity in culture supernatants. All virus isolates were found to replicate to high titers in the T-lymphoma cell lines (Table 4). The kinetics of replication were generally more rapid in HUT-78 than in C8166 cells for all isolates except G2B. U937 monocytic cells did not support replication of any of the isolates, although infection was clearly established by PCR analysis. HIV infection of 85HGB66 astrocytoma cells was not observed under these conditions.

These results indicate that HIV isolates from blood, CSF, or brain could not be distinguished by their ability to infect and replicate in different cell lines *in vitro*. This agrees with the assessment of growth properties of blood and CSF-derived isolates in PBMCs and primary macrophages.[15]

Table 4. Replication of HIV-1 isolates from CNS and blood in HIV-susceptible cell lines.

Source		Isolate	Target Cells							
			T-Lymphoma				Monocytic		Astrocytoma	
Patient	Tissue		HUT-78		C8166		U937		85IIG66	
			PCR	Repl.	PCR	Repl.	PCR	Repl.	PCR	Repl.
c	CSF	G1L	+++	+++(R)	+++	+++(S)	+	-	-	-
c	Blood	G2B	+++	+++(S)	+++	+++(R)	+	-	-	-
h	CSF	G3L	+++	+++(R)	+++	+++(S)	+	-	-	-
h	Blood	G4B	+++	+++(R)	+++	+++(S)	+	-	-	-
i	Brain	G5H	+++	+++(R)	+++	+++(S)	+	-	-	-

(R), (S): Rapid, slow replication kinetics; Repl. = replication; -: negative

CONCLUSIONS

Molecular analysis of the predominant HIV-1 variant in virus isolates from CSF or blood or directly in patient specimens from brain revealed that *nef* gene sequences cluster in a host-dependent rather than a tissue-dependent manner. HIV-1 *nef* genes from the CNS did not exhibit any common features segregating them from blood-derived sequences. These results were corroborated by analysis of *env*-V3 sequences of HIV-1 isolates from blood and CNS. Lack of a common genetic imprint for HIV-1 sequences from the CNS is supported by sequence analysis[3] of *env*-gp41, *env*-/CD4 binding regions[4] and *env*-V3 sequences.[5]

It has been suggested that HIV-1 isolates from the CNS can be distinguished from blood isolates by their capacity to grow to higher titer in macrophages.[29] This has been shown for some but not all HIV-1 isolates from the CSF or brain but by no means for all, and several isolates seem to possess dual tropism for T-lymphocytes and macrophages.[24,29,30] Since productive infection of HIV-1 in the brain is observed largely in macrophage-like cells,[31] ability for high-level replication in macrophages is thought to be a key force for the selection of HIV-1 variants in the CNS. We did not detect major differences in replicative capacities of isolates from CSF and blood in monocyte/macrophages or a glioma cell line (MG138)[15] or in T-lymphocyte cell lines or a monocytic cell line U937 (this study).

Analysis of *env* and *nef* gene sequence shows that blood and CNS within an individual patient contain distinct genotypes.[3-5] Analysis of molecular clones showed extensive intrapatient genetic variation of *env* gene sequences within the brain, comparable to genetic variation in the blood or spleen.[4,5] These results suggest that HIV-1 variants are sequestered in the CNS, where they evolve separately from blood-borne variants. Evidence of virus infection is found in the CSF of most asymptomatic seropositive individuals, indicating that virus invasion into the CNS occurs early after infection.[32-35] The population entering the CSF at this stage is likely to contain macrophage-tropic variants, because they are carried in the blood of the majority of HIV-1-infected asymptomatic individuals.[36] However, subsequent selection for neuropersistent viruses is probably not exclusively directed to macrophage-tropic variants. Although productive infection of HIV-1 in the brain is limited to brain macrophages and microglia,[31,37,38] HIV-producing cells are very few in number[39] and cannot account for the large amount of HIV DNA detected in some brains.[1,2,40] This indicates that HIV-1 can also enter and persists in nonmacrophage cells in the brain. HIV-infectibility of several cell types of neuroectodermal origin has been shown both *in vivo* and *in vitro* (reviewed in ref. 39). Glial cells especially have been found to be infectible with HIV-1 *in vitro* (reviewed in ref. 10), yielding a restricted infection phenotype with extremely low-level virus production.[9,12,13]

In conclusion, our study has indicated that neuropersistent HIV-1 isolates do not share common genetic or replicative properties which set them apart from blood-borne variants. This suggests that the capacity to invade and persist in the CNS may not be restricted to certain virus variants but rather may be a general feature of HIV-1.

Acknowledgements

We thank Dr. Weis, Institute of Neuropathology of the Ludwig Maximilian University of Munich, for brain samples. This work was supported by the Bundesgesundheitsamt, BGA III-002-89/FVP2.

REFERENCES

1. S. Pang, Y. Koyanagi, S. Miles, C. Wiley, H.V. Vinters, and I.S.Y. Chen. High levels of unintegrated HIV-1 DNA in brain tissue of AIDS dementia patients. *Nature* 343:85 (1990).
2. G.M. Shaw, M.E. Harper, B.H. Hahn, et al. HTLV-III infection in brains of children and adults with AIDS encephalopathy. *Science* 227:177 (1985).
3. H. Steuler, S. Munzinger, B. Wildemann, and B. Storch-Hagenlocher. Quantitation of HIV-1 proviral DNA in cells from cerebrospinal fluid. *J. AIDS* 5:405 (1992),
4. S. Pang, H.V. Vinters, T. Akashi, W.A. Obrien, and I.S.Y. Chen. HIV-1 *env* sequence variation in brain tissue of patients with AIDS-related neurologic disease. *J. AIDS* 4:1082 (1991).
5. L.G. Epstein, C. Kuiken, B.M. Blumberg, et al. HIV-1 V3 domain variation in brain and spleen of children with AIDS: tissue-specific evolution within host-determined quasispecies. *Virology* 180:583 (1991).
6. A.G. Hovanessian. On the HIV *nef* gene product. *Res. Virol.* 143:31 (1992).
7. B. Kohleisen, K. Gaedigk-Nitschko, T. Werner, et al. Biological properties of Nef and its pathogenic potential in HIV-1-related central nervous system dysfunction. *AIFO* 5:275 (1993).
8. H.W. Kestler, D.J. Ringler, K.I. Mori, et al. Importance of the *nef* gene for maintenance of high virus loads and for development of AIDS. *Cell* 65:6521 (1991).
9. R. Brack-Werner, A. Kleinschmidt, A. Ludvigsen, et al. Infection of human brain cells by HIV-1: restricted virus production in chronically infected human glial cell lines. *AIDS* 6:273 (1992).
10. R. Geleziunas, H.M. Schipper, and M.A. Wainberg. Pathogenesis and therapy of HIV-1 infection of the central nervous system. *AIDS* 6:1411 (1992).
11. B. Kohleisen, M. Neumann, R. Hermann, et al. Cellular localization of *nef* expressed in persistently HIV-1-infected low-producer astrocytes. *AIDS* 6:1427 (1992).
12. Y. Saito, L.R. Sharer, L.G. Epstein, et al. Overexpression of *nef* as a marker for restricted HIV-1 infection of astrocytes in postmoprtem pediatric tissues. *Neurology* 44:474 (1994).
13. C. Tornatore, R. Chandra, J.R. Berger, and E.O. Major. HIV-1 infection of subcortical astrocytes in the pediatric central nervous system. *Neurology* 44:481 (1994).
14. T. Werner, S. Ferroni, T. Saermark, et al. HIV-1 Nef protein exhibits struc-

tural and functional similarity for scorpion peptides interacting with K$^+$ channels. *AIDS* 5:1301 (1991).

15. B. Keys, J. Karis, B. Fadeel, et al. V3 sequences of paired HIV-1 isolates from blood and cerebrospinal fluid cluster according to host and show variation related to the clinical stage of disease. *Virology* 196:475 (1993).

16. P.G. Strauss, J, Schmidt, L. Pedersen, and V. Erfle. Amplification of endogenous proviral MuLV sequences in radiation-induced osteosarcomas. *Int. J. Cancer* 41:615 (1988).

17. M. Alizon, S. Wain-Hobson, L. Montagnier, and P. Sonigo. Genetic variability of the AIDS virus: nucleotide sequence analysis of two isolates from African patients. *Cell* 46:63 (1986).

18. K.R. Tindall, and T.A. Kunkel. Fidelity of DNA synthesis by the *Thermus aquaticus* DNA polymerase. *Biochemistry* 28:6008 (1988).

19. P. Simmonds, P. Balfe, J.F. Peutherer, et al. Human immunodeficiency virus-infected individuals contain provirus in small numbers of peripheral mononuclear cells and at low copy numbers. *J.Virol.* 64:864 (1992).

20. B. Chatterjee, W.Gimbel, T. Görblich, and T. Werner. HPLC purification of PCR products for direct PCR sequencing. *Trends Genet.* 9:406 (1993).

21. B.M. Blumberg, L.G. Epstein, Y. Saito, D. Chen, L.R. Sharer, and R. Anand. Human immunodeficiency virus type 1 *nef* quasispecies in pathological tissues. *J.Virol.* 66:5256 (1992).

22. G. Myers, A.B. Rabson, S.F. Josephs, et al. Human retroviruses and AIDS: A compilation and analysis of nucleic acid and amino acid sequences. Database by Los Alamos National Laboratory (1992).

23. R. Anand, R. Thayer, A. Srinivasan, et al. Biological and molecular characterization of human immunodeficiency virus (HIV-1 BR) from the brain of a patient with progressive dementia. *Virology* 168:79 (1989).

24. Y. Koyanagi, S. Miles, R.T. Mitsuyasu, et al. Dual infection of the central nervous system by AIDS viruses with distinct cellular tropisms. *Science* 236:819 (1987).

25. K. Cichutek, S. Norley, R. Linde, et al. Lack of HIV-1 V3 region sequence diversity in two haemophiliac patients infected with a putative biologic clone of HIV-1. *AIDS* 5:1185 (1991).

26. J. Kaminchik, N. Bashan, A. Itach, N. Sarver, M. Gorecki, and A. Panet. Genetic characterization of human immunodeficiency virus type 1 *nef* gene products translated *in vitro* and expressed in mammalian cells. *J.Virol.* 65:583 (1991).

27. B. Guy, Y. Rivière, K. Dott, A. Regnault, and M.P. Kieny. Mutational analysis of the HIV Nef protein. *Virology* 176:413 (1990).

28. K.P. Samuel, A. Seth, A. Konopka, J.A. Lautenberger, and T.S. Papas. The 3'-orf protein of human immunodeficiency virus shows structural homology with the phosphorylation domain of human interleukin-2 receptor and the ATP-binding site of the protein kinase family. *FEBS Lett.* 218:81 (1987).

29. C. Cheng-Mayer, C. Weiss, D. Seto, and J.A. Levy. Isolates of human immunodficiency virus type 1 from the brain may constitute a special group of the AIDS virus. *Proc. Natl. Acad. Sci. USA* 86:8575 (1989).

30. S. Gartner, P. Markovits, D.M. Markovits, M.H. Kaplan, R.C. Gallo, and M. Popovic. The role of mononuclear phagocytes in HTLV/LAV infection. *Science* 233:215 (1986).

31. S. Koenig, H.E. Gendelmann, J.M. Orenstein, et al. Detection of AIDS virus in macrophages in brain tissue from AIDS patients with encephalopathy. *Science* 233:1089 (1986).

32. L. Resnick, F. DiMarzo-Veronese, J. Schüpbach, et al. Intra-blood-brain-barrier synthesis of HTLV-III specific IgG in patients with neurological symptoms associated with AIDS or AIDS-related complex. *N. Engl. J. Med.* 313:1498 (1985).

33. D.D. Ho, T.R. Rota, R.T. Schooley, et al. Isolation of HTLV-III from cerebrospinal fluid and neural tissues of patients with neurologic syndromes related to the acquired immunodeficiency syndrome. *N. Engl. J. Med.* 313:1493 (1985).

34. L.G. Epstein, J. Goudsmit, D.A. Paul, et al. HIV expression in the cerebro-

spinal fluid of children with progressive encephalopathy. *Ann. Neurol.* 21: 396 (1987).

35. J.C. McArthur, B.A. Cohen, H. Farzedegan, et al. Cerebrospinal fluid abnormalities in homosexual men with and without neuropsychiatric findings. *Ann. Neurol.* 23:S34 (1988).
36. H. Schuitemaker, M. Koot, N.A. Kootstra, et al. Biological phenotype of human imnunodeficiency virus type I clones at different stages of infection: progression of disease is associated with a shift from monocytotropic to T-cell-tropic virus populations. *J. Virol.* 66:1354 (1992).
37. C.A. Wiley, R.D. Schrier, J.A. Nelson, et al. Cellular localization of human immunodeficiency virus infection within the brains of acquired immune deficiency syndrome patients. *Proc. Natl. Acad. Sci. USA* 83:7089 (1986).
38. R.W. Price, B. Brew, J. Sidtis, M. Rosenblum, A.C. Scheck, and P. Cleary. The brain in AIDS: central nervous system HIV-1 infection and dementia complex. *Science* 239:586 (1988).
39. D.C. Spencer, and R.W. Price. Human immunodeficiency virus and the central nervous system. *Annu. Rev. Microbiol.* 46:655 (1992).
40. R. Vazeux, C. Lacroix-Ciaudo, S. Blanche, et al. Low levels of human immunodeficiency virus replication in the brain tissue of children with severe acquired immunodeficiency syndrome encephalopathy. *Am. J. Pathol.* 140:137 (1992).

AN ORGAN MODEL FOR HIV INFECTION OF THE BLOOD-BRAIN BARRIER

Ashlee V. Moses and Jay A. Nelson

Department of Molecular Microbiology and Immunology
Oregon Health Sciences University
Portland, OR 97201-3098

INTRODUCTION

Neurologic complications are a common symptom in HIV-seropositive patients.[1,2] These neurologic disorders can occur at different frequencies and involve both the peripheral and central nervous systems. Between 10-25% of AIDS-related complex (ARC) or AIDS patients present with central nervous system (CNS) symptoms.[3-5] Approximately 50% of these individuals will develop an encephalopathy during the terminal phase of the disease.[2-5] Initial neurologic symptoms consist of impaired memory and concentration as well as behavioral and motor disorders.[1,4-6] The neurologic abnormalities progress to a subcortical dementia termed AIDS dementia complex (ADC).[5] While ADC has been the subject of intense study by many groups, the cause of the disease process is unknown.

Neuropathologic evaluation of brains from AIDS patients has revealed a variety of pathologic changes including white matter pallor and gliosis, multinucleated cell encephalitis, vacuolar myelopathy, and diffuse or focal spongiform change of the cerebral white matter.[2,7,8] Studies by our group[9] and others[10-14] of CNS tissue from AIDS patients by *in situ* hybridization and immunochemistry have identified cells of the macrophage lineage as the principal cellular target for HIV. Brain capillary endothelial cells were also found by several groups to be a cell type naturally infected by HIV[9,12,14,15]. Interestingly, macrophages and capillary endothelial cells were also the predominant cells infected by simian immunodeficiency virus (SIV) in the CNS of virally infected rhesus macaques.[16]. These observations suggest a role for these infected cell types in the development of HIV-induced CNS disease.

While HIV infection is clearly associated with pathologic changes in brain tissue and with behavioral manifestations, the relationship between cellular infection and the mechanisms of neurologic dysfunction remains unclear. CNS pathology could arise in part from direct infection of brain tissue by HIV. However, the level of viral abundance within the CNS does not correlate with the degree of tissue damage, suggesting that indirect mechanisms of tissue damage must play a role in viral pathogenesis. Indirect effects could be targeted against either neuronal soma or their unmyelinated and myelinated axonal processes. These indirect effects might be mediated by neurotoxic viral proteins such as tat and gp120, both of which are readily shed from infected cells, or virally induced cellular proteins or metabolites. Immunopathogenic processes

Technical Advances in AIDS Research in the Human Nervous System
Edited by E.O. Major and J.A. Levy, Plenum Press, New York, 1995

may also be induced by locally secreted cytokines from infiltrating inflammatory cells or resident CNS cells.

While physical breakdown of the blood-brain barrier (BBB) does not appear to be a clinical feature of AIDS neuropathy, more subtle alterations in the integrity of the BBB may contribute to neural dysfunction. The endothelial cells lining the cerebral capillaries are an integral part of the BBB. These brain capillary endothelial (BCE) cells possess unique structural and biochemical characteristics that distinguish them from endothelial cells lining the capillaries of other organs[17,18] and allow formation of the BBB. For example, they exhibit a low degree of pinocytic vesiculation, have no transcellular channels, and are joined together by continuous tight junctions.[19] The endothelium thus creates an effective barrier between the blood in the capillary lumen and the interstitial fluid of the brain, limiting the free passage of molecules across the capillary wall. Carrier-mediated and active transport systems within BCE cells maintain the volume and composition of the interstitial fluid by allowing the passage of select molecules such as essential amino acids, sugars and metabolites while excluding toxic compounds.

Several groups have reported BBB abnormalities in AIDS patients.[20-22] In two of these studies, perivascular immunoreactivity for IgG and fibrinogen, which are markers for vascular permeability, were consistently found in postmortem brains of AIDS patients compared to immunocompetent control brain tissues.[20-22] This diffuse leakage of serum proteins into the brain parenchyma was distinct from focal breakdown of the BBB associated with tissue necrosis. Since cerebral vessels are normally impermeable to these serum proteins because of tight junctions, these observations suggest that abnormal permeability may be an important process in the development of CNS disease in AIDS. HIV infection of human BCE (HBCE) cells may disrupt their barrier function, resulting in deficient transport of essential nutrients and amino acids required for neurotransmitter precursors and/or allowing entry of neurotoxic substances from the serum which could contribute to white matter injury or interfere with neuronal function. Enhanced vascular permeability may also facilitate entry of HIV-infected macrophages and T cells from the peripheral blood.

In addition to forming the BBB, endothelial cells are active participants in immune and inflammatory responses. They are a source of immunomodulatory and chemotactic cytokines,[23,24] and express MHC molecules and a spectrum of adhesion molecules including integrins (ICAM-1, ICAM-2, VCAM-1) and selectins (ELAM-1), on the cell surface. These adhesion molecules interact with circulating monocytes, T cells, and neutrophils to allow leukocyte adhesion and migration across vessel walls. Cytokines produced by leukocytes and endothelial cells themselves can induce or up-regulate these molecules.[25] Patterns of inducible and constitutive ligand expression allow differential regulation of leukocyte entry under normal physiologic conditions and during inflammatory or immune reactions.[26] Induction of endothelial adhesion molecules may facilitate entry of HIV into the CNS through virally infected macrophages and T cells. Interestingly, greatly elevated VCAM-1 has been observed on the majority of arteriolar, venular, and capillary endothelial cells in the encephalitic brains from SIV_{mac}-infected macaques.[27] VCAM-1 mediates the adhesion of lymphocytes and monocytes to activated endothelium, through a leukocyte integrin (VLA-4)-dependent pathway.[28-30]

In addition to disturbing the physiology of the endothelium, infection of HBCE cells may constitute an important mechanism whereby HIV enters the CNS. Endothelial cells express a differential polarity with respect to structure and function. Virus may preferentially enter HBCE cells from the luminal or apical surface and bud from the basal lamina allowing secondary spread to resident glial glands.

RETROVIRAL MODELS INVOLVING THE BLOOD-BRAIN BARRIER AND CNS DISEASE

Two different retroviral models with neurotropic viruses have been described in which brain endothelial cells may play a key role in the induction of neurologic disease.[31,32] In the first model, a highly neuropathogenic and lymphocytopathic mutant of the Moloney murine leukemia virus (ts-1) targets multiple cells types in the brain.[31] Cellular disintegration occurs in all cell types of neuroectodermal origin (astrocytes, oligodendrocytes, and neurons) whereas a cytopathic effect is not observed in microglial cells and vascular endothelial cells. Interestingly, vascular endothelial cells are the predominant site for virus replication. The primary neuropathogenic determinant of ts-1 maps to a single amino acid substitution (Va.25 Ile) in the precursor envelope protein gpr80env.

Another neuropathogenic mouse retrovirus, PVC-211 MuLV, was isolated after passage of Friend MuLV (F-MuLV) through F344 rats.[32] PVC-211 MuLV infection of newborn rats results in neurologic disease by 3 weeks of age in which animals develop extensive perivascular astrogliosis and neuropil vacuolation without inflammation. The primary target of virus infection is the brain capillary endothelial ((BCEC) cell whereas the presence of virus was not detected in astrocytes or neurons. Chimeric viruses constructed from PVC-211 MuLV and the non-neuropathogenic parental virus (F-MuLV) identified the *env* gene of PVC-211 MuLV as the determinant responsible for pathologic changes in the CNS. A direct correlation was established between the ability of virus to replicate in BCE cells with neuropathogenesis *in vivo*. The investigators speculate that virus-infected BCE cells may produce substances that stimulate astrocyte proliferation and/or neurotoxic substances.

ISOLATION AND CHARACTERIZATION OF HBCE CELLS

We have developed and characterized primary culture of HBCE cells and have established that they can be productively infected with HIV.[33] We are using this *in vitro* culture system to investigate the mechanisms and consequences of HIV infection of the brain endothelium and to serve as a model to examine mechanisms of viral entry into the CNS. This chapter describes the use of this primary system and evaluates the significance of our findings for AIDS dementia.

HBCE cells are isolated from brain tissue obtained from surgical temporal lobectomies. Within 4 hours of excision, >10 grams of brain tissue are minced, washed with RPMI media, and digested in RPMI containing 5 mg/ml of collagenase/dipase for 30 minutes at 37°C with intermittent shaking. Partially digested tissue is then forced through a 60-μm nylon mesh and centrifuged through a 25% BSA gradient. Brain capillaries which pellet through this gradient are resuspended in RPMI and pipetted onto a 6-mm glass-bead column in a 12-cc syringe. Brain capillaries possess the property of binding glass beads in contrast to other CNS cells. The column is rinsed thoroughly with RPMI media with the effluent containing a mixture of CNS cell types (oligodendrocytes, neurons, astrocytes, pericytes). Adherent capillaries are recovered from glass beads by gentle agitation followed by a brief trypsin wash and seeded on 35 mm² Primaria culture dishes. Pure endothelial cell cultures are derived by allowing endothelial cells to migrate out of capillary segments to form microcolonies in the presence of selective growth medium (RPMI plus 10% human serum, 50 μg/ml endothelial growth factor, 1% glutamine, 1% penicillin/streptomycin (Fig. 1A and 1B). Isolated microcolonies are trypsinized using cloning rings and subcultured. HBCE cells are identified by the presence of endothelial cell-specific factor VIII-related antigen, von Willebrand factor (vWf) (Fig. 1C) as well as binding to the lectin *Ulex europaens* agglutinin-1 (UEA-1) which is blocked by the addition of fucose. Purity of HBCE cell cultures is confirmed by the absence of staining for glial fibrillary acidic protein (GFAP) (astrocytes), vimentin (fibroblasts), galactocerebroside (oligodendrocytes), and a selection of macrophage (MAB 1219, MAB 1245) and T cell (CD3, CD4) markers (Table 1).

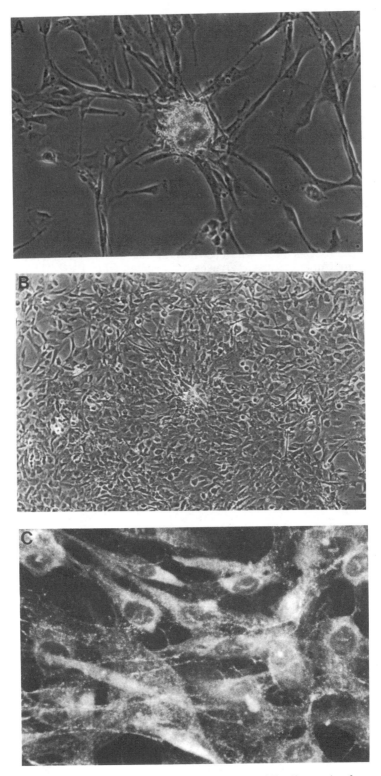

Figure 1. Isolation and characterization of HBCE cells. (A) HBCE cells growing from a capillary source at 2 weeks post infection. (B) Representative field of a confluent low-passage endothelial cell monolayer. (C) Indirect immunofluorescence showing positive staining for the endothelial cell-specific antigen vWf, using a MAB against vWf and a rhodamine conjugate.

In our HBCE cell cultures, we have observed induction of gamma-glutamyl transpeptidase (GTT) with astrocyte-spent media. Induction of GTT is a marker for activated brain epithelium.

Table 1. Antigenic phenotype of HBCE cells.

von Willebrand factor (VIII)	+
UEA 1	+
CD4	−
GFAP	−
Enolase	−
Desmin	−
Ham 56	−
Gal C	−
GTT	+

Characteristic endothelial cell ultrastructure was confirmed by electron microscopy.[34] In this study, the basement membrane was visible along the undersurface of the cell and pinocytotic vesicles characteristic of endothelial cells were apparent adjacent to the cytoplasmic membrane. Numerous dense granules suggestive of Weible-Palade bodies were observed and tight junctions were visible at intercellular junctions. Cell nuclei demonstrate a uniform euchromatic pattern with a central nucleolus.

HIV INFECTION OF HBCE CELLS

To determine the ability of HIV to productively infect HBCE cells, pure cultures of low-passage HBCE cells were infected with cell-free supernatants of the LAV-1 strain of HIV. Cells harvested at 7 days post infection (p.i.) were stained for the presence of p24 antigen. Approximately 40% of cells stained positive for the presence of antigen (Fig. 2). Double-staining for vWf and p24 antigen confirmed the endothelial cell lineage of HIV-infected cells. To evaluate the kinetics of HIV infection of HBCE cell cultures, expression of p24 antigen was assessed at various intervals p.i. HIV p24 was first detectable at day 2 p.i., and displayed a sequential increase in the percentage of infected cells as well as the accumulation of antigen per cell. By 4 weeks p.i., up to 90% of cells were p24-positive (Fig. 3). No cytopathic effects were detected in HIV-infected HBCE cells over a 6-week observation period. At this time, infected cells were repeatedly subcultured without altering their growth rate.

To assess the ability of HBCE cells to produce infectious HIV, cell-free supernatants were harvested from infected cultures at various times p.i., and assayed for the presence of virus. HIV titers were determine by a focal immuno-assay (FIA) which scores the formation of virus-induced syncytia on CD4-positive HeLa cells (HeLa CD4 cells).[35] Infectious virus was first detectable in HBCE cell supernatants at 2 days p.i., with a rapid increase in supernatant virus levels up to day 6 (Fig. 4). These results demonstrate that HIV infection if HBCE cells is productive and persists without cytopathic effect. This correlates with the findings that the BBB remains intact in AIDS patients.

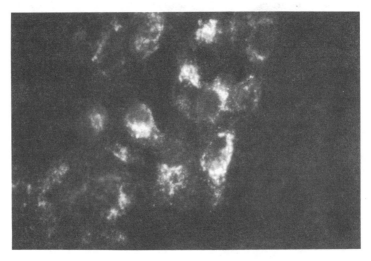

Figure 2. Representative field of infected HBCE cells fixed and stained with an anti-p24 MAB and an FITC conjugate at day 7 postinfection.

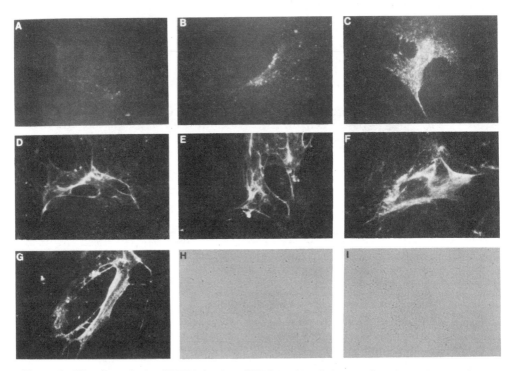

Figure 3. Kinetic analysis of HIV infection of HBCE cells. Cultures of HBCE cells were fixed and stained for p24 antigen as described for Fig. 1 on sequential days post infection (p.i.). (A-G) Expression of p24 on days 2, 4, 7, 10, 13, 21 and 24 days p.i. (H and I) Phase contrast of infected (H) and mock-infected (I) monolayers on day 21 p.i.

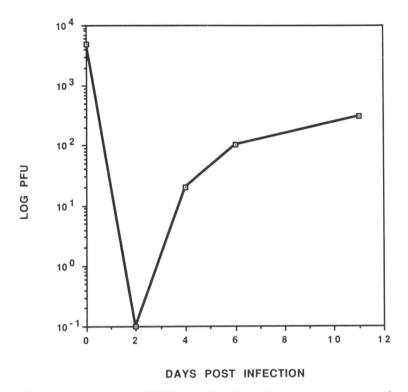

DAYS POST INFECTION

Figure 4. HIV productively infects HBCE cells. Cell-free culture supernatants were harvested from endothelial cells on sequential days p.i., and assayed for infectious virus by focal immuno-assay using HeLa CD4 cells as target cells. Briefly, HeLa CD4 cells were exposed to super-natants from mock- and HIV-infected endothelial cells for 4 hours. Virus inoculum was removed and HeLa cells were cultured for an additional 4 days before fixing and staining to allow scoring of HIV-induced syncytia.

ULTRASTRUCTURAL EXAMINATION OF HIV-INFECTED HBCE CELLS

Ultrastructural studies with HIV-infected HBCE cells were performed to examine characteristics of viral infection and confirm immunohistochemical and virus isolation studies described above. HIV-infected HBCE cell monolayers were examined by transmission electron microscopy (TEM). Typical lentivirus structures with a rod-like electron-dense core and a distinct viral envelope were observed in cells (Fig. 5). Virions were also seen intracellularly, budding from cells and in the extracellular spaces closely associated with the plasma membrane. The detection of budding HIV virions in HBCE cells confirms the ability of virus to productively infect these cells.

The binding properties of HIV to HBCE cells were also preliminarily examined by TEM. HBCE cells were infected by cell-free supernatant HIV at 4°C followed by incubation at 37°C for 60 minutes. HBCE cells absorbed with HIV exhibited numerous particles associated with the plasma membrane. Structures appearing to be virions fused to the plasma membrane were also observed in HIV-infected HBCE cell preparations. Endocytic vesicles with viral particles were not found, suggesting that the major mode of HIV entry into HBCE cells occurs via receptor-mediated fusion.

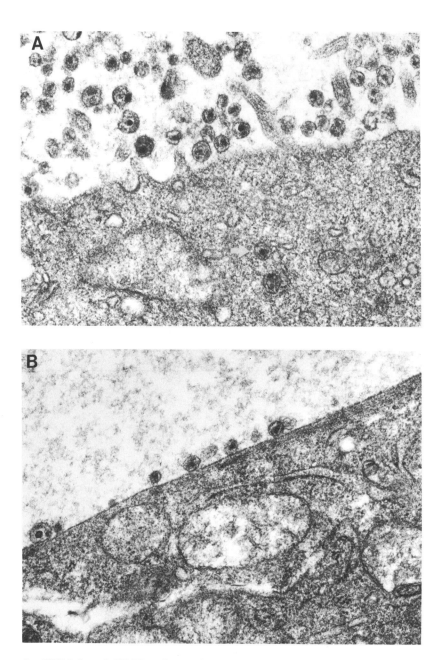

Figure 5. HIV-infected HBCE cell monolayers were examined by transmission electron microscopy. Virions demonstrated typical lentivirus structure with a rod-like electron-dense core and a distinct viral envelope. Virions were observed intracellularly, budding from cells and in the extracellular spaces closely associated with the plasma membrane. Figures (A) and (B) demonstrate virions closely associated with the plasma membrane. The arrow (A) indicates an intracellular virion.

HIV INFECTION OF LARGE-VESSEL ENDOTHELIAL CELLS

Since microvascular endothelial cells are biochemically and phenotypically distinct from large-vessel endothelial cells,[36,37] we tested the ability of HIV to infect large-vessel endothelial cells from human aorta and umbilical vein. Aortic and umbilical cord endothelial cells were infected with HIV and stained for the presence of p24 antigen at 7 and 14 days p.i. While viral antigen was readily detectable in control cultures of HIV-infected HBCE cells, aortic and umbilical endothelial cell cultures were consistently p24 negative (Fig. 6). Thus, HIV appears to specifically target endothelial cells originating from brain microvessels.

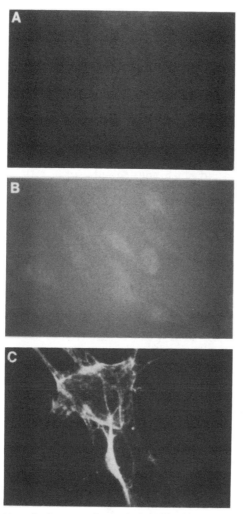

Figure 6. Selective infection of microvascular endothelium. Human aortic (A) , umbilical vein (B), and brain capillary (C) endothelial cells were exposed to HIV inoculum and fixed and stained for p24 at 2 weeks postinfection. Large-vessel endothelial cells showed no evidence of HIV infection whereas microvascular HBCE cells could be readily infected and stained for p24 antigen expression.

HIV INFECTION OF HBCE CELLS OCCURS THROUGH CD4- AND GalCer-INDEPENDENT PATHWAYS

CD4[38-40] and galactosyl ceramide (GalCer)[41,42] are the only two cellular moieties identified as cellular receptors for HIV. CD4 and GalCer were not detected on the surface of HBCE cells by immunofluorescence microscopy. This observation does not preclude the presence of these molecules on HBCE cells at levels sufficient to function as the receptor for HIV. HIV infection of HBCE cells was not blocked by incubating cell cultures with a monoclonal antibody (MAB) to CD4 (anti-Leu 3A), while this antibody successfully blocked viral infection of HeLa CD4 cells. Similarly, attempts to block HIV infection of HBCE cells with antibodies directed against GalCer were unsuccessful. Failure to neutralize HIV infection of HBCE cells with antibodies to the two known HIV receptors suggests that HIV utilizes an alternative pathway to infect endothelial cells which may be important for entry into the CNS.

SPECIFIC DOMAINS WITHIN THE HIV ENVELOPE MEDIATE ENTRY INTO HBCE CELLS

To map regions on gp120 that may be involved in the interaction between HIV and its receptor on HBCE cells, three MABs raised against defined epitopes on this glycoprotein were used in a series of neutralization experiments. MAB F105 is directed against an epitope within or topographically near the CD4-binding domain,[38] while MAB 0.5β[39] and MAB 902[43] recognize epitopes on the immunodominant hypervariable loop.[43] Incubation of viral inoculum with MAB F105 prior to infection did not hinder the ability of HIV to infect HBCE cells. The lack of HIV neutralization with antibodies against the CD4 domain of gp120 correlates with the failure of the anti-CD4 MAB (anti-Leu 3A) to block infection of HBCE cells. HIV infection of HBCE cells could, however, be reduced by incubation of virus with the two MABs directed against V3 loop epitopes. Relative to control cultures, MAB 0.5β allowed a 75% reduction in infection efficiency, while MAB 902 neutralized infection by up to 90%. The ability to neutralize infection of HBCE cells with MAB against specific gp120 epitopes provides further evidence that infection is mediated by a specific HBCE cellular receptor that is distinct from CD4.

HIV T CELL BUT NOT MACROPHAGE-TROPIC STRAINS INFECTED HBCE CELLS

HIV isolates can be distinguished by several biologic properties including *in vitro* growth in established T and macrophage cell lines, peripheral blood mononuclear (PBMN) cells, and primary macrophages as well as by cytopathic properties.[44] Previous studies of primary CNS isolates from autopsy tissue indicate that a key characteristic of the virus is macrophage tropism.[45-47] To determine whether tropic differences existed between HIV isolates, HBCE cells were infected with the T-cell tropic LAV strain utilized in previous experiments as well as a macrophage-tropic brain isolate JR-FL,[47] and a dual tropic CSF isolate JR-CSF[47] (Table 2). In these experiments, LAV but not JR-FL nor JR-CSF were able to efficiently infect the brain endothelial cells. However, all the HIV isolates productively infected PBMN cells and varied in their capacity to infect primary macrophage cultures as previously published.

Table 2. Relative infectivity of HIV strains.

HIV Strain	HBCE Cells[1]	Macrophage[2]	PBL[3]
LAV	+ + +	+	4.5×10^5
CSF	–	+ +	6.0×10^4
JR-FL	–	+ + +	5.7×10^4
MOCK	–	–	< 1,000

Relative degree of infection as assessed by:

[1]HBCE cells - p24 staining at day 10 p.i.
[2]Macrophages - % viability at day 21 p.i.
[3]PBL - RT activity (cpm/ml) at day 12 p.i.

This observation was unexpected since we anticipated primary macrophage-tropic brain isolates to be positive in HBCE cell cultures. However, since these HIV strains were acquired from autopsy specimens, this virus may represent HIV adapted to microglia and astroglia at late-stage disease. Early-stage CNS virus may be T-cell/HBCE cell-tropic in which virus must first traffic through the BBB to access and adapt to other cell types in the brain. Further analysis of other T cell and macrophage-tropic strains will be necessary to assess the importance of these observations.

DOES HIV INFLUENCE THE SURFACE PHENOTYPE OF HBCE CELLS?

The constitutive and inducible expression of the adhesion molecules ICAM-1 and VCAM-1 was examined using commercially available MAB (Becton-Dickinson). Both ICAM-1 and VCAM-1 were induced on the cell surface by IL-1 but undetectable in uninduced cells. Interestingly, ICAM-1 was selectively induced on HIV-infected HBCE cells in the absence of an additional induction stimulus (Fig. 7). These observations suggest that HIV can specifically alter phenotypic and hence functional properties of the brain endothelial cell surface. Up-regulation of leukocyte adhesion molecules may not only facilitate entry of leukocytes into the brain but also alter tight junction properties, since leukocyte binding to vessel walls has been shown to enhance vascular permeability.

DOES HIV INFLUENCE CYTOKINE PRODUCTION IN HBCE CELLS?

Cytokines produced by vascular endothelial cells participate in bidirectional interactions with leukocytes in the blood and cellular elements within organ compartments. Cytokines are thought to contribute to the pathogenesis of HIV encephalopathy. Studies on autopsy specimens have demonstrated enhanced cytokine expression in the brains of HIV-positive relative to HIV-negative individuals. Immunocytochemical staining of endothelial cells revealed elevated levels of IL-1, IL-6, TNF-α, and IFN-γ. Cytokines produced by HIV-infected HBCE cells could contribute to CNS damage via local release to the luminal or abluminal side of the brain microvasculature. For example, up-regulation of chemotactic cytokines or cytokines inducing expression of adhesion molecules and MHC antigens could enhance trafficking of inflammatory leukocytes to and through the vessel wall. Local production of cytokines could also enhance vascular permeability and disrupt the integrity of the BBB. Alternatively,

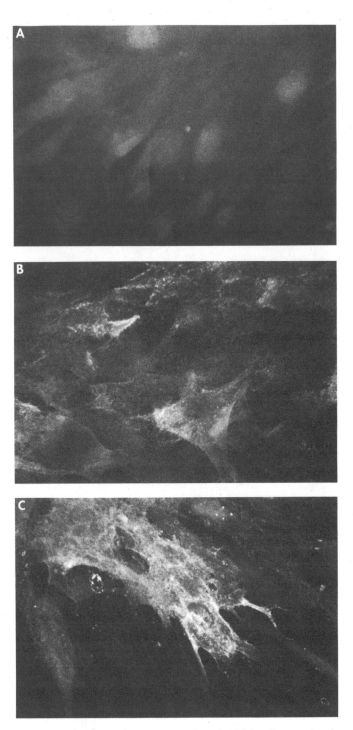

Figure 7. Induction of ICAM-1 on HBCE cells. Uninfected HBCE cells were incubated with normal growth medium (A) or medium supplemented with IL-1α (0.1 ng/ml) (B) for 12 hours prior to fixation. HIV-infected HBCE cells were incubated in normal growth medium and fixed at 7 days postinfection. HBCE cells were fixed in 3.5% p-formaldehyde and stained for the presence of ICAM-1 using commercial MAB (Becton-Dickinson) and an FITC conjugate. Uninfected HBCE cells demonstrated a low constitutive expression of ICAM-1 (A) which was strongly induced by IL-1α (B). HIV infection induced expression of ICAM-1 in the absence of IL-1α (C).

endothelial cytokines could damage CNS components involved in signal transduction (neurons, oligodendrocytes, myelin) either directly or indirectly via induction of neurotoxins from other CNS cells. In addition, cytokines may exacerbate immune activation within the CNS or induce HLA expression in infected brain macrophages/microglia and latently infected astrocytes.

CONCLUSIONS

In summary, we have demonstrated that HBCE cells unlike umbilical or aortic endothelial cells are permissively infected by HIV. HIV infection of HBCE cells is cytolytic and is mediated by a CD4- and GalCer-independent mechanism implying that HBCE cell-tropic strains utilize an unique receptor. T-cell but not macrophage-tropic HIV strains selectively infect brain endothelium and infectious viral strains are neutralized by antibodies directed against the V-3 loop but not the CD4 domain of gp120.

The observation that T-cell but not macrophage-tropic HIV strains infect HBCE cells is surprising since macrophage-tropic strains are readily isolated from brain tissue. The "brain-tropic" isolates, however, are commonly obtained from autopsy tissue. Therefore, the macrophage brain-tropic isolates may represent the adaptation of virus to microglia at end-stage disease. The tropism of HIV at early stages of CNS disease is unknown. Our HBCE model would predict that these isolates would primarily encompass T-cell-tropic strains. These observations suggest that T-cell tropism is important for HIV entry through the BBB and that as CNS disease progresses, the virus evolves into macrophage-tropic strains.

The ability of HIV to infect cells that compose the BBB implies that the virus may be directly involved in the BBB dysfunction observed in AIDS patients. Figure 8 illustrates several potential mechanisms in which HIV may mediate this process.

In the first model, HIV infection of HBCE cells may alter formation of tight junctions allowing the flow of either cytokines or toxic metabolites from the circulating blood into the brain parenchyma (model 1). Alternatively, viral infection of brain endothelium may allow the tight junctions to remain intact but alter the ability of the cell to regulate transport of these toxic substances across the BBB by transcytosis (model 2). Another mechanism may involve the production of abnormal amounts of cytokines or other cell metabolites from HIV-infected HBCE cells which are neurotoxic or cytotoxic (model 3). Finally, HIV infection of brain endothelium may result in endothelial cell-induced astrocytosis (model 4) by either release of cytotoxic substances as described above or alteration of abluminal surface antigens which by contact with astrocytic foot processes results in an apoptotic event. The establishment of our *in vitro* HIV-HBCE cell system will allow us to explore the above potential mechanisms which mediate AIDS dementia.

1. Tight Junction Leakage

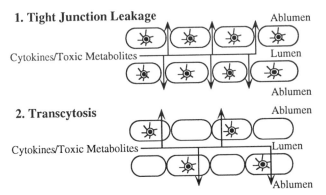

Cytokines/Toxic Metabolites

Ablumen

Lumen

Ablumen

2. Transcytosis

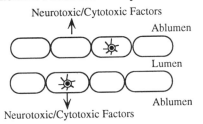

Cytokines/Toxic Metabolites

Ablumen

Lumen

Ablumen

3. Abnormal Production of Cytokines or Cell Metabolites

Neurotoxic/Cytotoxic Factors

Ablumen

Lumen

Ablumen

Neurotoxic/Cytotoxic Factors

4. Endothelial Induced Astrocytosis

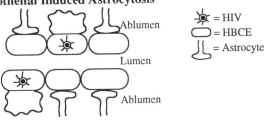

Ablumen

Lumen

Ablumen

= HIV
= HBCE
= Astrocyte

Figure 8. Models for HIV-induced BBB dysfunction.

ACKNOWLEDGEMENTS

We wish to express our sincere gratitude to Mary Lou Hall for the preparation of this manuscript. The work was supported by National Institutes of Health Grants AI 24178 and NIMH 47680. A.V.M. is a scholar for the American Foundation for AIDS Research.

REFERENCES

1. W.D. Snider, D.M. Simpson, S. Nielson, et al. Neurological complications of acquired immune deficiency syndrome: analysis of 50 patients. *Ann. Neurol.* 14:403 (1983).
2. R.W. Price, and B. Brew. Management of the neurologic complications of HIV-1 infection and AIDS. "The Medical Management of AIDS," W.B. Saunders, Philadelphia (1990).
3. S.L. Nielsen, C.K. Petito, C.D. Urmacher, and J.B. Posner. Subacute encephalitis in acquired immune deficiency syndrome: a postmortem study. *Am. J, Clin. Pathol.* 82:678 (1984).
4. J.A. Levy, J. Shimabukuro, H. Hollander, J. Mills, and L. Kaminsky. Isolation of AIDS-associated retrovirus from cerebrospinal fluid and brain of patients with neurologic symptoms. *Lancet* 2:586 (1985).
5. B.A. Navia, B.D. Jordan, and R.W. Price. The AIDS dementia complex. I. Clinical features. *Ann. Neurol.* 19:517 (1986).
6. D.D. Ho, T.R. Rota, J.C. Schooley, et al. Isolation of HTLV III from cerebrospinal fluid and neural tissues of patients with neurologic syndromes related to the acquired immunodeficiency syndrome. *N. Engl. J. Med.* 313:1493 (1985).
7. B.A. Navia, E.S. Cho, C.K. Petito, and R.W. Price. The AIDS dementia complex. II. Neuropathology. *Ann. Neurol.* 19:525 (1986).
8. G.M. Shaw, M.E. Harper, B.J. Hahn et al. HTLV-III infection in brains of children and adults with AIDS encephalopathy. *Science* 227:177 (1985).
9. C.A. Wiley, R.D. Schrier, F.J. Denaro, et al. Cellular localization of human immunodeficiency virus infection within the brains of acquired immune deficiency syndrome patients. *Proc. Natl. Acad. Sci. USA* 83:7098 (1986).
10. S.K. Koenig, H.E. Gendelman, J.M. Orenstein, et al. Detection of AIDS virus in macrophages in brain tissue from AIDS patients with encephalopathy. *Science* 233:1089 (1986).
11. M.H. Stoler, T.A. Eskin, S. Benn, R.C. Angerer, and L.M. Angerer. Human T-cell lymphotropic virus type III infection of the central nervous system: A preliminary *in situ* analysis. *J.A.M.A.* 256:2360 (1986).
12. D.H. Gabuzda, D.D. Ho, S.M. de la Monte, et al. Immunohistochemical identification of HTLV III antigen in brains of patients with AIDS. *Ann. Neurol.* 20:289 (1986).
13. T. Pumarola-Sune, B.A. Navia, C. Cordon-Cardo, E.S. Cho, and R.W. Price. HIV antigen in the brains of patients with AIDS dementia complex. *Ann. Neurol.* 21:490 (1987).
14. J.M. Ward, T.J. O'Leary, G.B. Baskin, et al. Immunohistochemical localization of human and immunodeficiency viral antigens in fixed tissue sections. *Am. J. Pathol.* 127:199 (1987).
15. S.W. Rostad, S.M. Sumi, C.M.Shaw, K. Olson, and J.K. McDougall. Human immunodeficiency virus (HIV) infection in brains with AIDS-related leukoencephalopathy. *AIDS Res. Human Retrovirus* 3:4 (1987).
16. A.A. Lackner, M.O. Smith, R.J. Munn, et al. Localization of simian immunodeficiency virus in the central nervous system of rhesus monkeys. *Am. J. Pathol.* 139:609 (1991).
17. F. Joo. The blood-brain barrier *in vitro*: ten years of research on microvessels isolated from the brain. *Neurochem. Int.* 7:1 (1985).
18. R. Turner, J.H. Beckstead, R.A. Warnke, and G.S. Wood. Endothelial cells

phenotypic diversity. *In situ* demonstration of immunologic and enzymatic heterogeneity that correlates with specific morphologic subtypes. *Am. J. Clin. Pathol.* 87:569 (1987).

19. G.W. Goldstein, and A. Lorris-Betz. Recent advances in understanding brain capillary function. *Sem. Neurol.* 14:389 (1983).

20. T.M. Lenhardt, and C.A. Wiley. Absence of humorally mediated damage within the central nervous system of AIDS patients. *Neurology* 39:378 (1989).

21. R.H. Rhodes. Evidence of serum-protein leakage across the blood-brain barrier in the acquired immunodeficiency syndrome. *J. Neuropathol. Exp. Neurol.* 50:171 (1991).

22. C.K. Petito, and K.S. Cash. Blood-brain barrier abnormalities in the acquired immunodeficiency syndrome: Immunohistochemical localization of serum proteins in postmortem brain. *Ann. Neurol.* 32:658 (1992).

23. P. Miossec, D. Cavender, and M. Ziff. Production of interleukin 1 by human endothelial cells. *J. Immunol.* 136:2486 (1986).

24. M. Sironi, F. Brevario, P. Prosperio, A. Biondi, and A. Vecchi. IL-1 stimulates IL-6 production in endothelial cells. *J. Immunol.* 142:549 (1989).

25. A. Montovani, F. Bussolino, and E. Dejana. Cytokine regulation of endothelial cell function. *FASEB J.* 6:2591 (1992).

26. Y. Shimizu, W. Newman, Y. Tanaka, and S.Shaw. Lymphocyte interactions with endothelial cells. *Immunol. Today* 13:106 (1992).

27. V.G. Sasseville, W.A. Newman, A.A. Lackner, et al. Elevated vascular cell adhesion molecule-1 in AIDS encephalitis induced by simian immunodeficiency virus. *Am. J. Pathol.* 141:1021 (1992).

28. D.W. Beck, H,.V. Vinters, M.N. Itart, and P.A. Cancilla. Glial cells influence polarity of the blood-brain barrier. *J. Neuropathol. Exp. Neurol.* 43:219 (1984).

29. G.G. Glenner, J.E. Folk, and P.J. McMillan. Histochemical demonstration of gamma-glutamyl transpeptidase-like activity. *J. Histochem. Cytochem.* 10:481 (1962).

30. G.E. Rice, J.M. Munro, and M.P. Bevilacqua. Inducible cell adhesion molecule 110 (INCAM-110) is an endothelial receptor for lymphocytes in a CD22/CD18-dependent adhesion mechanism. *J. Exp. Med.* 171:1369 (1990).

31. E.Shikova, Y-C. Lin, K. Saha, B.R. Brooks, and P.K.Y. Wong. Correlation of specific virus-astrocyte interactions and cytopathic effects induced by ts-1, a neurovirulent mutant of Moloney murine leukemia virus. *J. Virol.* 67:1137 (1993).

32. M. Masuda, P.M. Hoffman, and S.K. Ruscetti. Viral determinants that control the neuropathogenicity of PCV-211 murine leukemia virus *in vivo* determine brain capillary endothelial cell tropism of the virus *in vitro*. *J. Virol.* 67:1137 (1993).

33. A.V. Moses, F.E. Bloom, C.D. Pauza, and J.A. Nelson. HIV infection of human brain capillary endothelial cells occurs via a CD4-independent mechanism. *Proc. Natl. Acad. Sci. USA* 90:10474 (1993).

34. L.L. Lathey, C.A. Wiley, M.A. Verity, and J.A. Nelson. Cultured human brain capillary endothelial cells are permissive for infection by human cytomegalovirus. *Virology* 176:266 (1990).

35. B. Chesebro, and K. Wehrly. Development of a sensitive quantitative focal assay for human immunodeficiency virus infectivity. *J. Virol.* 62:3779 (1988).

36. K. Tsutomu, M. Takashi, K. Miyaka, and H,. Nagura. Phenotypic heterogeneity of vascular endothelial cells in the human kidney. *Cell. Tissue Res.* 256:27 (1989).

37. C. Page, M. Rose, M. Yacoub, and R. Pigott. Antigenic heterogeneity of vascular endothelium. *Am. J. Pathol.* 141:673 (1992).

38. A.G. Dalgleish, P.C.L. Beverley, P.R. Claphorn, et al. The CD4 (T4) antigen is an essential component of the receptor for the AIDS retrovirus. *Nature* 3123:763 (1984).

39. D. Klatzman, E. Champagne, S. Chamaret, et al. T lymphocyte T4 molecule behaves as the receptor for human retrovirus LAV. *Nature* 312:767 (1984).
40. P.J. Maddon, A.G. Dalgleish, J.S. McDougal, et al. The T4 gene encodes the AIDS virus receptor and is expressed in the immun system and the brain. *Cell* 47:333 (1986).
41. L. Pulliam, B.G. Herndier, N.M. Tang, and M.S. McGrath. Human immuno-deficiency virus-infected macrophages produce soluble factors that cause histological and neurochemical alterations in cultured human brains. *J. Clin. Invest.* 87:503 (1991).
42. S. Bhat, S.L. Spitalnik, F. Gonzalez-Scarano, and D.H. Silberberg. Galacto-syl ceramide or a derivative is an essential component of the neural receptor for human immunodeficiency virus type 1 envelope glycoprotein gp120. *Proc. Natl. Acad. Sci. USA* 88:7131 (1991).
43. S. Pincus, K. Wehrly, and B. Chesebro. Treatment of HIV tissue culture in-fection with monoclonal antibody-ricin A chain conjugates. *J. Immunol.* 142:3070 (1989).
44. J.A. Levy. Pathogenesis of human immunodeficiency virus infection. *Micro. Rev.* 57:183 (1993).
45. C. Cheng-Mayer, and J.A. Levy. Distinct biologic and serologic properties of HIV isolates from the brain. *Ann. Neurol.* 23:448 (1988).
46. C. Cheng-Mayer, C. Weiss, D. Sato, and J.A. Levy. Isolates of human immunodeficiency virus type 1 from brain may constitute a special group of the AIDS virus. *Proc. Natl. Acad. Sci. USA* 70:8575 (1989).
47. S. Koyanagi, S. Miles, R.T. Mitsyasu, et al. Dual infection of the central nervous system by AIDS viruses with distinct cellular tropisms. *Science* 236:819 (1987).

THE ROLE OF THE ASTROCYTE IN THE PATHOGENESIS OF THE AIDS DEMENTIA COMPLEX

Dale J. Benos,[1] James K. Bubien,[2] Beatrice H. Hahn,[2] George M. Shaw,[2] and Etty N. Benveniste[3]

[1]Department of Physiology and Biophysics
[2]Department of Medicine
[3]Department of Cell Biology
University of Alabama at Birmingham
Birmingham, AL 35294

INTRODUCTION

A chronic encephalopathy termed "AIDS dementia complex (ADC)" otherwise known as "HIV-associated cognitive/motor complex" afflicts up to 80% of adult AIDS patients.[1,2] ADC is characterized clinically by cognitive, motor, and behavioral dysfunctions. Manifestations include global cognitive defects, organic psychosis, and a variety of motor abnormalities. Pathologically, ADC presents with cerebral atrophy and abnormalities of the white matter and deep grey matter structures including the basal ganglia. These abnormalities include diffuse pallor and vacuolation of the white matter, and focal rarefaction accompanied by infiltration of macrophages, multinucleated cells, and lymphocytes. Infiltration of T-lymphocytes is limited in degree, and is primarily of the CD8+ phenotype. Discrete areas of demyelination are common, and are associated with reactive/hypertrophied astrocytes (astrogliosis), and the presence of microglia, blood-derived macrophages, and multinucleated giant cells.

ADC occurs in the absence of recognized opportunistic pathogens, and there is strong indication that direct infection of the central nervous system (CNS) by HIV-1 is responsible for ADC. HIV-1 DNA and RNA sequences are found in the CNS tissue of individuals with ADC in an abundance greater than that of lymphoid tissues.[3] HIV-1 has been isolated from both the brain and cerebrospinal fluid (CSF) of AIDS patients,[1,4] and anti-HIV-1 antibodies have been detected in the CSF of AIDS patients in levels indicating intracerebral CNS antibody production.[2] Much attention has been directed at determining which cells in the CNS are infected by HIV-1. A number of laboratories have conclusively determined by *in situ* hybridization coupled with immunocytochemistry that infiltrating monocytes/macrophages, as well as resident microglia, are infected by HIV-1.[5-8] Earlier reports suggested that brain capillary endothelial cells, astrocytes, oligodendrocytes, and neurons could occasionally be infected with HIV-1; however, these examples are rare and controversial.[6,8] The prevailing wisdom is that macrophages and microglia are the principal, and probably only, cell type productively infected with HIV-1 in the CNS. However, while it is clear that macrophages and microglia are the primary targets of HIV-1 infection, there is currently no satisfactory explanation for the extensive neurologic impairment observed clinically in ADC. The etiology of ADC is unknown, but undoubtedly a number of different cell types and cellular mech-

Technical Advances in AIDS Research in the Human Nervous System
Edited by E.O. Major and J.A. Levy, Plenum Press, New York, 1995

anisms contribute to its pathogenesis. Our hypothesis is that cytokine production and certain ion transport systems of the astrocyte are affected by HIV-1 infection of the brain.

Astrocytes are the largest and most numerous of the glial cells. They are essential for maintaining a proper CNS microenvironment by regulating extracellular pH and neuronal metabolite and neurotransmitter levels, and by structurally supporting neurons and the blood-brain barrier. Astrocytes function to regulate extracellular $K+$ by a process called $K+$ spatial buffering.[9] Astrocytes have well-defined ion transport systems: one for the coupled exchange of $Na+$ and $H+$ ions, one for the exchange of $Cl-$ and $HCO-_3$ ions, one for the cotransport of $Na+$ and $HCO-_3$, and a variety of ion channels.[10-14] These transport systems allow the astrocyte to exchange electrolytes with neighboring cells, including neurons, and the ion channels may function in cell signaling and ion homeostasis.[15] Astrocytes also have a role in neurotransmitter metabolism; for example, astrocytes possess a specific ATP and $Na+$-dependent uptake system that functions to remove the excitatory amino acid neurotransmitter glutamate from the extracellular medium.[16,17]

Although there has been controversy regarding HIV-1 infection and cytokine production *in vitro*, there are *in vivo* data demonstrating the association of certain cytokines with ADC. Studies have been performed on both CSF and brain material from HIV-1-infected patients. Elevated levels of interleukin-1 (IL-1) are present in the CSF of AIDS patients,[18,19] and IL-1 positive cells have been identified in the brains of these patients. The IL-1 positive cells are infiltrating macrophages, resident microglia, and astrocytes.[19,20] Elevated levels of tumor necrosis factor-α (TNF-α) have been demonstrated in the CSF of AIDS patients. TNF-α staining of brains from AIDS patients localizes with some endothelial cells and astrocytes, but primarily with macrophages/microglia.[19] Elevated levels of interferon-γ (IFN-γ) have also been detected in the CSF of HIV-1-infected individuals,[21] most likely the product of infiltrating CD8+ T-cells. Thus, there is precedence for a variety of cytokines to be present in the CSF and CNS of HIV-1-infected patients, and evidence that infiltrating lymphoid cells and macrophages, as well as endogenous astrocytes and microglia, can produce these cytokines. Most importantly, some of these cytokines act to enhance HIV-1 replication in macrophages. Although not normally produced endogenously within the CNS, IFN-γ has a wide range of influences on astrocytes including: (1) inducing proliferation of adult astrocytes; (2) inducing expression of class I and class II MHC antigens; (3) inducing expression of ICAM-1; (4) increasing PKC and $Na+/H+$ antiporter activity; and (5) priming astrocytes for subsequent cytokine (TNF-α, IL-6) release. Collectively, astrogliosis, demyelination, increased vascular permeability, inflammation, and CNS immunoglobulin production are all associated with ADC. IFN-γ has been shown to alkalinize murine macrophages, and produce a concurrent influx of $Na+$.[22] We have recently demonstrated that IFN-γ enhances $Na+/H+$ antiporter activity in primary cultures of rat astrocytes, and that this activity is required for IFN-γ-induced class II MHC gene expression in astrocytes.[23]

HYPOTHESIS

Because neurons are not directly infected with HIV-1, the severe pathophysiological manifestations of ADC are most likely mediated indirectly. Thus, our central hypothesis is that cytokines and/or viral proteins produced by HIV-1-infected macrophages/microglia directly alter normal astrocyte transport function, ultimately leading to neuronal cell injury. This working hypothesis is illustrated in Figure 1.

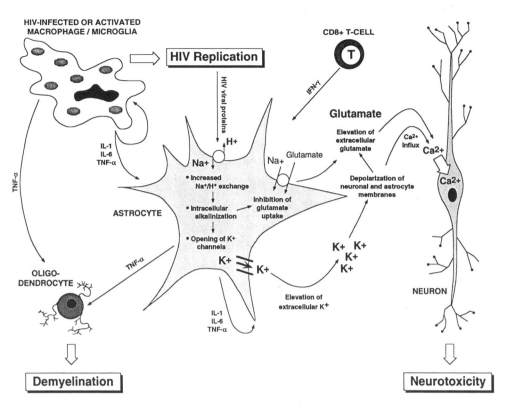

Figure 1. Hypothesis of HIV-1-induced changes in cytokine production and ion transport systems of the astrocyte leading to neurotoxicity and ADC.

HIV-1 infection of macrophages/microglia causes altered cytokine production and expression of HIV viral proteins. These polypeptides in turn are postulated to activate Na^+/H^+ exchange in the astrocyte. Likewise, exposure of astrocytes to specific HIV-1 proteins may also activate the astrocyte to produce cytokines. This cytokine and/or viral protein-induced increase in the activity of Na^+/H^+ exchange system will lead to intracellular alkalinization within the astrocyte which, in turn, can influence many other cellular processes, including the opening of various types of K^+ channels that are known to exist in the astrocyte membrane.[10,11,14,24-26] Intracellular alkalinization may also interfere with the astrocyte's primary function of buffering extracellular K^+, resulting in a net accumulation of K^+ in the extracellular space. This increase in extracellular K^+ will, in turn, produce a depolarization of both astrocyte and neuronal cell membranes. This depolarization can cause the opening of voltage-dependent Ca^{2+} channels in the neuron, producing a rise in neuronal intracellular free Ca^{2+} activity,[27] with subsequent onset of neural toxicity.[28,29] Dreyer *et al.*[29] have shown that gp120 treatment of cultured rat retinal ganglion cells and hippocampal neurons causes an increase in intracellular free Ca^{2+} and neural toxicity. More recent work has suggested that both gp120 and glutamate-related molecules are necessary for neuronal cell death, and that both voltage-dependent Ca^{2+} channels and NMDA receptor-operated channels are required for this form of HIV-related neurotoxicity.[30] Both of these channels are permeable to Ca^{2+}; therefore, both types of channels could contribute to the increased influx of Ca^{2+} associated with subsequent neuronal injury. In this regard, both elevated external K^+ and cytoplasmic alkalinization would lead to a diminution in glutamate uptake, as well as an enhancement of glutamate release.[16,17,31] Glutamate, in turn, can then activate receptors on both the neuronal and astrocyte membrane, further increasing Ca^{2+} entry. Importantly, glutamate activation of these receptors on the astrocyte membrane has been shown to depolarize the membrane potential, thus favoring K^+ loss from the cells into the extracellular compartment.[32] In addition to HIV-related neurotoxicity, glutamate has also been implicated as being responsible for neuronal degeneration *in vivo* and *in vitro* in another chronic progressive disease, namely, amyotrophic lateral sclerosis.[33,34] Wiley *et al.*[35] have observed that some neurons in the brains of ADC patients appear dystrophic, i.e., these neurons are tortuous, have a paucity of branches, and some of the neurons appear to be retracting. *In vitro*, this pattern of dystrophic neurons can be induced by treatment of cells with gp120 or sublethal concentrations of NMDA or glutamate,[36] and these effects depend upon Ca^{2+} influx into the neuron. Thus, in the CNS of ADC patients, neuronal injury may be mediated by a complex interaction of cytokines, HIV viral proteins, and neuronal toxic factors interacting with macrophages/microglia, astrocytes, and neurons.

RESULTS

The hypothesis presented in Figure 1 predicts certain experimental outcomes following exposure of astrocytes to cytokines, HIV-1 virions, or the envelope glycoprotein gp120. These involve: the Na^+/H^+ antiport system; glutamate transport systems; and K^+ conductance. A discussion of each of these follows in order.

Na^+/H^+ Antiport Activity

The Na^+/H^+ antiporter is present in most animal cells, and has been implicated in a variety of functions such as pH regulation, control of cell volume, gene transcription, and the initiation of proliferation and cellular differentiation (for review, see 37, 38). The Na^+/H^+ antiporter is a mechanism for H^+ extrusion and Na^+ uptake that is driven by the prevailing Na^+/H^+ electrochemical energy gradients. It has a tightly coupled stoichiometry of 1:1, and is inhibited by micro- to millimolar concentrations of the diuretic amiloride. This process does not directly require ATP or other forms of energy, and primarily functions to regulate intracellular pH. The resultant changes in intracellular pH and/or ionic environment appear to serve as triggers for subsequent cellular events. In many cells, this transport system is quiescent. It can be activated, however, by growth factors, phorbol esters, cytokines, cell volume changes, or acid load. As indicated earlier, the addition of IFN-γ to astrocytes enhances Na^+/H^+ antiporter activity.[23] We have found that two other cytokines, namely, TNF-α and IL-1, can also stimulate Na^+/H^+ exchange in astrocytes, while TGF-β and IL-6 do not. Our hypothesis predicts that amiloride-sensitive Na^+/H^+ exchange activity should be stimulated by heat-inactivated HIV-1 virion or gp120. This was, in fact, what we observed. Heat-inactivated HIV-1, in a concentration-dependent manner, stimulates amiloride-sensitive $^{22}Na^+$ influx into rat astrocytes; recombinant gp120 does the same. In fact, 25 nM gp120 stimulates Na^+ influx through this antiport system at a maximal rate (i.e., at a rate comparable to that observed when one lowers the intracellular pH to 6). Likewise, gp120 causes a significant intracellular alkalinization in both rat and human astrocytes. The effect of gp120 on intracellular pH was abrogated by incubating the cells in Na^+-free medium, in the presence of an inhibitor of Na^+/H^+ exchange, namely, amiloride or dimethylamiloride (DMA), or by first immunodepleting gp120 from the bathing solution with anti-gp120 antibodies. After 10 minutes of exposure to gp120, human astrocytes increased their intracellular pH (pH_i) to 7.26 from 6.99. On average, gp120 produced a 0.26 ± 0.06 increase in pH_i in human astrocytes, and a 0.14 ± 0.03 increase in pH_i in rat astrocytes. Thus, gp120 increases pH_i via activation of an amiloride-sensitive Na^+/H^+ exchange system in both rat and human astrocytes.

Glutamate Transport

The hypothesis presented in Figure 1 predicts that glutamate efflux should be stimulated by gp120 secondarily as a result of cytoplasmic alkalinization, and that glutamate efflux should also be increased by membrane depolarization. Again, both of these predictions have been borne out by experiment. If extracellular Na^+ is replaced by increasing amounts of K^+ in order to depolarize the astrocyte membrane, [3H]-D-aspartate efflux is stimulated in an amiloride-insensitive fashion. [Note: Aspartate is used as a nonmetabolized substrate for the glutamate transport system.] When the extracellular K^+ was raised from 4 to 40 mM, the efflux of aspartate was increased by a factor of 2. Exposure of astrocytes to 25 nM gp120 likewise increased the [3H]-D-aspartate efflux rate constant 2.5-fold, i.e., from 0.2 min^{-1} to 0.5 min^{-1}. This effect of gp120 could again be blocked by amiloride or Na^+-free solutions, indicating that the effect was mediated via Na^+/H^+ antiport-induced changes in intracellular pH. It is important to note that removal of external Na^+ (isosmotically replacing the Na^+ with the impermeant cation N-methyl-D-glucamine) or amiloride alone had no effect on aspartate efflux.

Similar effects were noted for [3H]-glutamate influx intro rat astrocytes. Elevation of extracellular K^+ to 25 or 40 mM depressed the uptake of [3H]-glutamate by approximately 20%. This effect of K^+ was independent of the presence or absence of amiloride, indicating that it most likely occurred because of membrane depolarization.[31] Treatment of astrocytes with gp120 (25 nM) likewise inhibited [3H]-glutamate uptake by 25%. However, in this case, amiloride could block this inhibitory effect of gp120. These results indicate that elevation of extracellular K^+ concentration (membrane depolarization) or the presence of gp120 both decrease glutamate uptake and increase the efflux of cytoplasmically located stores of glutamate, together leading to a net increase in the extracellular concentration of glutamate.

Astrocyte Membrane K+ Conductance

Our hypothesis that cytokine and/or HIV-1-induced stimulation of Na^+/H^+ exchange will lead to intracellular alkalinization within the astrocyte, which in turn can activate K^+ channels. We have performed whole-cell patch-clamp experiments on primary cultures of rat astrocytes to test this hypothesis. Figure 2 shows whole-cell patch-clamp measurements of an astrocyte bathed in Na^+ gluconate solution (K^+ gluconate was the patch pipette) under control conditions (A) and 3 minutes after treatment with IFN-γ (100 U/ml) (B). Note that the solution inside the pipette (and hence inside the astrocyte) was unbuffered. Thus, if Na^+/H^+ antiport was activated, the compartment bathing the cytoplasmic face of the astrocyte plasma membrane would alkalinize. The voltage-clamp protocol consisted of holding the membrane potential at -60 mV (outside = ground potential), stepping the voltage from -100 mV to +100 mV in 20 mV increments, and recording the resulting current at each potential. The voltage steps each lasted 1 second, and the membrane potential was returned to -60 mV between pulses. There is very little inward (i.e., Na^+) current before or after IFN-γ treatment. In the untreated cells, most of the resting membrane conductance is due to outward K^+ movement. After IFN-γ treatment, the K^+ conductance is significantly increased. This observation can better be appreciated by an examination of the steady-state current voltage (I-V) curves (Fig. 2C). First, the I-V curves are strongly outwardly rectified. Outward K^+ current increased by 39% and 62% after 1 and 3 minutes of IFN-γ treatment, respectively. The same effect fan be seen at the single-channel level (not shown). As further tests of the hypothesis that alterations in intracellular pH can directly influence K^+ conductance, several additional experiments have been performed. If amiloride, an inhibitor of Na^+/H^+ antiport, is present in the bathing medium, IFN-γ should not activate outward K^+ currents (even when the pipette solution has a low buffer capacity). This prediction is validated by the experiments shown in Figures 2D and E. Amiloride treatment of astrocytes has no effect on either inward or outward currents (data not shown). Likewise, outward K+ currents should not be activated by IFN-γ in the absence of amiloride if the pipette solution is highly buffered. That this is indeed the case is shown in Figures 2F and G.

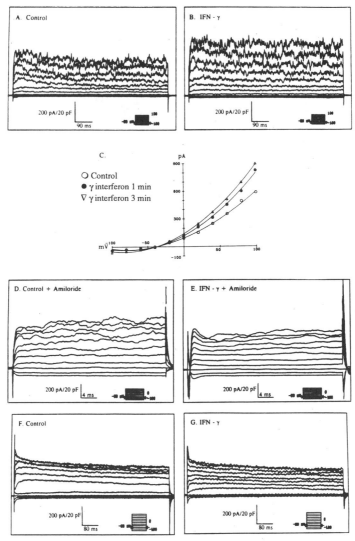

Figure 2. Whole-cell currents recorded from primary cultured rat astrocytes. The cells were cultured in serum-free medium for 24 hours prior to experimentation. The bath solution contained 150 mM Na+ gluconate, 6 mM HEPES (pH 7.25), 1 mM EGTA, and 2 mM CaCl₂. The pipette contained 30 mM KCl, 120 mM K+ gluconate, and 1 mM EGTA (pH 7.2; unbuffered). Control currents were stable for at least 1 hr. A. Control; B. 3 min after exposure to 100 U/ml IFN-γ; C. Steady-state I-V relations of control (0), and IFN-γ-treated [(•) - 1 min; (d) -3 min] rat astrocytes; D,E. Identical experiment as in A and B except that 0.2 mM amiloride was present in the external bathing solution throughout the experiment (amiloride had no effect on control current for up to 15 min); F, G. Identical experiment as in A and B except that the contents of the pipette solution were highly buffered with 50 mM HEPES (pH 7.2). This entire experimental protocol has been repeated five times with essentially the same results.

In other experiments, recombinant gp120, like IFN-γ also stimulated outward K+ currents via activation of Na+/H+ exchange. However, the stimulation produced by gp120 was significantly greater (by at least a factor of 2) than that produced by IGN-γ. Thus, our results are consistent with the hypothesis that activation of astrocyte Na+/H+ exchange (either by cytokines like IFN-γ or gp120) leads to intracellular alkalinization with a subsequent increase in membrane K+ conductance. Control experiments indicate that IGN-γ, gp120, or amiloride do not directly affect K+ conductance in the astrocyte (cf., Fig. 2G).

SUMMARY

It is undoubtedly true that the mechanisms operative in the pathogenesis of HIV-associated disease of the CNS will prove to be varied and interactive. Most workers in the field now agree that gp120 by itself is not neuronotoxic, i.e., gp120 does not directly kill neurons.[39] Therefore, brain cells other than neurons must also contribute to the etiology of the syndrome. Several groups have provided evidence that brain-derived mononuclear phagocytes infected with HIV release, in addition to cytokines, other substances that can act as neurotoxins. Recent work by Gendelman and colleagues[40] clearly demonstrates that HIV-infected human monocytes and astroglia secrete the cytokines TNF-α and IL-1, as well as large amounts of platelet-activating factor, arachidonic acid, and the arachidonic acid metabolites leukotriene B_4, leukotriene D_4, and lipoxin A_4. Importantly arachidonic acid has been shown to increase Ca^{2+} currents through NMDA receptors by increasing channel open probability.[41] Giulian et al.[42] show that HIV-infected or gp120-stimulated macrophages release small (<500 kDa), heat-stable, protease-resistant soluble factors that can promote neuronal killing. Dawson et al.[43] likewise report that gp 120 can indirectly kill neurons in primary rat mixed (i.e., neuronal, astrocyte, macrophage/microglia) cortical cultures. This toxicity requires glutamate and appears ultimately to result from Ca^{2+}-stimulated nitric oxide and superoxide anion production in the neuron. Heyes et al.[44] have shown that macrophages can synthesize and release quinolinic acid, an NMDA receptor agonist, and that the levels of quinolinic acid found in the CSF and HIV-positive patients correlate well with functional neurologic impairment.[45]

Nevertheless, many important and crucial questions remain. For example, can gp120 be detected in the brains of HIV-infected individuals, what concentrations are achieved, and can these concentrations be correlated with the severity of HIV-related neurologic disease?[45] What are the regional differences in concentration and/or sensitivities of neurotoxic substances, and do these correlate with the wide spatial variability observed in neuropathological specimens?[39] How does the metabolic state of the neuron impinge upon HIV-associated neurotoxicity?[46,47] Thus, in the CNS of patients infected with HIV, neuronal cell injury is probably mediated by an intricate interaction of cytokines, HIV-1 viral proteins, and soluble toxic factors.

It should be noted that the concentration of gp120 that we employed is several orders of magnitude higher than that achieved in plasma, given virion loads of 5 x 10^6 to 10^8 per milliliter. However, the concentrations of gp120 in the extracellular fluid surrounding an astrocyte may be much higher than in plasma. If we assume a 10 μm diameter circular region of an astrocyte separated from an associated neuron by 10-20 nm,[48] we can calculate the volume of that extracellular space, assuming a cylindrical geometry, to be 1.6 x 10^{-15} liters. According to Layne et al.,[49] 1 HIV virion contains 100-280 gp120 molecules; 100 gp120 molecules are equivalent to 1.66 x 10^{-22} moles. Therefore, if only a single HIV virus releases all of its gp120 in a volume of this size, the concentration of gp120 in the extracellular space between the astrocyte and the neuron would be 100 nM! In direct measurements of HIV p24 levels in CNS tissue obtained at autopsy from individuals with severe HIV encephalitis, p24 levels of around 1,000 pg/5mg tissue were found.[45] Assuming that 80% of brain tissue is water and that there are 1,200 p24 molecules per virion (to convert to an equivalent of gp120, namely, 420pg),[49] we can calculate a gp120 concentration of approximately 1 nM. This is a minimal concentration given that the computation presumed that gp120 was distributed throughout the entire (i.e., both intra- and extracellular) water space. Consequently, it is reasonable to conclude that the concentration of envelope glycoproteins employed could approximate those present in the interstitial spaces surrounding the astrocytes in the brain.

In conclusion, we hypothesize that the sustained presence of cytokines and/or viral proteins in the brain interfere with astrocyte K^+ and glutamate regulatory mechanisms. Because of the unique morphologic arrangement of astroglia and neurons in the CNS, the extracellular space separating these cell types is extremely small.[48] Making some simple geometric assumptions about this extracellular cleft (sometimes called the Frankenhaeuser-Hodgkin space), it can be estimated that large (40 mM) changes in $[K^+]$ can occur with only a small (<1%) less of K^+ from the astrocyte itself. This change in concentration can depolarize CNS neurons by more than 40 mV, seriously affecting conduction, and is of a magnitude sufficient to open voltage-dependent Ca^{2+} channels.[10,50] Orkland et al.[50] estimated that the half-time for $[K^+]$.in the extracellular space to fall from 20 to 4 mM was 6 seconds. Thus, interference of the K^+ buffering (i.e., uptake) systems of the astrocyte would, over time, adversely affect nerve conduction. Based upon the results presented in this chapter, we argue that the astrocyte itself plays a prominent role in the development of the AIDS-dementia complex. Therefore, we show that exposure of primary cultures of rat and human astrocytes to either cytokines, heat-inactivated HIV-1 virions, or to the purified envelope glycoprotein gp120 activates an amiloride-sensitive Na^+/H^+ exchange process. The resulting intracellular alkalinization stimulates astrocyte membrane K^+ conductance and glutamate efflux, and inhibits the uptake of glutamate from the extracellular space. As a result, we hypothesize that the subsequent rise in extracellular K^+ and glutamate concentrations produce a neuronal depolarization, thus activating both voltage-dependent and NMDA-operated Ca^{2+} channels. As a consequence, intraneuronal Ca^{2+} concentration increases, producing neuronotoxicity. Thus, our results implicate the astrocyte as a critical cell type involved in the pathogenesis of the HIV-associated cognitive/motor syndrome.[51]

ACKNOWLEDGMENT

This work was supported by funds from NIH Grant MH50421 and the NIH Center For AIDS Research at UAB.

REFERENCES

1. J.A. Levy, J. Shimabukuro, H. Hollander, J. Mills, and L. Kaminsky. Isolation of AIDS-associated retroviruses from cerebrospinal fluid and brain of patients with neurological symptoms. *Lancet* 9:586 (1985).
2. C.K. Petito, E.S. Cho, W. Lemann, B.A. Navia, and R.W. Price. Neuropathology of acquired immune deficiency syndrome (AIDS): an autopsy review. *J. Neuropathol. Exp. Neurol.* 45:635 (1986).
3. G.M. Shaw, M.E. Harper, B.H. Hahn, L.G. Epstein, D.C. Gajdusek, R.W. Price, B.A. Navia, C.K. Petito, C.J. O'Hara, J.E. Groopman, E.S. Cho, J.M. Oleske, F. Wong-Staal, and R.C. Gallo. HTLV-III infection in brains of children and adults with AIDS encephalopathy. *Science* 227:177 (1985).
4. D.D. Ho, R.R. Rota, R.T. Schooley, J.C. Kaplan, J. Davis-Allen, J.E. Groopman, L. Resnick, D. Felsenstein, C.A. Andrews, and M.S. Hirsch. Isolation of HTLV-III from the cerebrospinal fluid and neural tissues of patients with neurologic syndromes related to the acquired immune deficiency syndrome. *New Engl. J. Med.* 313:1493 (1985).
5. D.J. Eilbott, N. Peress, H. Burger, D. LaNeve, J. Orenstein, H.E. Gendelman, R. Seidman, and B. Weiser. Human immunodeficiency virus type I in spinal cords of acquired immune deficiency syndrome patients with myelopathy: expression and replication in macrophages. *Proc. Natl. Acad. Sci., USA* 86:3337 (1989).
6. D.H. Gabuzda, D.D. Ho, S.M. de la Monte, M.S. Hirsch, T.R. Rota, and R.A. Sobel. Immunohistochemical identification of HTLV-III antigen in brains of patients with AIDS. *Ann. Neurol.* 20:289 (1986).
7. S. Koenig, H.E. Gendelman, T.M. Orenstein, M.C. dal Canto, G.H. Pezeshkpour, M. Yungbluth, F. Janotta, A. Aksamit, M.A. Martin, and A.S. Fauci. Detection of AIDS virus in macrophages of brain tissue from AIDS patients with encephalopathy. *Science* 233:1089 (1986).
8. C.A. Wiley, R.D. Schreier, J.A. Nelson, P.W. Lampert, and M.B.A. Oldstone. Cellular localization of human immunodeficiency virus infection within the brains of acquired immune deficiency syndrome patients. *Proc. Natl. Acad. Sci. USA* 83:7089 (1986).
9. F.A. Henn, H. Haljamae, and A. Hamberger. Glial cell function: Active control of extracellular K+ concentration. *Brain Res.* 43L437 (1972).
10. B.A. Barres, L.L.Y. Chun, and D.P. Corey. Ion channels in vertebrate glia. *Annu. Rev. Neurosci.* 13:441 (1990).
11. Y. Berwald-Netter, A. Koulakoff, L. Nowak, and P. Ascher. Ionic channels in glial cells, *in:* "Astrocytes," S.S. Federoff and A. Vernadakis, eds., Academic Press, Orlando, 2:51 (1986).
12. L. Hertz. Regulation of potassium homeostasis by glial cells, *in:* "Differentiation and Functions of Glial Cells," G. Levi, ed., Wiley-Liss, New York 55:225 (1990).
13. L. Hertz, B. Soliven, E. Hertz, S. Szuchet, and D.J. Nelson. Channel-mediated and carrier-mediated uptake of K+ into cultured ovine oligodendrocytes. *Glia* 3:550 (1990).
14. W. Walz. Role of glial cells in the regulation of the brain ion microenvironment. *Prog. Neurobiol.* 33:309 (1989).
15. A.H. Cornell-Bell, S.M. Finkbeiner, M.S. Cooper, and S.J. Smith. Glutamate induces calcium waves in cultured astrocytes: Long-range glial signaling. *Science* 247:470 (1990).
16. H.K. Kimelberg, S.K. Goderie, S. Higman, S. Pang, and R.A. Waniewski. Swelling-induced release of glutamate, aspartate, and taurine from astrocyte cultures. *J. Neurosci.* 10:1583 (1990).
17. M. Szatkowski, B. Barbour, and D. Attwell. Nonvesicular release of glutamate from glial cells by reversed electrogenic glutamate uptake. *Nature* 348:443 (1990).

18. P. Gallo, K. Frei, C. Rordorf, J. Lazdins, B. Tavolato, and A. Fontana. Human immunodeficiency virus type 1 (HIV-1) infection of the central nervous system: an evaluation of cytokines in cerebrospinal fluid. *J. Neuroimmunol.* 23:109-116 (1989).

19. W.R. Tyor, J.D. Glass, J.W. Griffin, P.S. Becker, J.C. McArthur, L. Bezman, and D.E. Griffin. Cytokine expression in the brain during the acquired immunodeficiency syndrome. *Ann. Neurol.* 31:3499 (1992).

20. S. Griffin. Interleukin-1 expression in AIDS brain. *Neurological Consequences of Immune Dysregulation Workshop, Abstract* (1992).

21. D.E. Griffin. Cytokines in the CNS during HIV infection as assessed by CSF analysis, immunocytochemical staining of CNS tissue and PCR amplification mRNA from brain. *Neurological Consequences of Immune Dysregulation Workshop, Abstract* (1992).

22. V. Prpic, S.F. Yu, F. Figueiredo, P.W. Hollenbach, G. Gawdi, B. Herman, R.J. Uhing, and D.O. Adams. Role of Na^+/H^+ exchange of interferon-γ in enhanced expression of JE and I-A_b genes. *Science* 244:469 (1989).

23. E.N. Benveniste, M. Vidovic, R.B. Panek, J.G. Norris, A.T. Reddy, and D.J. Benos. Interferon-γ induced astrocyte class II major histocompatibility complex gene expression is associated with both protein kinase C activation and Na^+ entry. *J. Biol. Chem.* 266:18119 (1991).

24. S.Y. Chiu. Functional distribution of voltage-gated sodium and potassium channels with mammalian Schwann cells. *Glia* 4:541 (1991).

25. J.G. McLarnon and S.U. Kim. Ion channels in cultured adult human Schwann cells. *Glia* 4:534 (1991).

26. G.F. Wilson and S.Y. Chiu. Ion channels in axonal Schwann cell membranes at paranodes of mammalian myelinated fibers studied with patch clamp. *J. Neurosci.* 10:3263 (1990).

27. B.A. Macvicar, D. Hochman, M.J. Delay, and S. Weiss. Modulation of intracellular Ca^{2+} in cultured astrocytes by influx through voltage-activated Ca^{2+} channels. *Glia* 4:448 (1991).

28. D.E. Brenneman. Neuronal cell killing by the envelope protein of HIV and its prevention by vasoactive intestinal peptide. *Nature* 335:639 (1988).

29. E.B. Dreyer, P.K. Kaiser, J.T. Offermann, and S.A. Lipton. HIV-1 coat protein neurotoxicity prevented by calcium channel antagonists. *Science* 248:364 (1990).

30. S.A. Lipton, N.J. Sucher, P.K. Kaiser, and E.B. Dreyer. Synergistic effects of HIV coat protein and NMDA receptor-mediated neurotoxicity. *Neuron* 7:111 (1991).

31. J.S. Tabb, P.E. Kish, R. Van Dyke, and T. Ueda. Glutamate transport into synaptic vesicles. Roles of membrane potential, pH gradient, and intravesicular pH. *J. Biol. Chem.* 267:15412 (1992).

32. K.H. Backus, H. Kettenmann, and M. Schachner. Pharmacological characterization of the glutamate receptor in cultured astrocytes. *J. Neurosci. Res.* 22:274 (1989).

33. D.W. Choi. Glutamate neurotoxicity and diseases of the nervous system. *Neuron* 1:623 (1988).

34. Z.F. Rosenberg and A.S. Fauci. Immunopathogenesis of HIV infection. *FASEB J.* 5:2382 (1991).

35. C.A. Wiley, E. Masliah, M. Morey, C. Lemere, R. Deteresa, M. Grafe, L. Hansen, and R. Terry. Neocortical damage during HIV infection. *Ann. Neurol.* 29:651 (1991).

36. J. Offerman, K. Uchida, and S.A. Lipton. High-dose NMDA induces retraction and low-dose NMDA induces elongation of rat retinal ganglion cell (RGC) neurites. *Soc. Neurosci. Abst.* 17:927 (1991).

37. D.J. Benos, D.G. Warnock, and J.B. Smith. Amiloride-sensitive Na^+ transport mechanisms, *in:* "Membrane Transport in Biology," J.A. Schafer, G. Giebisch, eds., Academic Press, New York, Vol. 5:166 (1992).

38. W.F. Boron. Control of intracellular pH, *in:* "The Kidney: Physiology and Pathophysiology," Second Edition, D.W. Seldin and G.Giebisch, eds., Raven Press, New York (1992).

39. L.R. Sharer. Pathology of HIV-1 infection of the central nervous system. A review. *J. Neuropathol. Exp. Neurol.* 51:3 (1992).

40. P. Genis, M. Jett, E.W. Bernton, T. Boyle, H.A. Gelbard, K. Dzenko, R.W. Keane, L. Resnick, Y. Mizrachi, D.J. Volsky, L.G. Epstein, and H.E. Gendelman. Cytokines and arachidonic acid metabolites produced during human immunodeficiency virus (HIV)-infected macrophage-astroglia interactions: implications for the neuropathogenesis of HIV disease. *J. Exp. Med.* 176:1703 (1992).

41. B. Miller, M. Sarantis, S.F. Traynelis, and D. Attwell. Potentiation of NMDA receptor currents by arachidonic acid. *Nature (London)* 355:722 (1992).

42. D. Giulian, E. Wendt, K. Vaca, and C.A. Noonan. The envelope glycoprotein of human immunodeficiency virus type 1 stimulates release of neurotoxins from monocytes. *Proc. Natl. Acad. Sci. USA* 90:2769 (1993).

43. V.L. Dawson, T.M. Dawson, G.R. Uhl, and S.H. Snyder. Human immunodeficiency virus type 1 coat protein neurotoxicity mediated by nitric oxide in primary cortical cultures. *Proc. Natl. Acad. Sci. USA* 90:3256 (1993).

44. M.P. Heyes, B.J. Brew, A. Martin, R.W. Price, A.M. Salazar, J.J. Sidtis, J.A. Yergey, M.M. Mouradian, A.E. Sadler, J. Keilip, D. Rubinow, and S.P. Markey. Quinolinic acid in cerebrospinal fluid and serum in HIV-1 infection: Relationship to clinical and neurological status. *Ann. Neurol.* 29:202 (1991).

45. C.L. Achim, M.P. Heyes, and C.A. Wiley. Quantitation of human immunodeficiency virus, immune activation factors, and quinolinic acid in AIDS brains. *J. Clin. Invest.* 91:2769-2775 (1993).

46. A. Novelli, J.A. Reilly, P.G. Lysko, and R.C. Henneberry. Glutamate becomes neurotoxic via the N-methyl-D-aspartate receptor when intracellular energy levels are reduced. *Brain Res.* 451:205 (1988).

47. E. Chleide, J. Bruhwyler, and K. Ishikawa. Biochemistry of hypoxic damage in brain cells - roles of energy metabolism, glutamate, and calcium ion. *Neuroscience* 17:375 (1991).

48. J.G. Nicholls and S.W. Kuffler. Extracellular space as a pathway for exchange between blood and neurons in the central nervous system of the leech: ionic composition of glial cells and neurons. *J. Neurophysiol.* 27: 645 (1964).

49. S.P. Layne, M.J. Merges, M. Dembo, J.L. Spouge, S.R. Conley, J.P. Moore, J.L. Raina, H.Renz, H.R. Gelderblom, and P.L. Nara. Factors underlying spontaneous inactivation and susceptibility to neutralization of human immunodeficiency virus. *Virology* 189:695 (1992).

50. R.K. Orkland, J.G. Nicholls, and S.W. Kuffler. Effect of nerve impulses on the membrane potential of glial cells in the central nervous system of amphibia. *J. Neurophysiol.* 29:788 (1966).

51. D.J. Benos, B.H. Hahn, J.K. Bubien, S.K. Ghosh, N.A. Mashburn, M.A. Ch Chaikin, G.M. Shaw, and E.N. Benveniste. HIV-1 gp120 alters ion transport in astrocytes: implications for AIDS dementia complex. *Proc. Natl. Acad. Sci. USA* 91:494 (1994).

ALTERNATIVE RECEPTORS FOR HIV-1 IN NERVOUS SYSTEM TISSUES

Francisco González-Scarano,[1,2] Jacques Fantini,[3]
David G. Cook,[1] and Neal Nathanson[2]

[1]Department of Neurology
[2]Department of Microbiology
University of Pennsylvania Medical Center, CRB
422 Curie Boulevard
Philadelphia Pennsylvania, USA

[3]C.N.R.S., URA 1455
Faculté de Médecine Nord
Marseille, France

CD4 INDEPENDENT INFECTION

The CD4 molecule of lymphocytes, monocytes and microglia is the principal receptor molecule for HIV-1 and HIV-2.[1] Numerous studies have demonstrated that the HIV surface glycoprotein, gp120, binds this cell surface molecule with high affinity at its amino terminal immunoglobulin-like domain.[2,3] Furthermore, antibodies against certain epitopes on CD4, as well as soluble recombinant forms of the molecule, can inhibit HIV infectivity of many lymphoid cell lines and primary lymphoid cells.[4,5] Nevertheless, it is also clear that many cultured cells, both primary and immortalized, that do not express either CD4 protein or mRNA, can be infected with HIV-1, albeit at much lower efficiency than CD4-positive cells.[4,6-11] These findings suggest that HIV-1 can use alternative means of entry, possibly involving one or more alternative receptor molecules.

Table 1 lists a partial compilation of CD4 negative cell lines and primary cells that have been shown to be infectable with HIV-1 and/or HIV-2. In most instances where a CD4-independent infection has been documented, the presence of the provirus can only be detected by cocultivation with highly permissive cells or by assay for retroviral DNA with the polymerase chain reaction (PCR). (There are some exceptions, notably, the HT-29 colon adenocarcinoma cell line.[12]) In many studies, residual virus has been eliminated as a potential source of contamination by the judicious use of negative control cells and by frequent passage and trypsinization of the infected cells prior to cocultivation.

Although Table 1 illustrates the infectability of tissues from widely different sources, some cell lines (e.g., HeLa cells) and primary cells cannot be infected with HIV. This indicates that HIV enters CD4 negative cells through a specific mechanism characteristic of only some cell membranes. Furthermore, viruses that are taken up by nonspecific pinocytosis enter compartments where they do not uncoat or begin replication. Thus, it has been generally accepted that, at least in selected cultured cells, HIV is specifically bound and internalized by CD4-independent mechanisms.

Technical Advances in AIDS Research in the Human Nervous System
Edited by E.O. Major and J.A. Levy, Plenum Press, New York, 1995

Table 1. HIV-1 infectable, CD4 negative non-neural cells.*

Cell Type	Cocultivation[a]	Supernatant Virus[b]	Reference
Muscle	+		Clapham et al., (1989)[4]
Fibroblast	+		Tateno et al. (1989)[10]
Hepatoma	+	+	Cao et al. (1990)[13]
Fibroblast	+		Werner et al. (1990)[14]
Colon epithelium	+	+	Moyer & Gendelman (1991)[15]
Colon epithelium	+	+	Yahi et al. (1992)[16]
Adrenal	+	+	Barboza et al. (1992)[6]
Endothelial (umbilical)	+	+	Scheglovitova et al. (1993)[17]

*This table contains a partial list of CD4 negative nonneural cell lines that can be infected with HIV-1 and/or HIV-2.
[a]Provirus demonstrated by cocultivation.
[b]Virus present in supernatant.

Expression of the CD4 molecule through recombinant methods converts some CD4 negative cells, like HeLa, into cells able to replicate HIV to high levels.[1] That is not the case for all lines, as was shown by Chesebro and associates.[18] The restriction noted in some cell lines that have been engineered to express CD4 could be due to a requirement for an accessory molecule that is important for viral entry in conjunction with CD4. The existence of such a molecule has been speculated upon in many publications and a candidate molecule, CD26, has been proposed recently.[19] The presence of such an accessory molecule would determine whether CD4 expression was sufficient for converting a non-permissive to a permissive cell. Alternatively, there may be additional levels of restriction at many points beyond the entry process, at the steps of reverse transcription, integration or viral transcription/translation. As a number of CD4 negative neurally derived cells have been infected with HIV-1, some investigators have addressed this question on nervous system-derived cells directly (see below).

HIV INFECTION OF NEURAL CELLS

Since the pathogenesis of primary neurological complications of HIV-1 infection is still not understood, neurally-derived cells have been among the most important substrates for the investigation of alternative mechanisms for HIV entry. *In vivo* infection by HIV-1 in the CNS has been demonstrated primarily, although not exclusively, in microglia, but is the subject of continuing investigation using increasingly sensitive techniques. However, *in vitro*, a number of cell lines of neuronal and astrocytic origin, and primary cells from a few CNS and PNS sources, can be infected with HIV-1 (Table 2).

Table 2. Human neural cells infectable with HIV-1.[*]

Cell Type (Source)		CD4[a]	Cocultivation[b]	Viral Antigen[c]	GalCer/Sulf
Glioma	U138MG			+	?
	U373MG	No	+		Antibody blocks
	U489	No	+		?
	U251	No	+		?
	U87MG	No	+		?
	85HG-59			+	?
	86HG-63			+	?
	85HG-66			+	?
	85HG-64			+	?
Neuronal (PNS)	SK-N-MC	No		+	Antibody blocks
Neuronal (CNS)	HCN-1A	No		+	Present
Dorsal Root Ganglia	Primary	No		+	?
Astrocytes	Primary	No		+	?
Microglia	Primary	Yes		+ + +	
Endothelial	Primary	No		+	Antibody does not block
Adrenal	SW13	No	+		Antibody does not block

* The table contains a partial list of nervous system-derived cells and cell lines that have been described as infectable by HIV-1.

a The presence of CD4 protein or mRNA, as reported in the literature.

b Virus was only detected by cocultivation with highly permissive cells.

c Viral antigen was detected either by immunofluorescence or by assay of supernatant for p24.[8,11,24-26]

Primary Cells

Infection of dorsal root ganglia (DRG), astrocytes, microglia, and recently, cerebral endothelial cells has been documented by several investigators. Infection of DRG and primary astrocytes leads to transient antigenic expression, detected primarily with immunofluorescence for p24 and p17, appears to involve a significant proportion of the nonneuronal population, and does not lead to cytopathic changes.[20,21] Similarly, infection of a population of cells obtained from fetal brain which express glial fibrillary acidic protein (GFAP) leads to a persistent noncytopathic infection.[22] In this latter system, virus expression can be activated by exposure of the infected cell population to cytokines. More recently, Moses and coworkers[23] have reported that cerebral capillary endothelial cells, but not those obtained from peripheral tissues, could be readily infected with HIV-1. In this study, viral antigen was detected in a large proportion of the infected cells using indirect immunofluorescence, and modest level of virus were shed into the supernatant.

In contrast to these relatively nonproductive infections, the group headed by Dubois-Dalcq has been able to productively infect a cell population in cultured adult brain obtained at the time of surgical resection for the treatment of epilepsy.[27] When exposed to macrophage-tropic HIV-1 strains (see below), this population expresses intracellular viral antigens, and reasonably high levels of p24[gag] in the supernatant ($\geq$ 100 ng/ml). These cells express several cell markers normally associated with macrophages and monocytes (such as binding acetylated LDL), and it has been assumed that they represent microglia. However, they have not been shown to express specific microglial markers, and other investigators have questioned the infectability of 'true' microglial tissue.[28] In our experience, using a similar source of adult human brain, and with side-by-side comparison with monocyte-derived macrophages (MDM) grown in the same media supplemented with giant cell supernatant, there are distinct morphological differences between MDM and the microglial population (A. Albright and F. Gonzalez-Scarano, unpublished results). Thus, even if the origin of the cells cultured from adult brain is debatable, they are morphologically distinguishable from blood-derived macrophages.

Immortalized Cells

Many cell lines obtained from peripheral and central nervous system tissue are also easily infected with HIV-1 and HIV-2. However, as with primary cells from astrocytic or other glial origin, the infection is usually low level, although it can persist for several months in culture. A survey of the cells listed in Table 2 indicates that both cells expressing GFAP (astrocytic) and neuronal markers (neurofilament proteins) are infectable. There are no immortalized human cell lines that have distinct oligodendroglial features, accounting for their absence from these reports. With few exceptions (SK-N-MC, for example), these are very restrictive infections, although viral expression can be stimulated with exposure to cytokines and/or phorbol esters.[9,22]

Virus Strains

Most HIV strains can be divided into those that replicate primarily in cells of T-lymphocytic origin (lymphocyte-tropic) and those that can replicate in macrophages (macrophage-tropic). Cells of astroglial or neuronal derivation have been infected primarily with lymphocyte-tropic strains of HIV, like IIIb (LAI), RF or NL4-3. Although generally not reported, it is difficult to infect these cells with either primary or macrophage-tropic isolates. This is surprising, in view of the fact that most isolates obtained directly from brain are in fact macrophage-tropic. On the other hand, as the majority of experiments in the field have been performed with immortalized cell lines, it is possible that the absence of repli-cation noted with macrophage-tropic strains is a reflection of their general inability to replicate in continuous lines, rather than their 'macrophage-tropism'. It is also possible that the brain harbors a number of HIV strains that are not macrophage-tropic, but are underrepresented using current isolation methods. In contrast, microglial cells obtained from adult brain are infectable with macrophage-tropic viruses, and the ability to replicate appears to map to the *env* gene as does tropism for monocyte-derived macrophages.[29] Whether there are specific microglia-tropic virus strains is a current subject for experimentation.

Viral Entry into Neural Cells

In spite of initial reports indicating that CD4 is expressed in brain,[1] it has not been detected consistently within the nervous system. Most investigators agree that astrocytes, neurons and oligodendrocytes, as well as immortalized cells derived from such tissues, do not express CD4 protein or mRNA. Accordingly, *in vitro* HIV infection of astroglial and neuronal cells is not blocked by either recombinant soluble CD4 or by antibodies directed against epitopes of CD4 that are close to the HIV-1 binding site, for example, the site defined by OKT4A.[20] As it is unlikely that nonspecific uptake of virus could account for the infectability of some nervous system tissue, the potential role of alternative receptors has been the subject of experimentation. The role of glycolipids such as galactosylceramide (GalCer) and galactosylsulfatide (sulfatide) is discussed in more detail in sections that follow. Other investigators have suggested that cell surface glycoproteins may be responsible for HIV entry into glial lines, although the molecules have not been specifically identified.[29]

Several groups have used CD4 expression in glial cells as a mechanism for studying the role of entry in glial/neuronal tropism. A consensus opinion appears to be that the expression of CD4 in glial cells does not lead to a highly productive

HIV-1 infection, as it does in HeLa cells and some other cell lines. Harouse et al.[31] found that U373 glioblastoma cells expressing CD4 replicated virus initially, with p24gag levels reaching 2.5 ng/ml in the first week, but dropped to 1 ng or less chronically. In contrast, HeLa-CD4 cells produced up to 1 µg/ml p24gag in a parallel infection. Volsky and collaborators[32] similarly found that introduction of CD4 into a glioma line, H4, led to increased levels of intracellular p24gag production in comparison with the parent line. More recently, Harrington and Geballe[33] prepared a U373-CD4 line and showed minimal infection in either the U373 or the U373-CD4 cells. Using a fusion protocol with HeLa cells, they demonstrated increased levels of p24 production in some of the hybrids. However, in contrast to Volsky et al.[32] and Harouse et al.,[31] who interpreted their results as demonstrating a post-entry block, Harrington and Geballe suggested that their data are consistent with an entry block in either the U373 or U373-CD4 cells, arguing for the presence of a cofactor molecule important for either CD4 or alternate receptor-mediated entry. Although superficially it might appear that these results are discrepant, in fact, all three groups, as well as Chesebro[18] agree that glial cell lines have an additional level of restriction beyond the initial binding step.

In contrast to astroglial/neuronal infection, the entry process in microglial infection appears to be well defined. Although the presence of CD4 has not been directly demonstrated in microglia derived from adult brain, HIV-1 infection of these cells is inhibited by soluble CD4 and by antibodies against the CD4 molecule. This is usually sufficient evidence of CD4-mediated infection, particularly in view of the fact that direct demonstration of the presence of CD4 is difficult even in monocyte-derived macrophages, which are available in larger quantities and thus can be manipulated more extensively.[34]

Summary

In summary, the available evidence would indicate that *in vitro* infection of neural cells from a number of sources and with differing phenotypes is a well accepted phenomenon. Entry in glial or neuronal cells does not involve the CD4 molecule, which has not been found consistently in either of these cell types. Among potential entry mechanisms are alternative glycoproteins or glycolipids (see following section), but no single molecule is likely to be responsible for entry into all of the neural cell lines that have been described as infectable. A confounding problem is the clear evidence that there are additional levels of restriction to viral replication in glial cells, as several glial cell lines that have been engineered to express CD4 remain either only moderately permissive or nonpermissive to HIV infection. Whether this additional level of restriction is at the entry step or following entry is controversial.

GALACTOSYLCERAMIDE AND SULFATIDE: CANDIDATE RECEPTOR MOLECULES

As suggested in the previous section, it is unlikely that one receptor molecule is responsible for entry into all CD4 negative infectable cells. However, experiments from our laboratories have identified candidate receptor molecules, galactosylceramide (GalCer) and galactosylsulfatide (sulfatide), for a subset of glioblastoma and colonic epithelial cell lines. Two lines of evidence directed our attention to these glycolipids. First, antibodies raised against GalCer (and sulfatide) could inhibit HIV entry and infection in two neural cell lines SK-N-MC and U373, as well as the colonic epithelial line HT-29.[16,35] Most importantly, the HIV-1 receptor-binding glycoprotein, gp120, bound GalCer and sulfatide immobilized on a high-performance thin-layer chromatography (HPTLC) plate with high specificity, saturability and avidity.[35,36] GalCer is present in oligodendrocytes in the central nervous system, Schwann cells in the peripheral nervous system, and in colon epithelial cells. Sulfatide is also found in oligodendrocytes as well as neurons, and has also been found in kidney and sperm cells.

These results suggested, but by no means conclusively proved, that HIV-1 was utilizing these molecules as a means of entry. Subsequent studies have concentrated on identifying the region of gp120 involved in its interactions with GalCer/sulfatide, and in further correlating infectability of CD4 negative cells with the presence of GalCer/sulfatide on the cell surface.

Interaction Between HIV gp120 and GalCer/Sulfatide.
Biological Interactions

The interaction between gp120 and GalCer/sulfatide has been studied in our laboratory using HPTLC and ELISA, and confirmed with a liposome binding assay.[37] Binding of gp120 directly to cells expressing sulfatide has previously been reported by Schneider-Schaulies et al.[30] To determine whether gp120 molecules from different strains could bind GalCer equally effectively, selected recombinant gp120 molecules were used in a variation of the HPTLC

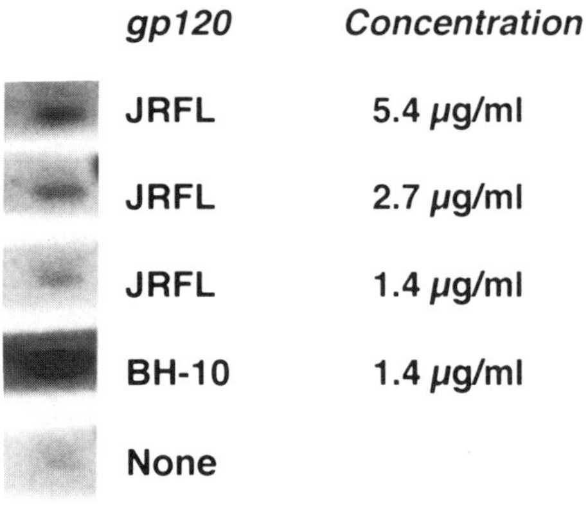

gp120	Concentration
JRFL	5.4 µg/ml
JRFL	2.7 µg/ml
JRFL	1.4 µg/ml
BH-10	1.4 µg/ml
None	

Figure 1. Binding of HIV-1 gp120 to GalCer. Recombinant gp120 from two HIV-1 strains, BH-10 (LAI) and JRFL were bound to GalCer immobilized on HPTLC, as previously described.[12] A 3.8-fold excess of JRFL gp120 did not bind GalCer as well as BH-10 gp120.

binding assay previously described.[36] Shown in Figure 1 are results of a comparison between HIV-1 BH-10 (LAI) gp120 and a similar recombinant protein from HIV-1 JRFL. In spite of a 3.8-fold excess of the JRFL gp 120 in comparison to BH-10 gp120, little was bound to the GalCer on the HPTLC plate. There were similar results when GalCer obtained from lipid extracts of human tissue culture cell lines was substituted for the commercial GalCer extracted from bovine brain.

Since there is a considerable difference between the ability of these two gp120 molecules to bind GalCer, a comparison between their amino acid sequences could provide clues to the region of gp120 involved in this interaction. In Figure 2, based on the two-dimensional representation of BH-10 gp120 described by Leonard et al.,[38] the amino acid differences between JRFL and BH-10 have been highlighted. As expected, amino acid differences between the two molecules are clustered around the variable regions, particularly V1 and V3, with only scattered changes elsewhere in the molecule. Previous HPTLC binding experiments, as well as biological data, had indicated that the CD4 binding region is not involved in gp120/GalCer binding. Thus, this comparison between the two strains narrowed the region of interest to the variable regions, particularly V1/V3.

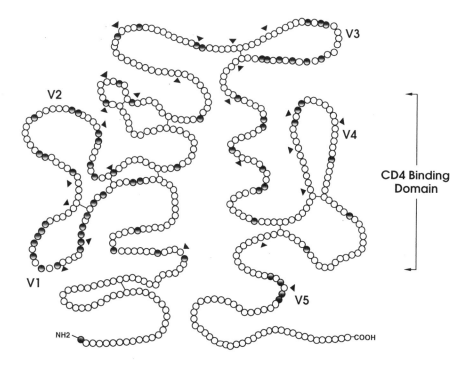

▼ ASN -GLYCOSYLATION

◉ JRFL CHANGES

Figure 2. Comparison between gp120 molecules from, HIV-1 LAI (BH-10) and HIV-1 JRFL. The deduced amino acid sequence from BH-10 was obtained from Myers,[39] and each amino acid is represented by a light circle, based on the two-dimensional representation of Leonard.[38] Differences between JRFL and BH-10 are indicated by the dark circles. Because of insertions and deletions, the figure can only approximate some of the changes, but all areas where there are changes have been highlighted.

A panel of 18 anti-gp120 monoclonal or monospecific antibodies representing most of the major regions of the molecule was then used to inhibit binding between gp120 and GalCer or sulfatide. Those antibodies directed against the V3 loop were particularly effective at blocking this interaction.[40] Figure 3 demonstrates such an experiment. Antibody 0.5β, directed against the V3 loop,[41] abolished the binding of gp120 to GalCer, whereas antibody AD3, which is directed against the amino terminal region,[42] had no effect.

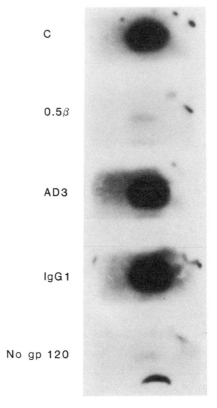

Figure 3. Antibodies against the V3 loop abolish binding of gp120 to GalCer. GalCer immobilized on HPTLC plates was reacted with recombinant gp120 (BH-10) followed by anti-gp120 and labelled anti-rabbit. Preincubation of the gp120 with AD3 (directed against the amino terminal half of gp120) had no effect on binding, in comparison with nonspecific mouse IgG. In contrast, antibody 0.5β, which is directed against the V3 loop, decreased binding to background levels.

Since gp120 binds sulfatide as well as GalCer, it was important to confirm that the V3 loop was also involved in this interaction. Since sulfatide is more soluble in methanol than GalCer, we could use an ELISA for these experiments. Peroxidase-labelled gp120 (ABT, Cambridge, MA) was used to bind sulfatide immobilized in 96-well plates, as previously described.[35] When this gp120 was preincubated with a mixture of anti-V3 loop antibodies, binding was virtually abolished, in contrast to preincubation with either an amino terminal antibody or antibodies directed against other glycoproteins (Fig. 4).

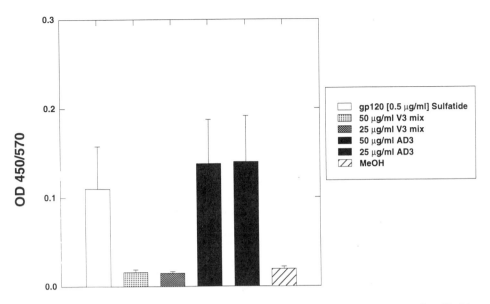

Figure 4. Antibodies against the V3 loop inhibit binding between gp120 and sulfatide. Peroxidase-conjugated BII-10 gp120 (ABT) was incubated with a combination of anti-V3 antibodies at either 50 μg/ml or 25 μg/ml, and then bound to sulfatide in ELISA. In comparison with an antibody directed against the amino terminal half of the molecule (AD3), there was marked inhibition of binding to sulfatide.

In other experiments,[40] gp120 already bound to either GalCer or sulfatide was incubated with a subset of the original panel of antibodies. These experiments indicated which areas of gp120 were exposed following the gp120 glycolipid interaction. As expected from the binding inhibition experiments, epitopes defined by the V3 loop antibodies were not exposed, whereas other regions, particularly the carboxy and amino terminal domains, were.

This series of experiments indicates that the V3 loop, or domains closely related to the V3 loop, are involved in the interaction between gp120 and GalCer or sulfatide. As the V3 loop is a principal determinant of tropism, the results are consistent with biological data which suggest that only some HIV-1 strains can infect cells that do not express CD4. Furthermore, the results are consistent with recent experiments that have shown that the V3 loop is exposed in the monomeric form of the molecule.[43]

Cellular Interactions

An experiment demonstrating that GalCer or sulfatide could convert a noninfectable cell line into one that could be infected with HIV-1 would offer definite confirmation of their role as receptors. Unfortunately, there are no molecular clones of galacosyl transferase with which to engineer such a cell line. To approximate the experimental paradigm, a series of cellular clones expressing varying levels of GalCer on their surface were obtained from a parent HT-29 colonic adenocarcinoma cell line. Expression of GalCer was defined by both immunofluorescence using anti-GalCer antibodies, and by extraction of lipids followed by resolution with HPTLC.[12] The selected clones, as well as clones of the noninfectable colon adenocarcinoma cell line CaCo-2, were then used in infection experiments, and a summary of the results is indicated in Table 3. The parent cell line, HT29, as well as clone HT29-A7, expressed GalCer at high levels, and were easily infectable with two HIV strains, LAI and NDK. Peak p24 levels following HIV-1 (NDK) infection were 7-11,000 pg/ml, and intracellular

Table 3. HIV-1 infection of human colon epithelial cells.

Cell Line[a]	GalCer[b]	HIV-1 NDK[c]	GalCer Block[d]	CD4 Block[e]
HT29	+ +	7312	Yes	No
HT29-A7	+ +	11,380	Yes	No
HT29-D4	+	654	ND	No
HT29-D9	±	$\leq 10^f$	ND	ND
CaCo-2	-	≤ 10	ND	ND

Table 3 was adapted from Fantini et al.[12]

[a] Human colon epithelial cells were selected from parental HT29 cells by limiting dilution.

[b] GalCer expression was determined by surface expression and HPTLC.

[c] HIV-1 NDK was used to infect the cells, and peak p24 levels (pg/ml) are represented.

[d] Infection was blocked by pretreatment of the cells with a monoclonal antibody against GalCer (R-Mab).

[e] Infection was blocked by pretreatment of the cells with monoclonal antibody OKT4a.

[f] HIV-1 was consistently rescued from these cells by cocultivation.

ND = not done.

antigen could be easily detected by indirect immunofluorescence.[12] As the level of GalCer on the surface decreased (clones HT29-D4 and HT29-D9), the infectability was correspondingly lower, with low or undetectable levels of p24 in the supernatant. The CaCo-2 cell line which does not express GalCer, was noninfectable.

In another series of experiments, virus was neutralized with a subset of antibodies directed against gp120 prior to infection of HT29 cells. Antibodies 0.5β and 924, both directed against the V3 loop,[41,44] abolished infection, in contrast to a number of antibodies directed against the carboxy and amino terminal regions of gp120.

Primary Cells

Oligodendrocytes in the central nervous system and Schwann cells in the peripheral nervous system express GalCer, and neurons have been reported to express sulfatide on the surface. None of these cell types have been reported to be infected with HIV *in vitro*, but one group of investigators has reported binding of gp120 to rat sensory ganglion neurons that was inhibited by an antibody against GalCer/sulfatide.[45] However, the investigators indicate that they believe that this antibody is cross-reacting with a glycoprotein(s), and not with the glyco-lipid. The relationship of a putative rat glycoprotein to HIV infection in human cells remains to be determined.

Fetal astrocytes can be infected with HIV, and virus production can be increased by exposure to cytokines.[22] To determine whether GalCer or sulfatide could be involved in entry into these cells, lipid extracts of fetal astrocytes were resolved in HPTLC and bound to either antibodies against GalCer or to recombinant gp120. No specific binding of gp120 to the lipid extracts was seen (Fig. 5). Furthermore, GalCer was not identified in these cells with either antibodies or by specific mobility on HPTLC.

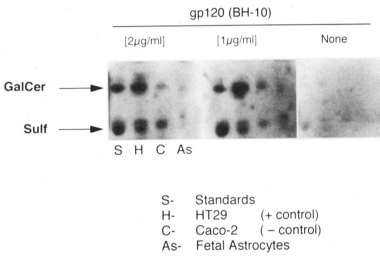

Figure 5. Lipid extracts of fetal astrocytes do not bind gp120. Neutral lipids were extracted from fetal astrocytes as previously described,[12] and equilibrated with extracts from HT29 or CaCo-2 colon adenocarcinoma cells, resolved on HPTLC, and bound to recombinant gp120. In comparison with either standards or extract from HT29, gp120 did not bind to extracts of fetal astrocytes.

SUMMARY AND CONCLUSIONS

A considerable body of data has established that many cells derived from the nervous system can be infected with HIV-1 and/or HIV-2. Infection of astroglial and neuronal elements is highly restrictive, but the presence of the provirus in infected cells has been established beyond question. Infection of neuronal and astroglial cells does not involve the CD4 molecule, the principal cellular receptor for the primate immunodeficiency viruses, and recombinant expression of CD4 in such cells does not result in high levels of virus production, suggesting that there are levels of restriction to viral replication beyond binding at the cell surface. Microglial cells appear to be infected via CD4, and replicate macrophage-tropic HIV strains to high levels.

Galactosylceramide and/or galactosyl sulfatide are potential alternative receptors in some cells of neural origin, as well as in colon epithelial cells, as antibodies against these glycolipids inhibit their infection. The V3 loop, an important region of the viral surface glycoprotein, gp120, appears to be significant in binding to GalCer/sulfatide. Antibodies against the V3 loop inhibit both binding between gp120 and GalCer and infection of GalCer-expressing colon epithelial cell lines.

It is likely that other HIV receptors will be identified, both for neural and other CD4 negative cells, and several investigators have suggested that glycoproteins may be involved in entry into some neural cell lines. These could function independently, or in conjunction with the aforementioned glycolipids. Interestingly, the V3 loop appears to be involved in entry in one system where neither CD4 nor GalCer is involved, that of primary brain capillary endothelial cells. This may suggest that the V3 loop, already a candidate for mediating binding to accessory molecules working in conjunction with CD4, may also be responsible for binding to alternative receptors.

Acknowledgements

Supported by PHS grants NS30606, NS31067, and NS27405. DGC was supported by PHS training grant AI07324.

REFERENCES

1. P.J. Maddon, A.G. Dalgleish, J.S. McDougal, et al. The T4 gene encodes the AIDS virus receptor and is expressed in the immune system and the brain. *Cell* 47:333 (1986).
2. L.A. Lasky, G. Nakamura, D.H. Smith, et al. Delineation of a region of the human immunodeficiency virus type 1 gp120 glycoprotein critical for interaction with the CD4 receptor. *Cell* 50:975 (1987).
3. R.W. Sweet, A. Truneh, and W.A. Hendrickson. CD4: its structure, role in immune function and AIDS pathogenesis, and potential as a pharmacological target. *Curr. Opin. Biotechnol.* 2:622 (1991).
4. P. Clapham, J. Weber, D. Whitby, et al. Soluble CD4 blocks infectivity of diverse strains of HIV and SIV for T-cells and monocytes but not for brain and muscle cells. *Nature* 337:368 (1989).
5. Q.J. Sattentau, A.G. Dalgleish, R.A. Weiss, and P.C.L. Beverley. Epitopes of the CD4 antigen and HIV infection. *Science* 243:1120 (1986).
6. A. Barboza, B.A. Castro, M. Whalen, et al. Infection of cultured adrenal cells by different strains of the human immunodeficiency virus, types 1 and 2. *AIDS* 6:1437 (1992).
7. C. Cheng-Mayer, J.T. Rutka, M.L. Rosenblum, et al. Human immunodeficiency virus can productively infect cultured human glial cells. *Proc. Natl. Acad.Sci. USA* 84:3526 (1987).
8. F. Chiodi, S. Fuerstenberg, M. Gidland, B. Asjo, and E.M. Fenyo. Infection of brain-derived cells with the human immunodeficiency virus. *J. Virol.* 61:1244 (1987).
9. J.M. Harouse, C. Kunsch, H.T. Hartle, et al. CD4-independent infection of human neural cells by human immunodeficiency virus type 1. *J. Virol.* 63:2527 (1989).
10. M. Tateno, F. Gonzalez-Scarano, F., and J.A.Levy. Human immunodeficiency virus can infect CD4-negative human fibroblastoid cells. *Proc. Natl. Acad. Sci. USA* 86:4287 (1989).
11. J. Weber, P.Clapham, J. McKeating, et al. Infection of brain cells by diverse human immunodeficiency virus isolates: role of CD4 as receptor. *J. Gen. Virol.* 70:1653 (1989).

12. J. Fantini, D.G. Cook, N. Nathanson, S.L. Spitalnik, and F. Gonzalez-Scarano. Infection of colonic epithelial cells lines by type 1 human immunodeficiency virus is associated with cells surface expression of galactosylceramide, a potential alternative gp120 receptor. *Proc. Natl. Acad. Sci. USA* 90:2700 (1993).

13. Y. Cao, A.E. Friedman-Kien, Y. Huang, et al. CD4-independent, productive human immunodeficiency virus type 1 infection of hepatoma cell lines in vitro. *J. Virol.* 64:2553 (1990).

14. A. Werner, G. Winskowsky, K. Cichutek, et al. Productive infection of both CD4+ and CD4- human cell lines with HIV-1, HIV-3, and SIV$_{agm}$. *AIDS* 4:537 (1990).

15. M.P. Moyer and H.E. Gendelman. HIV replication and persistence in human gastrointestinal cells cultured *in vitro*. *J. Leuk. Biol.* 49:499 (1991).

16. N. Yahi, S. Baghdiguian, H. Moreau, and J. Fantini. Galactosyl ceramide (or a closely related molecule) is the receptor for human immunodeficiency virus type 1 on human colon epithelial HT29 cells. *J. Virol.* 66:4848 (1992).

17. O. Scheglovitova, M.R. Capobianchi, G. Antonelli, D. Guanmu, and F. Dianzani. CD4-positive hymphoid cells rescue HIV-1 replication from abortively infected human primary endothelial cells. *Arch. Virol.* 132:267 (1993).

18. B. Chesebro, R. Buller, J. Portis, and K. Wehrly. Failure of human immunodeficiency virus entry and infection in CD4-positive human brain and skin cells. *J. Virol.* 64:215 (1990).

19. C. Callebaut, B. Krust, E. Jacotot, and A.G. Hovanessian. T cell activation antigen, CD26, as a cofactor for entry of HIV in CD4+ cells. *Science* 262:2045 (1993).

20. C. Kunsch, H.T. Hartle, and B. Wigdahl. Infection of human fetal dorsal root ganglion glial cells with human immunodeficiency virus type 1 involves an entry mechanism independent of the CD4 T4A epitope. *J. Virol.* 63:5054 (1987).

21. B. Wigdahl, R. Guyton, and P.S. Sarin. Human immunodeficiency virus infection of the developing human nervous system. *Virology* 159:440 (1987).

22. C. Tornatore, A. Nath, K.Amemiya, and E.O. Major. Persistent human immunodeficiency virus type 1 infection in human fetal glial cells reactivate by T-cell factors or by the cytokines tumor necrosis factor alpha and interleukin-1 beta. *J. Virol.* 65:6094 (1993).

23. A.V. Moses, F.E. Bloom, C.D. Pauza, and J.A. Nelson. Human immunodeficiency virus infection of human brain capillary endothelial cells occurs via a CD4/galactosylceramide-independent mechanism. *Proc. Natl. Acad. Sci. USA* 90:10474 (1993).

24. R. Brack-Werner, A. Kleinschmidt, A. Ludvigsen, et al. Infection of human brain cells by HIV-1: restricted virus production in chronically infected human glial cell lines. *AIDS* 6:273 (1992).

25. C. Dewhurst, K. Sakai, J. Bresser, et al. Persistent productive infection of human glial cells by HIV and by infectious molecular clones of HIV. *J. Virol.* 61:3774 (1987).

26. M.E. Truckenmiller, H. Kulaga, M. Coggiano, et al. Human cortical neuronal cell line: a model for HIV-1 infection in an immature neuronal system. *AIDS Res. Hum. Retrovir.* 9:445 (1993).

27. C.A. Jordan, B.A. Watkins, C. Kufta, and M. Dubois-Dalcq. Infection of brain microglial cells by human immunodeficiency virus type 1 is CD4 dependent. *J., Virol.* 64:736 (1991).

28. S. Peudenier, C. Hery, J. Montagnier, and M. Tardieu. Human microglial cells: characterization in cerebral tissue and in primary culture, and study of their susceptibility to HIV-1 infection. *Ann. Neurol.* 29:152 (1991).

29. N.E. Sharpless, W.A. O'Brien, E. Verdin, et al. Human immunodeficiency virus type 1 tropism for brain microglial cells is determined by a region of the env glycoprotein that also controls macrophage tropism. *J.Virol.* 66:2588 (1992).

30. J. Schneider-Schaulies, S. Schneider-Schaulies, R. Brinkman, et al. HIV-1 gp120 receptor on CD4-negative brain cells activates a tyrosine kinase. *Virology* 191:7645 (1992).
31. J.M. Harouse, M.A. Laughlin, C. Pletcher, H.M. Friedman, and F. Gonzalez-Scarano. Entry of HIV-1 into glial cells proceeds via an alternate, efficient pathway. *J. Leukocyte Biol.* 49:605 (1991).
32. B. Volsky, K. Sakai, M.M. Reddy, and D.J. Volsky. A system for the high efficiency replication of HIV-1 in neural cells and its application to antiviral evaluation. *Virology* 186:303 (1992).
33. R.D. Harrington, and A.P. Geballe. Cofactor requirement for HIV type entry in a CD4-expressing human cell line. *J. Virol.* 67:5939 (1993).
34. R. Collman, B. Godfrey, J. Cutili, et al. Macrophage-tropic strains of human immunodeficiency virus type 1 utilize the CD4 receptor. *J. Virol.* 64: 4468 (1990).
35. J. Harouse, S. Bhat, S. Spitalnik, et al. HIV-1 infection of neural cells is inhibited by antibodies against galactosyl-ceramide. *Science* 253:320 (1991).
36. S. Bhat, S.L. Spitalnik, G. Gonzalez-Scarano, and D.H. Silberberg. Galactosyl ceramide or a derivative is an essential component of the neural receptor for human immunodeficiency virus type 1 envelope gp120. *Proc. Natl. Acad. Sci. USA* 88:7131(1991).
37. D. Long, J.F. Berson, D.G. Cook, and R.W. Doms. Characterization of human immunodeficiency virus type 1 gp120 binding to liposomes containing galactosylceramide. *J. Virol.* 68: 5890 (1994).
38.. C. Leonard, M. Spellman, L. Riddle, et al. Assignment of intrachain disulfide bonds and characterization of potential glycosylation sites of the type 1 recombinant HIV envelope glycoprotein. *J. Biol. Chem.* 265:10373 (1990).
39. G. Myers, S. Wain-Hobson, B. Korber, and R.F. Smith. "Human Retroviruses and AIDS. Theoretical Biology and Biophysics," Los Alamos, New Mexico (1993).
40. D.G. Cook, J. Fantini, S.L. Spitalnik, and F. Gonzalez-Scarano. Binding of human immunodeficiency virus type 1 (HIV-1) gp120 to galactosylceramide (GalCer): relationship to the V3 loop. *Virology* 210:206 (1994).
41. S. Matsushita, M. Robert-Guroff, K.J. Rusche, et al. Characterization of a human immunodeficiency virus neutralizing monoclonal antibody and mapping of the neutralizing epitope. *J. Virol.* 62:2107 (1988).
42. K.E. Ugen, Y. Refaeli, U. Ziegner, et al. Generation of monoclonal antibodies against the amino terminus of gp120 that elicit antibody-dependent cellular cytotoxicity,. *Vaccines* 93:215 (1993).
43. J.P. Moore, Q.T. Sattentau, R. Wyatt, and J. Sodroski. Probing the structure of the human immunodeficiency virus surface glycoprotein gp120 with a panel of monoclonal antibodies. *J. Virol.* 68:469 (1994).
44. S.H. Pincus, R.L. Cole, E.M. Hersh, et al. *In vitro* efficacy of anti-HIV immunotoxins targeted by various antibodies to the envelope protein. *J. Immunol.* 146:4315 (1993).
45. S. Apostolski, T. McAlarney, A. Quattrini, et al. The gp120 glycoprotein of human immunodeficiency virus type 1 binds to sensory ganglion neurons. *Ann. Neurol.* 856:855 (1993).

MOLECULAR TECHNOLOGY FOR THE DETECTION AND ANALYSIS OF HIV-1 IN NERVOUS SYSTEM TISSUE

DETECTION OF HIV-1 GENE SEQUENCES IN BRAIN TISSUES BY IN SITU POLYMERASE CHAIN REACTION

Omar Bagasra,[1] Thikkavarapu Seshamma,[1] Joseph P. Pestaner,[2] and Roger J. Pomerantz[1]

[1]Section of Molecular Retrovirology
Infectious Diseases Division, Department of Medicine
Jefferson Medical College - Thomas Jefferson University
Jefferson Alumni Hall
Philadelphia, PA 19107

[2]Department of Pathology and Laboratory Medicine
The Fairfax Hospital
Falls Church, VA 22046

ROLE OF HIV-1 IN THE AIDS DEMENTIA COMPLEX (ADC)

Central nervous system (CNS) neuropathology is a common manifestation of the acquired immunodeficiency syndrome (AIDS). CNS malfunction of the brain in individuals with HIV-1 infection may result from a number of causes including primary infection with the human immunodeficiency virus 1 (HIV-1).[1-8] Secondary infections with opportunistic pathogens,[8-10] due to various neoplasms,[10-14] or secretory toxic factors from infected monocytes, gp120-induced neuronal growth factor inhibition or cytotoxicity induced by HIV-1 Tat can also be present.[15-32] Recently, abnormal induction of L-arginine-nitric oxide pathways has been implicated as one of the mechanisms of AIDS.[31,32] Furthermore, it has been demonstrated by Dawson et al.[31] that HIV-1 gp120 is neurotoxic via nitric oxide pathways.

The study of HIV-1 infection and replication in the CNS and its targeted cell types has been an active area of investigation since the beginning of the AIDS epidemic. ADC affects more than 60% of patients with AIDS and pathological findings of HIV-1 infection of the CNS may be found in 90% of HIV-1-infected individuals at postmortem examination (ref. 33 for review). The mechanism(s) are, as yet, poorly understood. This noninflammatory syndrome, characterized by microglial nodules,[33] may be secondary to neurotoxins or tumor necrosis factor alpha (TNF-α) secreted from HIV-1-infected microglia; neurotoxicity secondary to the HIV-1 envelope glycoprotein gp120, or other factors.[34-36] Of note, the level of HIV-1 in the brain correlates with the degree of CNS dysfunction.[37] Studies utilizing *in situ* hybridization and immunohistochemical techniques suggest that more productive HIV-1 infection in the CNS is in the monocyte/macrophage derivative, the microglial cell.[1-4,38] These data do not, however, address the hypothesis that other cell types (especially astrocytes) may be latently infected with HIV-1. Of particular note, murine retroviruses

Technical Advances in AIDS Research in the Human Nervous System
Edited by E.O. Major and J.A. Levy, Plenum Press, New York, 1995

251

have been demonstrated as leading to abortive infection in spongiform CNS degeneration, and are difficult to detect using standard methodologies.[39] Small numbers of astrocytes and endothelial cells have also been demonstrated to be infected with HIV-1.[1,40] A recent study has demonstrated that *in vitro* production of interleukin-6 (IL-6) by astrocytes can stimulate HIV-1 expression from latently infected monocytic cells, and may thus play an indirect role, at least in part, in the development of ADC.[41] It is also noteworthy that macrophage-tropic strains of HIV-1 have been cloned from the CNS and high levels of unintegrated HIV-1 DNA reside in CNS macrophage/microglial cells in infected individuals.[42-44]

Astrocytic Glial Cell Lines

Such cell lines have been studied *in vitro* in relation to HIV-1 infection, since the role of astrocytes in ADC remains controversial. A variety of astrocytic glial cell lines (e.g., U373MG, U251MG, U138MG, U87MG) have been infected with HIV-1 in cell culture.[45-48] Although some have been demonstrated to allow highly productive infection,[48] many produce low levels of HIV-1 and may be latently infected, as recently demonstrated using the polymerase chain reaction (PCR).[49]

The concept of proviral latency in astrocytic glial cells is complex. Human fetal glial explants have been demonstrated to pass through an early phase of productive HIV-1 infection and then remain in a state of low-level persistent infection.[50] Of note, the viral RNA expression patterns in these cells were not reported.[50] In a preliminary study, it was suggested that latent HIV-1 infection in astrocytic cells may be secondary to increased Nef expression.[51] Nevertheless, in an important study, stable CD4 antigen transfections into neuroglioma cells led to high levels of HIV-1 expression in these cells.[52] Thus, at least in some astrocytic lines, the spread and penetration of the virus within a culture may be a primary determinant of viral production.

Unlike microglial cells,[53] most astrocytic glial cell lines are infected by HIV-1 in a CD4-independent manner.[54-56] In addition, it remains controversial whether glial cell-tropic strains of HIV-1 exist.[46-49] As with many cell types which can be infected *in vitro* (e.g., CD8 lymphocytes, B-lymphocytes, and fibroblasts), the precise documentation of HIV-1 infection of astrocytic glial cells *in vivo* requires further study.[54] With few neuronal cells, apparently infected with HIV-1 *in vivo*,[1,40] although a novel receptor, galactosyl ceramide, has been recently demonstrated on neuronal and some glial cell lines,[58] astrocytic glial cells remain an intriguing and critical area of investigation.

As such, studies of the molecular mechanism of HIV-1 replication, and their possible *in vivo* correlations in astrocytic glial cells, will lead to both a better understanding of the increasingly complex cell-specific controls of HIV-1 virion production and the possible mechanisms of HIV-1-induced CNS disease states.

In situ Polymerase Chain Reaction (IS-PCR) for Detection of HIV-1 in the CNS

PCR has proven to be a valuable tool for amplifying defined DNA sequences, even if they are available in only minute amounts, to obtain quantities which can be analyzed and/or sequenced. Using a variety of thermostable DNA polymerase enzymes (e.g., Taq, Vent, etc.), the PCR can quickly and efficiently amplify a genetic sequence utilizing an automated thermocycler.[59] Thus, genes or virus sequences[60-62] present in only small samples of cells, or in a small fraction of cells in a heterogeneous population can be traced. A specific area of study especially important for PCR has been in the area of HIV-1/AIDS research, as the actual percentage of HIV-1-infected cells in the peripheral blood has been the subject of controversy.[61-63] Since HIV-1 was first described as the etiologic agent of AIDS,[64] the number of cells infected *in vivo* with HIV-1 have been evaluated in patients in various clinical stages of disease.[63] These studies have sought to correlate levels of HIV-1 infection with the pathogenesis and clinical course of the disease. Various modifications of the PCR method have been used to quantitatively or semiquantitatively assess the relative frequency of HIV-1-infected cells in peripheral blood mononuclear cells (PBMCs), lymph nodes, and other cell types.[61-65] One of the major drawbacks of the currently used standard DNA-PCR method is that the procedure does not allow the association of amplified signals of a specific genetic segment with the histologic cell type(s). The ability to identify individual cells carrying a specific gene(s) or a portion of a genetic element under the microscope or by automated signal sensor (e.g., FACS or image analyzer), would be extremely useful in delineating various aspects of normal and pathologic conditions. For example, this technique could be used in various leukemias and lymphomas, where specific aberrant gene sequences are associated with certain types of malignancy. As such, the HIV-1 virus has been demonstrated to infect both CD4-positive and CD8-positive lymphocytes, monocytes, B-lymphocytes, fibroblasts, and glial cells in cell culture.[61-66] The ability to demonstrate nonproductive HIV-1 infection in different cell types, *in vivo*, will be critical to further understand the pathogenesis of HIV-1.

Determination of HIV-1-Infected Cells Before the Development of IS-PCR

In order to determine the percentage of PBMCs and lymph nodes infected with HIV-1, the initial studies of Harper et al.[61] demonstrated that with the use of *in situ* hybridization for HIV-1-specific RNA, only 1 in 10,000 to 1 in 100,000 PBMCs and lymph node cells could be identified as positive for HIV-1 *in vivo*. Of course, these findings did not exclude the possibility that HIV-1 may be present in a higher proportion of PBMCs as a nonreplicating provirus. However, these data made it difficult to understand how such a low number of HIV-1-infected cells could cause such a severe depletion of CD4-positive lymphocytes. Data from Ho et al.[62] and Lewis et al.[67] suggested that the number of PBMCs containing HIV-1-specific RNA is higher than initially demonstrated in patients infected with HIV-1 using limiting dilution assays. These investigators showed that infectious HIV-1 can be isolated from an average of 1 in 400 PBMCs obtained from patients with AIDS. Much higher levels were detected during acute seroconversion to HIV-1 by Clark et al.[68] and Darr et al.[69] Schnittman et al.,[63] using a combination of cell sorting and quantitative DNA-PCR techniques, observed that in patients with AIDS, at least 1% of CD4-positive lymphocytes were infected with HIV-1. In asymptomatic persons seropositive for HIV-1, the range of CD4-positive lymphocytes harboring HIV-1 is broad (1 in 100 to 1 in 100,000). Hsia and Spector,[70] using a "booster" PCR method, calculated that at least 10% of CD4-positive lymphocytes carry HIV-1 provirus in AIDS and symptomatic HIV-1 infection. Nevertheless, relatively lower proportions of CD4-positive lymphocytes are positive for the provirus in asymptomatic HIV-1 infection. Thus, DNA-IS-PCR for proviral sequences of HIV-1 is an important next step in precisely quantifying the proviral load in infected individuals.

Development of *in situ* PCR Techniques

As noted above, a current limitation of PCR with isolated DNA is that the results of amplification cannot be directly associated with a specific cell type, nor can the percentage of cells that carry the target sequences be easily measured. However, CD4-positive lymphocytes may be the primary reservoir of HIV-1 in the bloodstream,[63] and the monocyte/macrophage may be the principal reservoir in solid tissues (reviewed in 33). It is highly desirable to identify all cell types that carry the virus *in vivo*, as well as the cells that allow active replication of HIV-1. It would, therefore, be greatly advantageous if gene sequences could be amplified and traced *in situ* within intact cells. Recently, other investigators have been successful in developing a DNA-IS-PCR method for the sheep lentivirus, visna, using cell suspensions.[72-73] Importantly, smears or tissue sections are readily available and are often stored for long periods of time, allowing reevaluation, whereas cell pellets or even viable frozen cells are rarely preserved for DNA isolation. If the DNA-IS-PCR procedure could be performed directly on slides, visualization of altered or foreign DNA directly in the cells would allow morphological and cytochemical characterization of the cells containing the sequences in question, which would be especially helpful in heterogeneous cellular populations.[72-75]

We have designed a procedure to apply PCR to cell preparations on slides. We have demonstrated not only that it is possible to sufficiently amplify single copy genes to be visualized by microscopy or microautoradiography, but also that this reaction is highly specific and allows distinguishing cells containing defined gene sequences. It can be hypothesized that an intact fixed cell may function as an ultrasmall chamber for amplification. Once cells are heat-fixed and then permeabilized by paraformaldehyde, and DNA-binding proteins are digested by proteinase K, the entrance of DNA polymerase, PCR primers, and other agents can be accomplished. It appears that in our DNA-IS-PCR method, after heat fixation, amplification products are retained by the nuclear and/or cytoplasmic membranes within the cell.[76,77]

The current standard DNA-PCR method in which one isolates DNA from many cells, usually 1 mg of DNA (or about 1.5×10^5 cells) for amplification, has several limitations. As stated above, one of the limitations of standard DNA-PCR is that with isolated DNA, one cannot generally link the amplification signal to a specific cell type or easily quantify the percentage of cells which carry the target gene(s) or genetic sequence(s). One of the other main concerns of investigators, using the standard DNA-PCR method, is false-positive results due to contamination of samples by HIV-1-positive amplified genetic segments.[59,68] However, with the use of DNA-IS-PCR, such concerns are less significant. Using the DNA-IS-PCR, the intracellular DNA is amplified and remains localized in the intranuclear/intracellular areas. Therefore, even if a small fragment of DNA enters the cell, it probably will not contaminate nuclear DNA. Even in the worst case scenario, the contamination would only involve a few cells instead of providing totally false-positive results as in the case of the standard DNA-PCR method, where amplified results are measured as absolute positives or negatives.

Studies of Retroviruses Using *in situ* PCR

The technique of DNA-IS-PCR, which allows amplification of a specific DNA fragment within an intact cell, has many potentials. For example, it can be used in determining the actual peripheral blood or tissue proviral or viral load in various stages of many infections (e.g., cytomegalovirus, Epstein-Barr virus) and in evaluating the efficacy of various therapeutic interventions. One of its many potential uses is to determine the tumor load, especially in various human leukemias and lymphomas where selective chromosomal rearrangements and genetic alterations are known to be associated with a specific malignancy. In addition, early intracellular viral events, especially in the case of a retrovirus, can be quantified during the course of viral infections.

One of the important uses of the DNA-IS-PCR technique may be in evaluating retroviral entry and replication. Currently, there are several hypotheses regarding the early molecular events following HIV-1 entry into target cells. An hypothesis was forwarded to Zack et al.[78] who postulated that HIV-1 entry is unrestricted into CD4-positive T-lymphocytes, but completion of reverse transcription and proviral integration is limited only to cells which are stimulated whereas in nonstimulated primary T-lymphocytes, HIV-1 is not completely reverse transcribed. This partial HIV-1 DNA intermediate can persist in these quiescent cells for a short period of time. In immortalized T-lymphocytic cell lines, a full-length HIV-1 provirus is reverse transcribed but viral latency is regulated by temporal programming of HIV-1-specific RNA species.[79] Similarly, Burkinsky et al.[80] have demonstrated full-length unintegrated HIV-1 proviral DNA in unstimulated PBMCs which integrate only after cellular activation. Utilizing various specific primer pairs and probes, studies are underway to investigate the molecular pathogenesis of HIV-1 infection *in vivo*, using DNA-IS-PCR technology.

By adapting a modified PCR *in situ*, we have demonstrated the percentage of PBMCs infected with HIV-1. In these experiments, the cells used were PBMCs isolated from whole blood using Ficoll-Hypaque gradient centrifugation, as well as various cell lines. U1 is a subclone[81] of the monocytoid U937 cells[82] which is chronically infected with HIV-1 and carries two copies of the integrated proviral HIV-1 per cell. The ACH-1 cell line[83] is a subclone of a variant of the CEM T-lymphocyte cell line which carries a single copy of HIV-1 provirus per cell. SUP-T_1/HIV-1 is a chronically infected derivative of the SUP-T_1 cell line, a T-lymphocytic cell line which expresses a very high density of CD4 antigen.[84]

To perform DNA-IS-PCR on glass slides (Fig. 1), cells (1 x 10^6 cell/ml) to be examined are seeded into the wells (1 x 10^5 cells/well) of specifically designed heavy teflon-coated (HTC) slides and allowed to settle through sedimentation via gravity. In case of paraffin tissue sections, they can be placed in the slide-well and then can be deparaffinized by sequential treatment with xylene, ethanol and then incubating at 80°C for 4-6 hours. Cells (either tissue sections or cells) are fixed first on a heat block at 105°C for 90 seconds and then in 2% paraformaldehyde for 1 hour or longer. Paraformaldehyde is inactivated by washing the slides, with 3X PBS, then endogenous peroxidase activity is removed by quenching the specimens with 3% hydrogen peroxide overnight at 37°C and then treating with proteinase K for 2 hours at 55°C.

Proteinase K is inactivated by placing the slides on a heat block at 96°C for 2 minutes, and finally the slides are washed in distilled water, air-dried, and the PCR reaction mixture, with Taq polymerase, is added to the top two wells of each slide. A PCR mixture lacking the primers is added to the bottom well. These slides are covered with coverslips, which are sealed with a clear nail polish, and then placed on an automatic thermocycler. The amplification is carried out at 94°C/45°C/72°C for 1 minute for 30 cycles. After PCR, the slides are placed in 100% alcohol for 2 hours, the coverslips are removed, and the slides are washed with 2X SSC. Amplification products are detected by a biotinylated oligonucleotide according to *in situ* hybridization method. For HIV-1, the primers and probe can be from various sections of the HIV-1 genome.[76,77] After hybridization, the slides are thoroughly washed, then incubated with streptavidin-peroxidase complex for 1 hour at 37°C. After incubation, the color is developed with 3'-amino-9'-ethylene carbozone in the presence of 0.3% hydrogen peroxide in 50 mM acetate buffer. Positive staining cells, using biotinylated probes, stained brownish-red, whereas negative cells usually appeared colorless or slightly pink. Of note, these fixation and amplification conditions corrected our initial problem with leakage of amplified products from cells. In addition, we have recently demonstrated similar results utilizing fluoresceinated and ^{32}P-labelled probes.[76,77]

The sensitivity of the DNA-IS-PCR technique was further tested with the ACH-2 and U1 cells. When ACH-2 and U1 cells were subjected to DNA-IS-PCR, all cells were positive at the same degree of intensity. When the ACH-2 cells were mixed in varying proportions with uninfected CEM cells, the results were those expected and no leakage of amplified products with contamination of uninfected cells was demonstrated.[71,75-77]

In addition, experiments using DNA-IS-PCR were conducted to evaluate the theoretical possibility that HIV-1 virions may encapsulate some proviral DNA, which could contaminate uninfected cells during DNA-IS-PCR. Cells from a productively HIV-1-infected T-lymphocytic cell line, SUP-T_1, were mixed in various ratios with uninfected cells from a T-lymphocytic cell line H9,[76] as the ACH-2 cells and uninfected CEM cells had been mixed, and the predicted ratios of infected-to-uninfected cells were observed after DNA-IS-PCR. Thus, if there was virion-associated proviral DNA, it did not contaminate HIV-1 negative cells during this procedure.[71,75-77]

These experiments demonstrated that *in situ* amplification can be accomplished in cell populations known to carry only one copy of the HIV-1 provirus per cell. This modification of gene amplification makes DNA-IS-PCR more sensitive than many standard PCR methods for examining DNA.[59,63] The reason(s) for

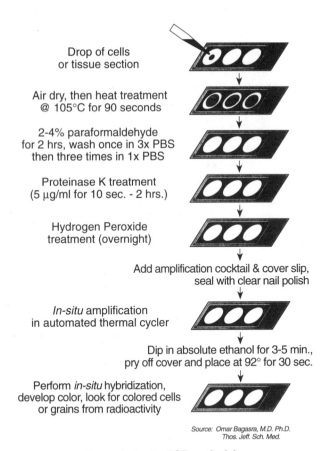

Drop of cells
or tissue section

Air dry, then heat treatment
@ 105°C for 90 seconds

2-4% paraformaldehyde
for 2 hrs, wash once in 3x PBS
then three times in 1x PBS

Proteinase K treatment
(5 µg/ml for 10 sec. - 2 hrs.)

Hydrogen Peroxide
treatment (overnight)

Add amplification cocktail & cover slip,
seal with clear nail polish

In-situ amplification
in automated thermal cycler

Dip in absolute ethanol for 3-5 min.,
pry off cover and place at 92° for 30 sec.

Perform *in-situ* hybridization,
develop color, look for colored cells
or grains from radioactivity

Source: Omar Bagasra, M.D. Ph.D.
Thos. Jeff. Sch. Med.

Figure 1. *In situ* PCR methodology.

the unusually high sensitivity of the DNA-IS-PCR is not fully clear. It is possible that in the standard DNA-PCR, one is diluting the positive genetic element in a sea of nucleic acids. As such, poorly described cellular factors may inhibit amplification.[85] In addition, these data demonstrated that with this technique, amplified DNA does not leak out of infected cells and contaminate uninfected cells. In the other DNA-IS-PCR techniques, where signal leakage was described (reviewed in 76-77), it usually manifests as nonspecific, perimembranous staining. Utilizing our technique, such staining has not been observed.

Frequency of Peripheral Blood Mononuclear Cells (PBMCs) Positive for HIV-1 Sequences Assessed by DNA-IS-PCR

Using this DNA-IS-PCR technique, we reported the percentages of peripheral blood mononuclear cells (PBMCs) infected with HIV-1.[76] We demonstrated that relatively higher percentages of PBMCs (10-15%) carry HIV-1 in infected individuals, than previously demonstrated by some other groups.[61-65] Our observation that the numbers of PBMCs harboring HIV-1 provirus are significantly higher than the levels of infectious HIV-1 cells per mononuclear cell in coculture assays,[62] suggest that some copies of the HIV-1 provirus may be either defective or maintained in cells that are not activated in cell cultures to produce virions. As such, the evaluation of proviral latency and defective viral genomes *in vivo* remains an important area in the study of the complex pathogenesis of HIV-1 infection. Certainly, as the sensitivity to detect HIV-1 *in vivo* has improved, understanding its molecular pathogenesis has continued to evolve. Most recently, several laboratories have independently confirmed our initial report that up to 13% of PBMCs are infected in the late stages of HIV-1 infection.[70,86,88]

Utilizing our IS-PCR technique, we have recently demonstrated HIV-1 in low levels of PBMCs (mean: 1%) of HIV-1-infected individuals. Although tissue-bound macrophages in HIV-1-infected persons are known to harbor HIV-1 proviral DNA *in vivo*, it is quite controversial whether the PBMCs contain provirus (reviewed in 71). Using the IS-PCR technique, we have now demonstrated HIV-1 provirus in eight of the 11 HIV-1-infected subjects evaluated. Monocytes from four HIV-1-seronegative hosts were not positive for provirus. Of note, the morphology of the proviral positive cells in these preparations was classic for monocyte/macrophages.[71]

To further address the issue of proviral-positive cells in PBMCs of HIV-1-infected individuals, using IS-PCR, we have recently carried out subset analyses. Fluorescent cell sorting (FACS) could not be utilized because our IS-PCR required nonfixed cells to be applied and heat-fixed to special slides; additionally, live HIV-1-infected cells cannot be used in most FACS equipment. Thus, cell-panning was inefficient and distorted the cellular morphology. Nevertheless, we could utilize immunomagnetic bead separation to give highly specific separation of CD4+ lymphocytes from other PBMCs. Of note, mixing experiments using HIV-1-infected and uninfected Sup-T1 cells, as described for the initial studies,[76,77] utilizing CD4-immunomagnetic beads and IS-PCR, yielded expected results. Thus, leakage of amplified products was not a problem if immunomagnetic beads were used prior to IS-PCR (specificity control). IS-PCR could be used to evaluate cells after beads were dissociated or with beads still attached, since beads are easily distinguished from cells and did not alter the IS-PCR procedure.[75-77]

We evaluated PBMCs from 42 HIV-1-infected individuals, using IS-PCR both before and after bead separation. These are different patients from those used in our initial studies. Seronegative controls were evaluated in all experiments. Importantly, the mean levels of HIV-1-positive unfractionated PBMCs were similar, in each stage of disease, among patients in this recent series of experiments, as compared to the previous study.[76] Only rare cells in the unbound fraction, using immunomagnetic beads for CD4, were positive (<1%) in PBMCs *in vivo*, with the exception of low levels in some monocyte populations, is the CD4+ lymphocyte. The CD4+ lymphocyte fraction revealed HIV-1-positive cells in the range of 0.2% to 69%. The mean levels of CD4+ lymphocytes in Stages 2 and 4 patients were statistically different (Student's t -Test: $p < 0.001$). All studies were done blinded and at least twice. Thus, these important new data further point to the utility of IS-PCR in investigating HIV-1 levels *in vivo*.[77]

Detection of HIV-1 in Brain Tissues

Since most standard techniques which determine HIV-1 infection of cells either are not sensitive enough (e.g., *in situ* hybridization and immunohistochemistry) to detect low abundance of signal or latent infections or do not measure HIV-1 infection in specific intact cells (e.g., standard DNA-PCR), our laboratory has begun to evaluate autopsy brain tissues using our *in situ* PCR technique. Using brain tissue obtained at The Fairfax Hospital (Fairfax, VA) from several HIV-1-infected individuals with severe ADC, we have preliminary data regarding HIV infection of CNS cell types *in vivo*.

As demonstrated in Figure 2, numerous CNS cells were positive for HIV-1-specific DNA by *in situ* PCR. Brain tissue from an HIV-1-seronegative individual revealed no positively staining cells. Although immunochemistry is planned to allow better identification of histological typing of cells infected with HIV-1, certain cells in these samples revealed a morphology which may be more consistent with infection of astrocytes, oligodendrocytes, microglial cells, and microvascular endothelial cells. Multinucleated cells are also seen in these patients. These data are quite preliminary and require further study. Of note, though, the *in situ* PCR revealed a 100-fold higher level of HIV-1-positive CNS cells, in these samples, as compared to standard *in situ* hybridization.

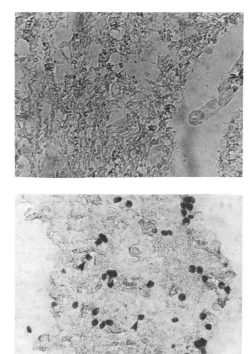

Figure 2. *In situ* PCR of CNS tissue. (A) *In situ* PCR of brain tissue from an HIV-1 seronegative individual. (Magnification 400 X).

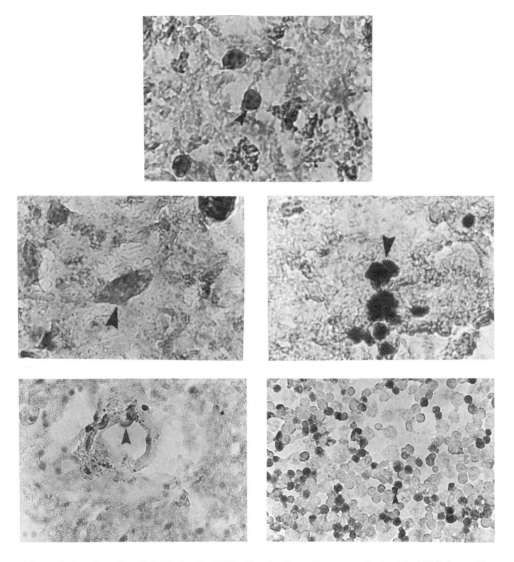

Figure 2. (continued). (B & F) *In situ* PCR of brain tissue from a patient with AIDS-dementia complex. (B) HIV-1-positive cells, morphologically similar to oligodendrocytes; (C) cells which appear to be neuronal cells; (D) cells appearing to be astrocytic in morphology; (E) multi-nucleated cells and neuronal-like cells positive for HIV-1; (F) microvascular endothelial cells positive for HIV-1; (G) positive controls for IS-DNA-PCR -- a 1:10 mixture of ACH-2 cells with CEM cells.

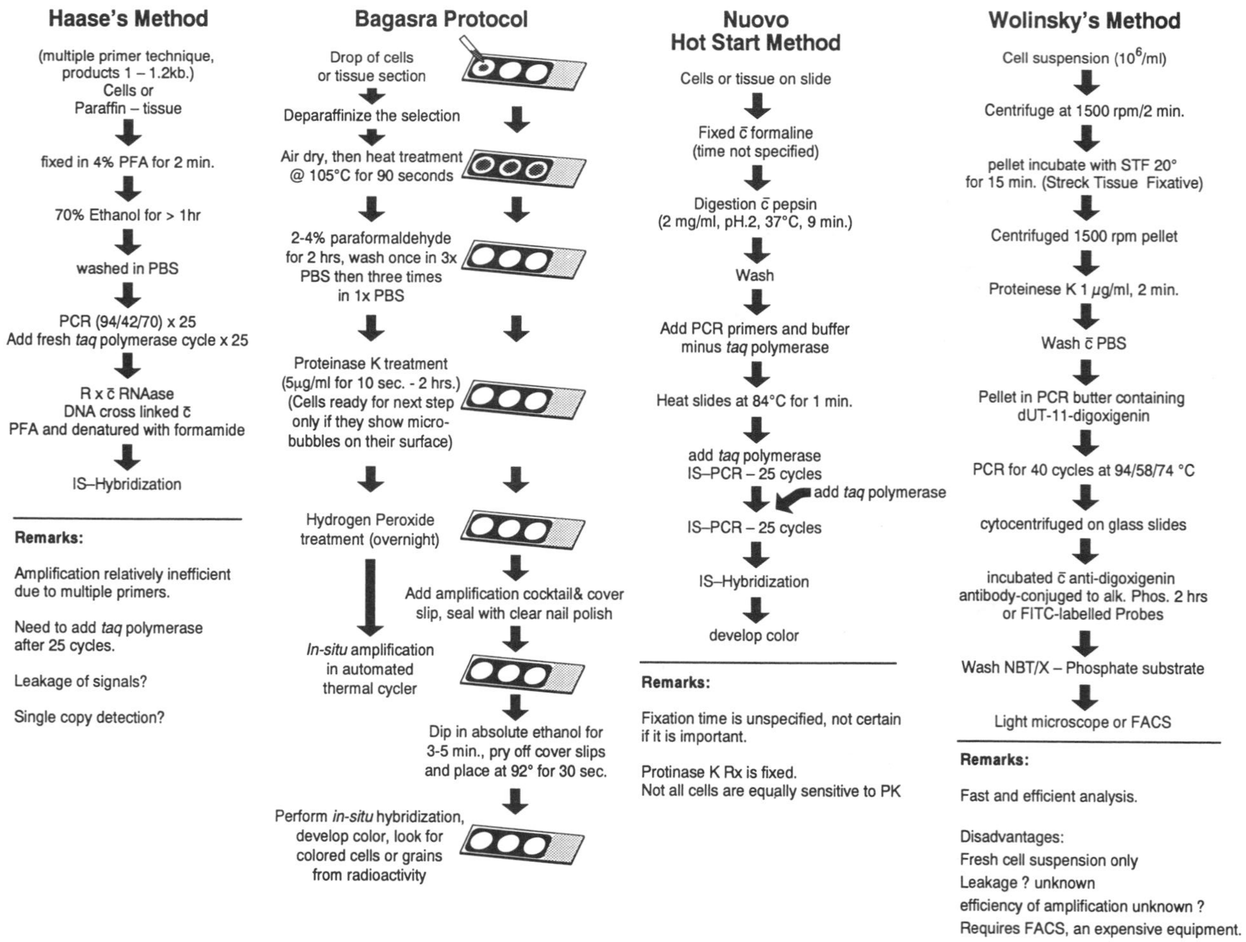

Haase's Method

(multiple primer technique, products 1 – 1.2kb.)
Cells or
Paraffin – tissue

↓

fixed in 4% PFA for 2 min.

↓

70% Ethanol for > 1hr

↓

washed in PBS

↓

PCR (94/42/70) x 25
Add fresh *taq* polymerase cycle x 25

↓

R x δ RNAase
DNA cross linked δ
PFA and denatured with formamide

↓

IS-Hybridization

Remarks:

Amplification relatively inefficient due to multiple primers.

Need to add *taq* polymerase after 25 cycles.

Leakage of signals?

Single copy detection?

Bagasra Protocol

Drop of cells or tissue section

↓

Deparaffinize the selection

↓

Air dry, then heat treatment @ 105°C for 90 seconds

↓

2-4% paraformaldehyde for 2 hrs, wash once in 3x PBS then three times in 1x PBS

↓

Proteinase K treatment (5μg/ml for 10 sec. - 2 hrs.) (Cells ready for next step only if they show micro-bubbles on their surface)

↓

Hydrogen Peroxide treatment (overnight)

→ Add amplification cocktail & cover slip, seal with clear nail polish

↓

In-situ amplification in automated thermal cycler

↓

Dip in absolute ethanol for 3-5 min., pry off cover slips and place at 92° for 30 sec.

↓

Perform *in-situ* hybridization, develop color, look for colored cells or grains from radioactivity

Nuovo
Hot Start Method

Cells or tissue on slide

↓

Fixed δ formaline (time not specified)

↓

Digestion δ pepsin (2 mg/ml, pH.2, 37°C, 9 min.)

↓

Wash

↓

Add PCR primers and buffer minus *taq* polymerase

↓

Heat slides at 84°C for 1 min.

↓

add *taq* polymerase
IS-PCR – 25 cycles

→ add *taq* polymerase

↓

IS-PCR – 25 cycles

↓

IS-Hybridization

↓

develop color

Remarks:

Fixation time is unspecified, not certain if it is important.

Protinase K Rx is fixed.
Not all cells are equally sensitive to PK

Wolinsky's Method

Cell suspension (10^6/ml)

↓

Centrifuge at 1500 rpm/2 min.

↓

pellet incubate with STF 20° for 15 min. (Streck Tissue Fixative)

↓

Centrifuged 1500 rpm pellet

↓

Proteinese K 1 μg/ml, 2 min.

↓

Wash δ PBS

↓

Pellet in PCR butter containing dUT-11-digoxigenin

↓

PCR for 40 cycles at 94/58/74 °C

↓

cytocentrifuged on glass slides

↓

incubated δ anti-digoxigenin antibody-conjuged to alk. Phos. 2 hrs or FITC-labelled Probes

↓

Wash NBT/X – Phosphate substrate

↓

Light microscope or FACS

Remarks:

Fast and efficient analysis.

Disadvantages:
Fresh cell suspension only
Leakage ? unknown
efficiency of amplification unknown ?
Requires FACS, an expensive equipment.

Figure 3. IS-PCR: Comparison of Various Methods.

These studies are analogous to our investigations of HIV-1 proviral-positive cells in peripheral blood. It is critical to note that immunohistochemistry measures only highly productive infections leading to high levels of viral protein expression, while standard *in situ* hybridization techniques measure HIV-1-specific RNA or DNA. As has recently been demonstrated in PBMLs,[75-77,86,87] using standard DNA-PCR and now using *in situ* PCR technique, standard *in situ* hybridization grossly underestimates the number of HIV-1-infected cells. These findings may have significant implications for HIV-1 infection of the CNS. As such, our laboratory has begun to utilize the *in situ* PCR technique to investigate which cells in the CNS of individuals, in various clinical HIV-1 disease states, harbor the HIV-1 provirus.

CONCLUSIONS

The technique of DNA-IS-PCR allows a specific DNA fragment to be amplified within the intact cell. This technique has great potential for determining the actual proviral load in peripheral blood and CNS tissues at various stages of HIV infection, and for evaluating the efficacy of various therapeutic interventions. This technique should allow for the direct localization of other viruses and DNA sequences present in one to a few copies per cell. Although great strides have been made in the last few years, the technology of DNA-IS-PCR is clearly still in its infancy. Further modifications of this powerful technique will allow a continued increase in the sensitivity, specificity and reproducibility of DNA-IS-PCR. Although a variety of genetic sequences, such as papillomavirus, cytomegalovirus, visna virus, HIV-1, HLA-DQα and various cellular genes, have been studied using DNA-IS-PCR, unlimited others await investigation. Thus, DNA-IS-PCR should allow the study of various key aspects of disease pathogenesis, especially in infectious diseases and oncology.

ACKNOWLEDGEMENTS

The authors thank Drs. Gerald Nuovo and Ashley Haase for helpful discussions; Ms. P. Saikuman for technical assistance; and Ms. Rita M. Victor for excellent secretarial assistance.

REFERENCES

1. S.Koenig, H.E. Gendelman, J.M. Orenstein, et al. Detection of AIDS virus in macrophages in brain tissue from AIDS patients with encephalopathy. *Science* 233:1089 (1986).
2. C.A. Wiley, R.D. Schrier, J.A. Nelson, P.W. Lampert, and M.A. Oldstone. Characterization of human immunodeficiency virus infection within brains of AIDS patients. *Proc. Natl. Acad. Sci. USA* 83:7089 (1986).
3. S. Gartner, P. Markovitz, D.M. Markovitz, R.F. Betts, and M. Popovic. Virus isolation from and identification of HTLV-III/LAV-producing cells in brain tissue from a patient with AIDS. *J.A.M.A.* 256:2365 ((1986).
4. F. Gyorkey, J.L. Melnick, and P.Gyorkey. Human immunodeficiency virus in brain biopsies of patients with AIDS and progressive encephalopathy. *J. Infect. Dis.* 155:870 (1987).
5. D.D. Ho, T.R. Rota, R.T. Schooley, et al. Isolation of HTLV-III from cerebrospinal fluid and neural tissues of patients with neurologic syndromes related to the acquired immunodeficiency syndrome. *N. Engl. J. Med.* 313:1493 (1985).
6. G.M. Shaw, M.E. Harper, B.H. Hahn, et al. HTLV-III infection in brains of children and adults with AIDS encephalopathy. *Science* 227:177 (1985).
7. J.A. Levy, J. Shimabukuro, H. Hollander, J. Mills, and L. Kaminsky. Isolation of AIDS-associated retroviruses from cerebrospinal fluid and brain of patients with neurological symptoms. *Lancet* 11:586 (1985).
8. E. Bishburg, R.H. Eng, J. Slim, G. Perez, and E. Johnson. Brain lesions in patients with acquired immunodeficiency syndrome. *Arch. Intern. Med.* 149:941 (1989).
9. S.L. Neilson, C.K. Petito, C.D. Urmacher, and J.B. Posner. Subacute encephalitis in acquired immune deficiency syndrome: A postmortem study. *Am. J. Clin. Pathol.* 82:678 (1984).
10. W.D. Snider, D.M. Simpson, S. Nielson, et al. Neurological complications of acquired immune deficiency syndrome: analysis of 50 patients. *Ann. Neurol.* 14:403 (1983).
11. R.M. Levy, R.S. Janssen, T.J. Bush, and M.L. Rosenblum. Neuroepidemiology of acquired immunodeficiency syndrome. *J. AIDS* 1:31 (1988).
12. R. Vazeux, N. Brousse, A. Jarry, et al. AIDS subacute encephalitis. Identification of HIV-infected cells. *Am. J. Pathol.* 126:403 (1987).
13. H.E. Gendelman, J.M. Orenstein, M.M. Martin, et al. Efficient isolation and propagation of human immunodeficiency virus on recombinant colony-stimulating factor A-treated monocytes. *J. Exp. Med.* 167:1428 (1988).
14. S. Gartner, P. Markovits, D.M. Markovits, et al. The role of mononuclear phagocytes in HTLV-III/LAV infection. *Science* 233:215 (1986).
15. P.D. Smith, K. Ohura, H. Masur, et al. Monocyte-macrophage function in the acquired immunodeficiency syndrome: defective chemotaxis. *J. Clin. Invest.* 74:2121 (1984).
16. S.M. Wahl, J.B. Allen, S. Gartner, et al. Human immunodeficiency virus-1 and its envelope glycoprotein down-regulate chemotactic ligand receptors and chemotactic function of peripheral blood monocytes. *J. Immunol.* 143:3553 (1989).
17. J.B. Allen, N. McCartney, P.D. Smith, et al. Expression of IL-2 receptors by monocytes from patients with acquired immunodeficiency syndrome and induction of monocyte IL-2 receptors by human immunodeficiency virus *in vitro. J. Clin. Invest.* 85:192 (1990).
18. S. Roy, and M.A. Weinberg. Role of the mononuclear phagocyte system in the development of acquired immunodeficiency syndrome. *J. Leukocyte Biol.* 43:91 (1988).
19. J.E. Merrill, Y. Koyanagi, and I.S.Y. Chen. Interleukin-1 and tumor necrosis factor-α can be induced from mononuclear phagocytes by human immunodeficiency virus type 1 binding to the CD4 receptor. *J. Virol.* 63:4404 (1989).
20. K.W. Selmaj, and C.S. Raine. Tumor necrosis factor mediates myelin and oligodendrocyte damage *in vitro. Ann. Neurol.* 23:339 (1988).

21. D.S. Robbins, Y. Shirazi, B. Drysdale, et al. Promotion of cytotoxic factor for oligodendrocytes by stimulated astrocytes. *J. Immunol.* 139:2593 (1987).
22. S.M. Wahl, D.A. Hunt, L.M. Wakefield, et al. Transforming growth factor beta (TGF-β) induces monocyte chemotaxis and growth factor production. *Proc. Natl. Acad. Sci. USA* 84:5788 (1987).
23. S.M. Wahl, N. McCartney-Francis, and S.E. Mergenhagen. Inflammatory and immunomodulatory role of transforming growth factor beta. *Immunol. Today* 10:258 (1989).
24. S.M. Wahl, D.A. Hunt, G. Bansal, et al. Bacterial cell wall induced immuno-suppression: role of transforming growth factor beta. *J. Exp. Med.* 168:1403 (1988).
25. E.C. Breen, A.R. Rezai, K. Nahjima, et al. Infection with HIV is associated with elevated IL-6 levels and production. *J. Immunol.* 144:4809 (1990).
26. L.M. Wahl, M.L. Corcoran, S.W. Pyle, L.O. Arthur, and W.L. Farrar. Human immunodeficiency virus glycoprotein (gp120) induction of monocyte arachidonic acid metabolites. *Immunol. Today* 10:258 (1989).
27. D.E. Brenneman, G.L. Westbrook, S.P. Fitzgerald, et al. Neuronal cell killing by the envelope protein of HIV and its prevention by vasoactive intestinal peptide. *Nature (Lond.)* 335:639 (1989).
28. M.-M. Sabatier, E. Vives, K. Mabrouk, et al. Evidence for neurotoxic activity of tat from human immunodeficiency virus type 1. *J. Virol.* 65:961 (1991).
29. L. Pulliam, B.G. Herndier, N.M. Tang, and M.S. McGrath. Human immunodeficiency virus-infected macrophages produce soluble factors that cause histological and neurochemical alterations in cultured human brain. *J. Clin. Invest.* 87:503 (1991).
30. D. Giulian, J. Vaca, and C.A. Noonan. Secretion of neurotoxins by mononuclear phagocytes infected with HIV-1. *Science* 240:1593 (1991).
31. V.L. Dawson, T.M. Dawson, G.R. Uhl, and S.H. Snyder. Human immunodeficiency virus type 1 coat protein hemotoxicity mediated by nitric oxide in primary cortical cultures. *Proc. Natl. Acad.Sci., U.S.A.* 90:3256 (1993).
32. S. Moncada, and A. Higgs. The arginine-nitric oxide pathway. *N. Engl. J. Med.* 329:2002 (1993).
33. R.W. Price, B. Brew, J. Sidtis, et al. The brain in AIDS: central nervous system HIV-1 infection and AIDS dementia complex. *Science* 239:586 (1988).
34. D. Giulian, K, Vaca, and C.A. Noonan. Secretion of neurotoxins by mononuclear phagocytes infected with HIV-1. *Science* 250:1593 (1990).
35. E.B. Dreyer, P.K. Kaiser, J.T. Offermann, and S.A. Lipton. HIV-1 coat protein neurotoxicity prevented by calcium channel antagonists. *Science* 248:364 (1990).
36. L. Pulliam, B.G. Herndier, N.M. Tang, and M.S. McGrath. Human immunodeficiency virus-infected macrophages produce soluble factors that cause histological and neurochemical alterations in cultured human brains. *J. Clin. Invest.* 87:503 (1991).
37. B. Weiser, N. Peress, D. La Neve, et al. Human immunodeficiency virus type 1 expression in the central nervous system correlates directly with extent of disease. *Proc. Natl. Acad. Sci. USA* 87:3997 (1990).
38. B.A. Watkins, H.H. Dorn, W.B. Kelly, et al. Specific tropism of HIV-1 for microglial cells in primary human brain cultures. *Science* 249:549 (1990).
39. A.H. Sharpe, J.J. Hunter, P. Chassler, and R. Jaenisch. Role of abortive retroviral infection of neurons in spongiform CNS degeneration. *Nature* 246:181 (1990).
40. F. Gyorkey, J.L. Melnick, and P. Gyorkey. Human immunodeficiency virus in brains of patients with AIDS and progressive encephalopathy. *J. Infect. Dis.* 155:870 (1987).
41. L. Vitkovic, G.P. Wood,E.)O. Major, and A.S. Fauci. Human astrocytes

stimulate HIV-1 expression in chronically infected promonocyte clone via interleukin-6. *AIDS Res. and Human Retroviruses* 7:723 (1991).

42. S. Pang, Y. Koyanagi, S. Miles, et al. High levels of unintegrated HIV-1 DNA in brain tissue of AIDS dementia patients. *Nature (Lond.)* 343:85 (1990).

43. Y. Koyanagi, S. Miles, R.T. Mitsuyasu, et al. Dual infection of the central nervous system by AIDS viruses with distinct cellular tropisms. *Science* 236:819 (1987).

44. W.A. O'Brien, Y. Koyanagi, A. Namazie, et al. HIV-1 tropism for mononuclear phagocytes can be determined by regions of gp120 outside the CD4-binding domain. *Nature (Lond.)* 348:69 (1990).

45. F. Chiodi, S. Fuerstenberg, M. Gidlund, B. Asjo, and E.M. Fenyo. Infection of brain-derived cells with the human immunodeficiency virus. *J. Virol.* 61:1244 (1987).

46. C. Cheng-Mayer, J.T. Rutka, M.L. Rosenblum, et al. Human immunodeficiency virus can productively infect cultured human glial cells. *Proc. Nat,. Acad. Sci. USA* 84:3526 (1987).

47. S. Dewhurst, K. Sakai, J. Bresser, et al. Persistent productive infection of human glial cells by human immunodeficiency virus (HIV) and by infectious molecular clones of HIV. *J.Viol.* 61:3774 (1987).

48. S. Dewhurst, K. Sakai, Z.H. Zhang, A. Wasiak, and D.J. Volsky. Establishment of human glial cel lines chronically infected with the human immunodeficiency virus. *Virology* 62:151 (1988).

49. B. Keys, J. Albert, J. Kovamees, and F. Chiodi. Brain-derived cells can be infected with HIV-1 isolates derived from both blood and brain. *Virology* 183:834 (1991).

50. C. Tornatore, A. Nath, K. Amemiya, and E.O. Major. Persistent human immunodeficiency virus type 1 infection in human fetal glial cells reactivated by T-cell factor(s) or by the cytokines tumor necrosis factor alpha and interleukin-1 beta. *J. Virol.* 65:6094 (1991).

51. R. Brack-Werner, A. Kleinschmidt, A. Ludvigsen, et al. Infection of human brain cells by HIV-1: restricted virus production in chronically infected glial cell lines. *AIDS* 6:273 (1992).

52. B. Volsky, K. Sakai, M.M. Reddy, and D.J. Volsky. A system for the high efficiency replication of HIV-1 neural cells and its application to antiviral evaluation. *Virology* 186:303 (1992).

53. S. Swingler, A. Easton, and A. Morris. Cytokine augmentation of HIV-1 LTR-driven gene expression in neural cells. *AIDS Res. and Human Retroviruses* 8:487 (1992).

54. M. Shahabuddin, B. Volsky, H. Kim, K. Sakai, and D. Volsky. Regulated expression of human immunodeficiency virus type 1 in human glial cells: induction of dormant virus. *Pathobiology* 60:195 (1992).

55. C.A. Jordan, B.A. Watkins, C. Kufta, and M. Dubois-Dalcq. Infection of brain microglial cells by human immunodeficiency virus type 1 is CD4-dependent. *J. Virol.* 65:736 (1991).

56. C. Kunsch, H.T. Hartle, and B. Wigdahl. Infection of human fetal dorsal root ganglion cells with human immunodeficiency virus type 1 involves an entry mechanism independent of the CD4 T4A epitope. *J. Virol.* 63:5054 (1989).

57. J.M. Harouse, C. Kunsch, H.T. Hartle, et al. CD4-independent infection of human neural cells by human immunodeficiency virus type 1. *J. Virol.* 63:2527 (1989).

58. X. Ling, T. Moudgil, H.V. Vinters, and D.D. Ho. CD4-independent, productive infection of a neuronal cell line by human immunodeficiency virus type 1. *J. Virol.* 6:1383 (1990).

59. J. Bell. The polymerase chain reaction. *Immunol. Today* 10:351 (1989).

60. F.F. Chehab, X. Xiao, Y.W. Kan, and T.S. Yen. Detection of cytomegalovirus infection in paraffin-embedded tissue specimens with the polymerase chain reaction. *Med. Pathol.* 2:75 (1989).

61. M.E. Harper, L.M. Marselle, R.C. Gallo, and F. Wong-Staal. Detection of

lymphocytes expressing human T-lymphotropic virus type III in lymph nodes and peripheral blood from infected individuals by *in situ* hybridization. *Proc. Natl. Acad. Sci. USA* 83:772 (1986).

62. D.D. Ho, T. Moudgil, and M. Alam. Quantitation of HIV-1 in the blood of infected persons. *N. Engl. J. Med.* 321:1621 (1989).

63. S.M. Schnittman, J.J. Greenhouse, M. C. Psallidoupoulos, and A.S. Fauci. Increasing viral burden in CD4 T-cells from patients with HIV infection reflects rapidly progressive immunosuppression and clinical disease. *Ann. Intern. Med.* 113:438 (1990).

64. J. Barre-Sinoussi, J.C. Chermann, F. Rey, et al. Isolation of a T-lymphotropic retrovirus from a patient at risk for acquired immunodeficiency syndrome (AIDS). *Science* 220:868 (1983).

65. G.H. Keller, D.P. Huang, and M.D. Manak. A sensitive nonisotopic hybridization assay for HIV-1 DNA. *Anal. Biochem.* 177:23 (1989).

66. L. Montagnier, J. Gruest, and S. Chamasret. Adaptation of LAV to replication in EBV-transformed B-lymphoblastoid cell lines. *Science* 225:63 (1984).

67. D.E. Lewis, M. Minshall, N.P. Wray, et al. Confocal microscopic detection of human immunodeficiency virus RNA-producing cells. *J. Infect. Dis.* 162:1373 (1990).

68. S.J. Clark, M.S. Saag, W.D. Decker, et al. High titers of cytopathic virus in plasma of patients with symptomatic primary HIV-1 infection. *N. Engl. J. Med.* 324:954 (1991).

69. E.S. Daar, T. Mougdil, R.D. Meyer, and D.D. Ho. Transient high levels of viremia in patients with primary human immunodeficiency virus type 1 infection. *N. Engl. J. Med.* 324:961 (1991).

70. K. Hsia, and S.A. Spector. HIV DNA is present in a high percentage of CD4+ lymphocytes of seropositive individuals. *J. Infect. Dis.* 164:470 (1991).

71. O. Bagasra, and R.J. Pomerantz. Human immunodeficiency virus 1 provirus is demonstrated in peripheral blood monocytes *in vivo*; a study utilizing an *in situ* polymerase chain reaction. *AIDS Res. and Human Retroviruses* 9:69 (1993).

72. A.T. Haase, E.F. Retzel, and K.A. Staskus. Amplification and detection of lentiviral DNA inside cells. *Proc. Natl. Acad. Sci. USA* 87:4971 (1990).

73. K.A. Staskus, L. Couch, P. Herman et al. *In situ* amplification of visna virus DNA in tissue sections reveals a reservoir of latently-infected cells. *Microbiol. Pathogen.* 11:67 (1991).

74. G.J. Nuovo, M. Margiotto, P,. MacConnell, and J. Becker. Rapid *in situ* detection of PCR-amplified HIV-1 DNA. *Diag. Mol. Pathol.* 1:98 (1992).

75. O. Bagasra, T. Seshamma, and R.J. Pomerantz. Polymerase chain reaction *in situ*: intracellular amplification detection of HIV-1 proviral DNA and other specific genes. *J. Immunol. Meth.* 158:131 (1993).

77. O. Bagasra, T. Seshamma, J.W. Oakes, and R.J. Pomerantz. High percentages of CD4-positive lymphocytes harbor the HIV-1 provirus in the blood of certain infected individuals. *AIDS* 7:1419 (1993).

78. J.A. Zack, S.R. Weistman, A.S. Go, A. Haislip, and I.S.Y. Chen,. Incompletely reverse transcribed HIV-1 genomes in quiescent cells can function as intermediates in the viral life-cycle. *Cell* 61:212 (1990).

79. S. Kim, R. Byrn, J. Groopman, and D. Baltimore. Temporal aspects of DNA and RNA synthesis during HIV infection. *J. Virol.* 63:3708 (1989).

80. M.I. Bukrinsky, T.L. Stanwick, M.P. Dempsey, and M. Stevenson. Quiescent T-lymphocytes as an inducible virus reservoir in HIV-1 infection. *Science* 243:423 (1989).

81. T. Folks, J. Justement, A. Kinter, C.A. Dinarello, and A.S. Fauci. Cytokine induced expression of HIV-1 in chronically infected promonocyte cell lines. *Science* 238:800 (1987).

82. C. Sundstrom, and K. Nilsson. Establishment and characterization of human histocyclic lymphoma cell line (U237). *Int. J. Cancer* 17:565 (1976).

83. K.A. Clouse, D. Powell, I. Washington, et al. Monokine regulation of HIV-1

expression in a chronically infected human T-cell clone. *J. Immunol.* 142:431 (1989).

84. J.A. Hoxie, J.D. Alpers, J.L. Rackowsk, et al. Alterations in T4 protein and mRNA synthesis in cells infected with HIV. *Science* 234:1123 (1986).

85. J.P. Clewley. The polymerase chain reaction: A review of the practical limitations for HIV diagnosis. *J.Virol. Meth.* 245:179 (1986).

86. J. Embretson, M. Zupancic, J.L. Ribas, et al. Massive covert infection of helper T lymphocytes by HIV during the incubation period of AIDS. *Nature (Lond.)* 263:359 (1992).

87. B.K. Patterson, M. Till, P. Otto. Detection of HIV-1 DNA and messenger RNA in individual cells by PCR-driven *in situ* hybridization and flow. *Science* 260:976 (1993)..

THE UTILITY OF PCR *IN SITU* HYBRIDIZATION FOR THE DETECTION OF HIV-1 DNA AND RNA

Gerard J. Nuovo

Department of Pathology
SUNY at Stony Brook
Stony Brook, New York 11794

INTRODUCTION

Although the primary manifestation of AIDS is severe immunosuppression and associated opportunistic infections and malignancies, other systems are often involved. Many patients with AIDS will show symptoms indicative of central nervous system (CNS) or skeletal muscle involvement.[1-3] Further, given that homosexual and heterosexual transmission are primary modes of spread of the virus, it is evident that HIV-1 must be able to proliferate at certain sites in the anogenital tract.

Much work has focused on detecting HIV-1 in the peripheral blood, lymph nodes, CNS, skeletal muscle, and lower genital tract.[4-8] Viral DNA and RNA have been detected at each of these sites, primarily by polymerase chain reaction (PCR). *In situ* hybridization and quantitative PCR and reverse transcriptase PCR (RT-PCR) analyses have led to estimates that about 1 per every 1,000 CD4 lymphocytes are infected by HIV-1 early in the disease process.[9,10] It is difficult to reconcile such estimates with the severe lymphocyte dysfunction characteristic of AIDS. Further, although PCR can amplify part of the viral genome, because DNA extraction is necessary, one cannot identify the cellular distribution of the virus.

A critical molecular event for HIV-1-induced pathogenesis and the clinical disease state is the shift from latent infection to the production of the multiple-spliced and full-length genomic transcripts.[11] Although HIV-1 RNA can be detected by standard *in situ* hybridization in actively infected cells, those latently infected by HIV-1 with the characteristic 1 to few integrated copies may not be detected by *in situ* analysis as the copy number is below the detection threshold of the assay.[5,12,13]

A major advance in the last two years has been the ability to combine the extreme sensitivity of PCR with the cell-localizing ability of *in situ* hybridization.[14,15] Several groups have published data based on the detection of HIV-1 by PCR *in situ* hybridization. These studies have agreed on the following points: (1) the percentage of CD4 lymphocytes in the peripheral blood and lymph nodes infected by HIV-1 is much higher than originally estimated, ranging from 1-20% early in the disease (being higher in the lymph node) to over 80% at the end stage of AIDS; (2) early in the disease process, many of the lymphocytes are latently infected; (3) the detection rate of the provirus increases dramatically with PCR *in situ* hybridization as compared to standard *in situ* hybridization; (4) macrophages that contain transcriptionally active HIV-1 are routinely detected in the transformation zone of the uterine cervix.[4,5-8,12,13] Several groups have

Technical Advances in AIDS Research in the Human Nervous System
Edited by E.O. Major and J.A. Levy, Plenum Press, New York, 1995

267

also published data on the detection of RNA with PCR *in situ* by incorporating a reverse transcriptase (RT) step (RT *in situ* PCR). By combining PCR *in situ* hybridization and RT *in situ* PCR, one can readily differentiate latently versus actively infected cells.[5,8,12] It has been suggested that the HIV-1 DNA/HIV-1 RNA ratio may serve as an *in vitro* system to test the efficacy of possible anti-retroviral drugs.[12,15]

The purpose of this chapter is two-fold: (12) to describe the protocols for the detection of PCR-amplified HIV-1 DNA and cDNA; and (2) to demonstrate the utility of these analyses for the study of HIV-1 infection in the peripheral blood, lymph nodes, cervix, skeletal muscle, and CNS.

MATERIALS AND METHODS

Specimen Selection

The HIV-1-infected cell lines were CR10 cells and pooled normal lymphocytes and macrophages infected with HIV-1. The cervical tissues were obtained from 21 women with AIDS being evaluated for an abnormal Papanicoloau smear.[5] The peripheral blood cells were obtained from 15 patients with AIDS.[12] The lymphocytes were isolated with a Ficoll gradient, and about 2,500 cells were placed onto a silane-coated glass slide using a cytocentrifuge. The lymph nodes were biopsies (5) obtained from seropositive patients with lymphadenopathy early in their disease process (CD4 count from 350 to 900). The skeletal muscle tissues (8) were from patients with clinical evidence suggestive of myositis. The CNS tissues were from 7 patients who died of AIDS. Three of these individuals had clinical and pathologic evidence of AIDS/dementia encephalitis whereas the remaining 4 had no or minimal CNS-related clinical findings or pathologic changes. All cells and tissues were fixed in 10% buffered formalin. Cross-linking fixatives such as buffered formalin are required to optimize the signal with PCR *in situ* in part by inhibiting migration of the amplified product from the site of synthesis.[16]

Standard *in situ* Hybridization

Standard *in situ* hybridization analysis was done for sequences homologous to HIV-1. The probes used for HIV-1 detection were SK19 and SK102 (Perkin-Elmer Corporation, Norwalk, CT). These were labeled with digoxigenin-dUTP using the 3' tailing method according to the manufacturer's recommendations (Genius 5 kit, Boehringer-Mannheim, Indianapolis, IN). The standard *in situ* hybridization protocol used for these oligoprobes has been previously published.[5,15] Briefly, after protease digestion (2 mg/ml of trypsin at 37°C for 10-15 minutes), the probe (50 ng/ml in a solution of 10% formamide, 5% dextran sulfate, and 300 mM NaCl) and target DNA are simultaneously denatured by heating to 100°C for 5 minutes. After a 2-hour hybridization at 37°C, the slides are washed in a solution of 1% bovine serum albumin and 300 mM NaCl for 10 minutes at 47°C. The slides are then incubated in the anti-digoxigenin-alkaline phosphatase conjugate (1:50 dilution) at 37°C for 30 minutes and the probe/target complex detected by incubation in the chromagen NBT/BCIP (ONCOR Corporation, Gaithersburg, MD). A hybridization signal is evident as a dark bluish precipitate whereas the counterstain nuclear fast red stains nuclei and cytoplasm pale pink.

PCR *in situ* Hybridization and RT *in situ* PCR

Our procedure for detecting PCR-amplified HIV-1 DNA has already been published.[5,15] The primers SK38 and SK39 plus SK145 and SK431 are used with the probes SK19 and SK102, respectively. The procedure for RT *in situ* PCR has three modifications: (1) after protease digestion, the tissue is treated overnight in a RNase-free DNase solution (Boehringer-Mannheim, 10 units/section at 37°C) which eliminates nonspecific mis-priming and DNA repair; (2)

RT employing the downstream primer (SK39 and SK431) is done at 42ºC for 30 minutes according to the manufacturer's recommendations (Perkin-Elmer); (3) direct incorporation of digoxigenin dUTP into the PCR product is accomplished by using 10 µM of the reporter molecule in the amplifying solution. Thus, detection of RNA was not done with a probe but rather with direct incorporation of the digoxigenin reporter molecule into the PCR product (hence called RT *in situ* PCR) whereas detection of PCR-amplified DNA was done by hybridization with a digoxigenin-labeled internal probe and not by incorporation of the molecule into the PCR product (hence called PCR *in situ* hybridization). Other checks on the specificity of the signal with RT *in situ* PCR included the use of nonsense (HPV-specific) primers, the omission of the RT step, and a pretreatment in an RNase solution.[5,15,17]

Immunohistochemistry

After PCR or RT *in situ* PCR, sections were incubated overnight at 4ºC with either a mouse p24, leukocyte common antigen (LCA-lymphocytes and macrophages), Mac 387 (macrophages), GFAP (astrocytes), neuron-specific enolase (neurons) monoclonal antibody (DAKO, Carpinteria, CA), rabbit anti-galactose cerebroside (oligodendroglial cells) (Sigma), or biotin-labeled RCA-1 (microglial cells/macrophages) (Sigma). It was demonstrated that the antigenicity of these epitopes was either not affected or, at most, minimally decreased by the protease digestion and heating from the cycling and hybridization steps. Our detection procedure, which uses the Stravigin kit (Biogenics, San Ramon, CA) and fast red as the chromagen, has been published.[5,15]

RESULTS

Detection of HIV-1 in Infected Cells, PBMs, and Lymphocytes in Lymph Nodes

CR10 cells infected by HIV-1 as well as pooled lymphocytes and macrophages infected by HIV-1 were available for study. These data are compiled in Table 1 and representative photomicrographs are presented in Figure 1. Note that the detection rate of HIV-1 DNA by standard *in situ* hybridization ranged from 0 to 2%. The rate increased to over 90% if *in situ* hybridization was preceded by PCR. Also note that only about 5-10% of the proviral positive lymphocytes contained HIV-1 RNA as determined by RNA *in situ* hybridization using a ^{35}S probe cocktail as compared to a rate of 76% for the infected macrophages.[12,15]

PBMs from 15 AIDS patients were analyzed next. HIV-1 DNA was not detected in any of the peripheral leukocytes using standard *in situ* analysis. However, in each of the 15 cases, HIV-1 DNA was detected *in situ* after PCR amplification. The range of HIV-1 DNA-positive leukocytes relative to the total peripheral CD4 cells was 1-80%; with the low percentages for patients with advanced AIDS with CD4 counts from 1-3%. Co-labeling of the HIV-1 DNA-positive cells demonstrated that most were CD4+ as previously reported and illustrated.[12] Each of the PBMs from 10 controls were negative for HIV-1 using the *in situ* technique.

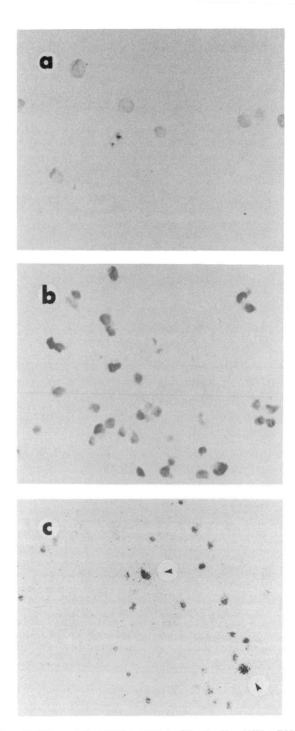

Figure 1. Detection of PCR-amplified HIV-1 DNA in CR 10 cells. HIV-1 DNA was not detected in these viral infected cells by standard in situ hybridization (a). Most of the cells had detectable provirus if the in situ hybridization was preceded by PCR (b; dark is positive due to action of alkaline phosphatase on NBT/BCIP). About 10% of the cells had viral transcripts as detected by RNA in situ hybridization (c; ^{35}S probe).

Table 1. Detection of HIV-1 DNA and RNA in various infected cell lines.

Cell Lines	ISH-DNA*	PCR ISH-DNA	ISH-RNA
CR10	0%	90%	10%
Macrophages**	2%	74%	76%
Lymphocytes**	1%	98%	5%
Lymphocytes, sham	0%	0%	0%

*ISH = *In situ* hybridization for either DNA or RNA as stated.
**The macrophages and lymphocytes were normal cells pooled from several donors and then infected *in vitro* with HIV-1.

HIV-1 DNA was detected in each of the 5 lymph nodes in patients with asymptomatic HIV-1 infection by *in situ* hybridization only after PCR amplification. Most viral infected cells were CD21+ dendritic cells and CD4+ lymphocytes. From 5-80% of the CD4+ cells in these lymph nodes contained HIV-1 DNA as compared to 1-5% of the PBMC (Figure 2). The infection in most cells was latent in the asymptomatic group as defined by the lack of viral RNA. However, there was marked variability in the asymptomatic HIV-1-infected group in their ratio of HIV-1 DNA to HIV-1 RNA-positive cells in the lymph nodes, although for each patients, HIV-1 RNA was very rarely detected in peripheral blood lymphocytes. In contrast, the lymph nodes of patients with advanced AIDS showed almost total loss of dendritic cells and marked depletion of CD4+ cells. Virtually all the remaining CD4+ cells in the lymph nodes and blood contained both HIV-1 DNA and RNA, indicating robust active viral replication in the advanced AIDS group (Nuovo, submitted for publication).

Uterine Cervix

Cervical biopsies from 21 women with AIDS were available for study, and 10 biopsies from women without evidence of HIV-1 infection served as the controls.[5] HIV-1 was detected by standard *in situ* hybridization in 40% of the biopsies. HIV-1 DNA was detected in each of 21 cervical biopsies with the PCR *in situ* hybridization technique and in none of the 10 controls. The viral nucleic acids were most abundant in the endocervical aspect of the transformation zone at the interface of the glandular epithelium and the submucosa and in the deep submucosa around microvessels. This localized signal was lost if PCR *in situ* hybridization was done on serial sections on the same glass slide without the Taq DNA polymerase or with the enzyme but with "nonsense" (HPV-specific) primers. Eight cervical tissues from children who had acquired HIV *in utero* were available for study and only 1 had detectable *in situ* PCR-amplified DNA.

The histologic distribution of viral DNA was compared to the distribution of PCR-amplified HIV-1 cDNA in serial sections as determined by RT *in situ* PCR. Viral cDNA was noted in the 21 seropositive cases and the distribution was identical to the amplified HIV-1 DNA. The number of cells infected by HIV-1 ranged from about 20 to about 1,000. The cDNA-based signal was eliminated if RT PCR was preceded by a 2-hour digestion in RNase, if the RT step was omitted, or if nonsense primers were substituted for the RT and PCR steps.

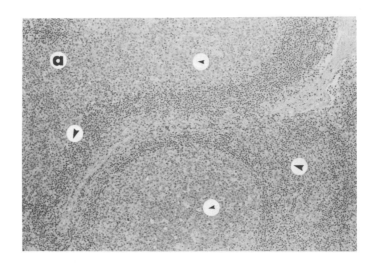

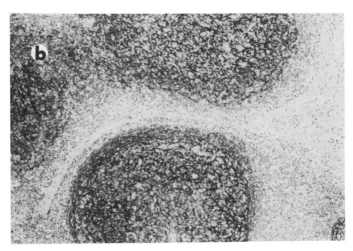

Figure 2. Detection of PCR-amplified HIV-1 DNA in the lymph nodes of a patient with asymptomatic HIV-1 infection. Routine histologic analysis showed expanded germinal centers (small arrow) and prominent parafollicular zones (large arrow) (a). The CD21+ dendritic cells are located in the germinal centers (b). HIV-1 DNA positive cells were detectable by PCR *in situ* hybridization and not standard DNA *in situ* hybridization; the viral infected cells localized to the germinal center and parafollicular zones which is where the CD4+ cells are located (c). (Figure 2c is on the following page).

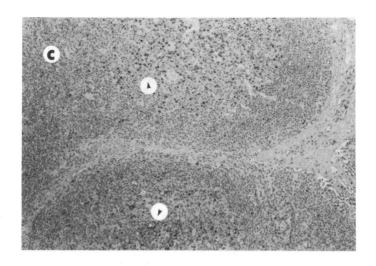

Figure 2c.

In order to determine the phenotype of the HIV-1-infected cells, directly adjacent sections were analyzed from LCA, CD4, and Mac387 by immunohisto-chemistry. Epitopes cross-reactive to the LCA and Mac387 antibodies had a distribution similar to the amplified viral nucleic acids. This finding suggests that most of the infected cells were macrophages. To determine whether the macrophages were activated, serial sections were assayed for TNF mRNA using RT *in situ* PCR. Amplified TNF cDNA was detected in most of the HIV-1 DNA and cDNA-positive cells.[5]

Skeletal Muscle

Eight muscle biopsies from patients infected by HIV-1 and 6 negative controls were tested for HIV-1 DNA and RNA using PCR *in situ* hybridization and RT *in situ* PCR. HIV-1 DNA was detected in rare cells in only 1 case by standard *in situ* hybridization. However, after PCR amplification, HIV-1 DNA was detected in 6 of 8 muscle tissues from AIDS patients and in none of the controls. The number of cells with detectable provirus in the 1 case positive by standard *in situ* analysis increased up to 100-fold amplification. Most of the HIV-1-infected cells were macrophages as determined by co-labeling experiments and these cells were located mainly in the areas of myocyte necrosis (Figure 3). Myocyte nuclei that contained amplified HIV-1 nucleic acids were also noted. Most viral infected cells contained HIV-1 transcripts as determined by RT *in situ* PCR (Nuovo, submitted for publication).

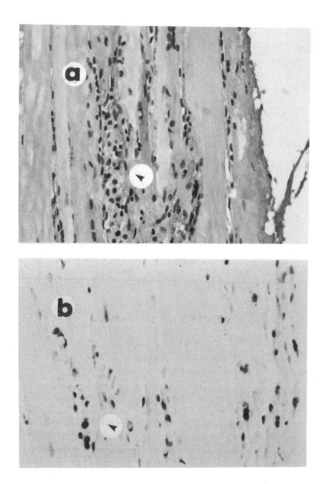

Figure 3. Detection of PCR-amplified HIV-1 DNA in skeletal muscle. This muscle biopsy from an AIDS patient with myopathy showed foci of myocyte necrosis and inflammation (a). HIV-1 DNA was not detected by standard *in situ* hybridization but was detected by PCR *in situ* hybridization in the areas of myocyte necrosis (b).

Central Nervous System

Fourteen tissues from the CNS of 7 AIDS patients and 7 tissues from 7 patients without evidence of HIV-1 infection were studied. Three of the AIDS patients had evidence of dementia whereas the other 4 patients had either no or minimal CNS-related symptoms. The CNS pathologic changes which included neuronal loss evident on routine histologic staining, demyelination, and the microglial nodules and multinucleated giant cells were seen in the 3 patients with CNS symptomatology. HIV-1 DNA was detected in 6/14 tissues by standard *in situ* hybridization and only in the patients with AIDS dementia. The detection rate increased to 14/14 if *in situ* hybridization was preceded by PCR and the number of positive cells in the tissues with a hybridization signal with standard *in situ* hybridization increased by 10- to 100-fold after PCR amplification (Figure 4). Analysis of adjacent serial sections demonstrated a similar distribution of the PCR-amplified signal using the SK19 and SK102 probes with their respective primers. Amplified viral DNA was not detected in any of the 7 negative controls. In patients with minimal clinical and pathologic CNS involvement, only rare HIV-1 DNA-positive perivascular microglial cells were noted. In the 3 patients with AIDS dementia, many infected neurons and astrocytes as well as microglial cells were detected as demonstrated by co-labeling with the appropriate phenotypic marker (Figure 4). PCR-amplified TNF cDNA and HIV-1 cDNA were detected by RT *in situ* PCR only in the tissues of the 3 patients with dementia in a distribution similar to that for HIV-1 DNA. The SK38/39 and SK145/431 primer pairs cannot distinguish between genomic HIV-1 RNA and spliced transcripts. A primer pair which either does not or poorly amplifies a product in genomic viral RNA due to its large size of 3,500 bp and robustly amplified a 250-bp segment after splicing in the rev and tat exons (kindly provided by Dr. R. Pomerantz) produced an intense signal after RT *in situ* PCR in most of the cells which showed a signal using the other primer pairs; similar results were obtained with the cervical tissues. Cells positive for p24 were identified in tissues from the patients with dementia, but in far fewer cells that had detectable viral DNA or transcripts (Nuovo, submitted for publication).

DISCUSSION

The central theme of this chapter is that the *in situ* localization of HIV-1 DNA is greatly enhanced after PCR amplification. HIV-1 DNA was detected by only a few percent of cells infected *in vitro* by the virus by standard *in situ* hybridization. Over 90% of these cells contained viral DNA as demonstrated by PCR *in situ* hybridization. Similarly, most cervical biopsies, lymph nodes, PBMs, skeletal muscle, and CNS tissues from patients with AIDS were negative for HIV-1 by standard *in situ* analysis. The virus was routinely localized in these cells/tissues if the *in situ* hybridization was preceded by PCR. It follows that if the provirus is present in amounts below 10 copies per cell, one must use PCR *in situ* hybridization to accurately assess the histologic distribution of HIV-1 DNA.

HIV-1, like other retroviruses, can have an extended latent period manifested by one to a few copies of integrated DNA with no or minimal transcriptional activity.[11] Interactions between the host cell and virus can lead to an activated infection recognized by the presence of multiply spliced and full-length genomic transcripts. By combining PCR *in situ* hybridization with RT *in situ* PCR, one could differentiate cells that apparently contain only HIV-1 DNA from those in which viral DNA and a variety of mRNAs that characterize the wild type infection are detected. It was shown in this study that most of the CD4+ PBMs and CD4+ plus CD21+ (dendritic) cells in the peripheral blood and lymph nodes, respectively, that contain HIV-1 are latently infected early

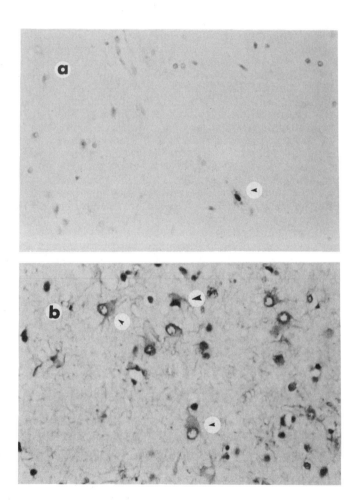

Figure 4. Detection of PCR-amplified HIV-1 DNA in the CNS. PCR-amplified HIV-1 DNA was detected in rare cells in and around the small blood vessels in this patient who had no evidence of AIDS dementia (a); these cells co-labeled with markers for microglia/macrophages. In patients with dementia, many more HIV-DNA positive cells were detected by PCR *in situ* hybridization. These cells were most common in the gray matter and were shown by co-labeling experiments to be microglia, neurons, and astrocytes (b). Panel b is a co-label for GFAP (marks astrocytes); note the HIV-1 DNA negative astrocytes with their branching cytoplasmic processes (small arrow) and the HIV-1 DNA positive astrocyte (large arrow).

in the disease process. This is in agreement with other studies as is the assessment that as many as 20% of T helper cells contain the virus early in the infection and over 50% at the end stage of AIDS.[4,7,8,12,13] These numbers are much higher than has been suggested by standard *in situ* hybridization and quantitative PCR analyses which may reflect the limitations of the latter technique where copy number, mis-priming, and primer oligomerization can affect the accuracy of the results.[9,10,18] The observation by a variety of researchers that many T helper cells are infected by the virus even early in the disease process helps explain a controversial aspect of AIDS, namely, the severe immunosuppression in the setting of relatively few infected cells.

Activation of viral transcription is prerequisite for the evolution of the clinical disease state. It has been postulated that certain viral products may be directly toxic to cells, such as gp120 for neurons, as may be the shift of the cellular machinery to synthesis of viral products in general.[19,20] An intriguing finding in this study is that certain well-defined clinical manifestations of AIDS, namely dementia and myopathy, are associated with a marked increase in the number of infected cells and wild type (i.e., production) viral transcription pattern. Alternatively, in patients without dementia, rare cells with viral DNA were identified and viral RNA was not detectable. These findings suggest a model for HIV-1-induced pathogenesis in which the percentage of infected target cells and state of viral activation are two key variables. PCR *in situ* and RT PCR *in situ*, by permitting the determination of the ratio of latent to active infection, may serve as a useful *in vitro* assay for testing prospective drugs for anti-HIV-1 activity.

In only one site of those included in this study did most of the HIV-1 DNA-positive cells contain spliced and full-length transcripts irrespective of the patient's disease state - the cervix.[5] One may speculate that this represents an adaptation of the virus to increased productive infection to enhance the probability of sexual transmission. It is unclear if the cervical infection is a primary event or represents hematogenous spread. However, the inability to detect HIV-1 at other sites such as the endometrium and esophagus in women with AIDS suggest that viral proliferation in the cervix represents a primary event. The localization in macrophages both at the transformation zone and around the deep lymphatics suggests a possible mode of spread from the cervix to the lymph nodes (Figure 5).

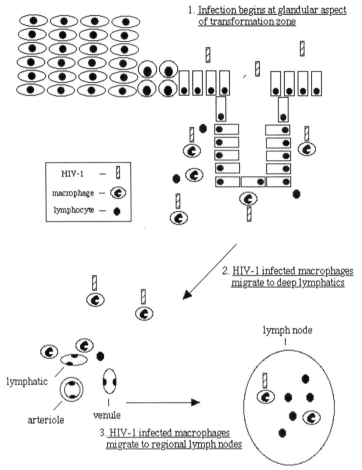

Figure 5. Graphic representation of the distribution of HIV-1 in cervical tissues. The localization of IIIV-1 PCR-amplified nucleic acids to the endocervical aspect of the transformation zone and around the deep microvessels is depicted as is a proposed model for the systemic spread of HIV-1 infection from heterosexual transmission via the cervical macrophages.

Acknowledgements

The author greatly appreciates the technical and material assistance from Dr. John Snisnky (Roche Molecular Systems), John Atwood and Dr. Larry Haff (Perkin-Elmer Corporation), and Dr. Roger Pomerantz. Ms. Phyllis MacConnell provided expert technical and editorial assistance and Dr. Harold Ginsburg and Roy Steigbigel kindly provided the HIV-1-infected cells. This work was supported by grants from the Lewis Foundation, ONCOR, and Perkin-Elmer Corporation to GJN.

278

REFERENCES

1. H. Budka. Neuropathology of human immunodeficiency virus infection. *Brain Pathol.* 1:163 (1991).
2. R.W. Price, B. Brew, J. Sidti, M. Rosenblum,. A.C. Scheck, and P. Cleary. The brain in AIDS: Central nervous system HIV-1 infection and AIDS demen dementia complex. *Science* 239:586 (1988).
3. M.A. Wrzolek, J.H. Sher, P.B. Kozlowski, and C.Rao. Skeletal muscle pathology in AIDS: An autopsy study. *Muscle & Nerve* 13:508 (1990).
4. J. Embretson, M. Zupancic, J. Beneke, M. Till, S.Wolinsky, J.L. Ribas, A. Burke, and A.T. Haase. Analysis of human immunodeficiency virus infected tissues by amplification and *in situ* hybridization reveals latent and permissive infections at single cell resolution. *Proc. Natl. Acad. Sci., USA* 90:357 (1993).
5. G.J. Nuovo, M. Margiotta, P. MacConnell, and J. Becker. Rapid *in situ* detection of PCR-amplified HIV-1 DNA. *Diagn. Mol. Pathol.* 1:98 (1992).
6. G. Pantaleo, C. Graziosi, J.F. Demarest, L. Butini, M. Montroni, C.H. Fox, J.M. Orenstein, D.P. Kotler, and A.S. Fauci. HIV infection is active and progressive in lymphoid tissue during the clinically latent stage of the disease. *Nature* 362:355 (1993).
7. O. Bagasra, S.P. Hauptman, H.,W. Lischer, M. Sachs, and R.J. Pomerantz. Detection of human immunodeficiency virus type 1 provirus in mononuclear cells by *in situ* polymerase chain reaction. *New Engl. J. Med.* 326:1385 (1992).
8. B.K. Patterson, M. Till, P. Otto, C. Goolsby, M.R. Furtado, L.J. McBride, and S.M.Wolinsky. Detection of HIV-1 DNA and messenger RNA in individual cells by PCR-driven *in situ* hybridization and flow cytometry. *Science* 260:976 (1993).
9. M.E. Harper, L.M. Marselle, R.C. Gallo, and F. Wong-Staal. Detection of lymphocytes expressing human T-lymphotropic virus type III in lymph nodes and peripheral blood from infected individuals by *in situ* hybridization. *Proc. Natl. Acad. Sci., USA* 83:772 (1986).
10. P. Shapshak, N.C.J. Sun, L. Resnick, M.Y.K. Hsu, W.W. Tourtellotte, P., Schmid, A. Conrad, M. Fiala, and D.T. Imagawa. The detection of HIV by *in situ* hybridization. *Mod. Pathol.* 3:146 (1990).
11. R.J. Pomerantz, D. Trono, M.B. Feinberg, and D. Baltimore. Cells nonproductively infected with HIV-1 exhibit an aberrant pattern of viral RNA expression: A molecular model for latency. *Cell* 61:1271 (1990).
12. G.J. Nuovo, M. Margiotta, P. MacConnell, and J. Becker. Rapid *in situ* detection of PCR-amplified HIV-1 DNA. *Diagn. Mol. Pathol.* 1:98 (1992).
13. J. Embretson, M. Zupancic, J.L.Ribas, A. Burke, P. Racz, T. Tenner-Racz, and A.T. Haase. Massive covert infection of helper T lymphocytes and macrophages by HIV during the incubation period of AIDS. *Nature* 362:359 (1993).
14. A.T. Haase, E.F. Retzel, and K.A. Staskus. Amplification and detection of lentiviral DNA inside cells. *Proc. Natl. Acad. Sci., USA* 84:4971 (1990).
15. G.J. Nuovo. "PCR Methods and Applications." Raven Press, New York (1992).
16. G.J. Nuovo, F. Gallery, R. Hom, P. MacConnell, and W. Block. Importance of different variables for optimizing *in situ* detection of PCR-amplified DNA. *PCR Meth. Applic.* 2:305 (1993).
17. G.J. Nuovo, K. Lidonocci, P. MacConnell, and B. Lane. Intracellular localization of PCR-amplified hepatitis C cDNA. *Am. J. Pathol.* 17:68 (1993).
18. F.Clayton, E.B. Klein, and D.P. Kotler. Correlation of *in situ* hybridization with histology and viral culture in patients with acquired immunodeficiency syndrome with cytomegalovirus. *Arch. Pathol. Lab. Med.* 113: 1124 (1989).
19. G. Pantaleo, C. Graziosi, and A.S. Fauci. The immunopathogenesis of human immunodeficiency virus infection. *N. Engl. J. Med.* 328:327 (1993).
20. D.D. Ho, R.J. Pomerantz, and J.C. Kaplan. Pathogenesis of infection with human immunodeficiency virus. *N. Engl. J. Med.* 321:278 (1987).

ELECTROCHEMILUMINESCENCE-BASED DETECTION SYSTEM FOR THE QUANTITATIVE MEASUREMENT OF ANTIGENS AND NUCLEIC ACIDS: APPLICATION TO HIV-1 AND JC VIRUSES

John J. Oprandy,[1] Kei Amemiya,[2] John H. Kenten,[1]
Richard G. Green,[1] Eugene O. Major, [2] and Richard Massey[1]

[1]IGEN, Inc.
1530 East Jefferson Street
Rockville, Maryland 20852

[2]Laboratory of Molecular Medicine and Neuroscience
National Institute of Neurological Disorders and Stroke
National Institutes of Health
Bethesda, Maryland 20892

ABSTRACT

A system for quantitative measurements based on electrochemilumi-nescence (ECL) has recently been developed. ECL is the generation of light through a series of chemical reactions at an electrode surface using a label that is a chelate of ruthenium(II) tris(2,2'-bipyridine) (Rubpy). ECL is ideally suited for analytic procedures involving antigens or nucleic acids because of the precision, sensitivity, and accuracy of the system. In addition, assay formats which elim-inate wash steps and have rapid kinetics have been developed.

Applications of the ECL system which produce significant advantages over conventional methods are DNA probe assays and the quantitation of PCR pro-ducts. Assay measurements produce a linear log-log plot (signal vs. concentra-tion of analyte), facilitating quantitation over the wide dynamic range. Several assay formats have been developed. Sandwich hybridizations have been per-formed using biotinylated capture probes for the immobilization of analyte onto magnetic beads. Biotinylated primers can be used for this purpose, in polymerase chain reaction (PCR) amplification. The biotinylated PCR elongated strand or capture probe was bound to streptavidin-coated magnetic beads for detection by a Rubpy-labeled oligo probe. Oligonucleotide probe assays were performed in one step, 15-minute incubation time test formats. Experimental data indicated a sensitivity of 10^5 molecules per 10 µl sample of HIV-1 gag gene DNA and a five-order of magnitude linear dynamic range. The sensitivity and quantitative efficiency of the ECL system was demonstrated. The application of this system to the quantitation of the input copy number in competitive PCR amplification, using internal standards of JC virus, is also discussed.

Technical Advances in AIDS Research in the Human Nervous System
Edited by E.O. Major and J.A. Levy, Plenum Press, New York, 1995

INTRODUCTION

Electrochemiluminescence (ECL) is a sensitive new technology to detect molecular species such as proteins (antigens and antibodies) and nucleic acids. This technology has several advantages over existing methods: no radioisotopes or enzymes are used; there is no substrate reaction; and detection limits are extremely low (fmol). The instrumented system has a seven-order of magnitude dynamic range. The ECL label has a molecular weight of 1,054 and can be covalently bound to proteins and nucleic acids via an N-hydroxysuccinimide (NHS) linkage. This technology has been used to develop clinical diagnostic immunoassays and oligonucleotide probe assays.[1]

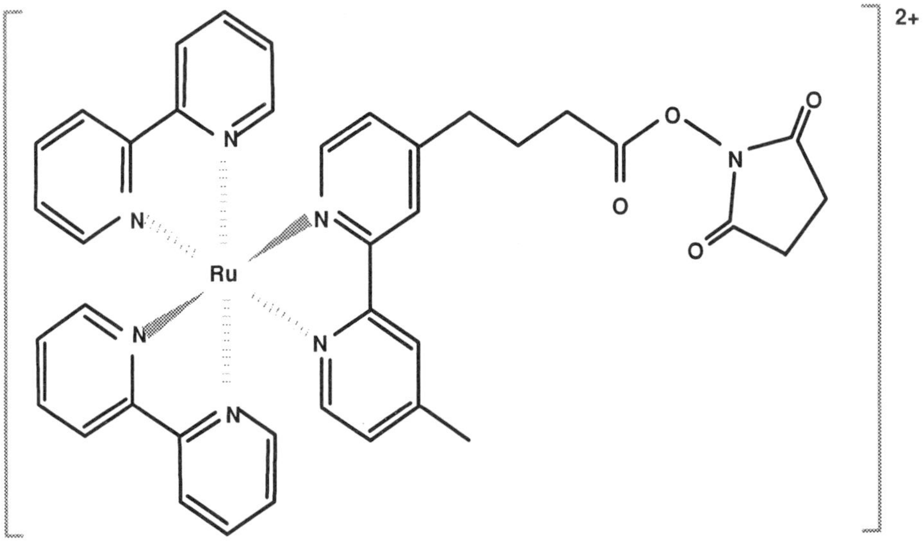

Figure 1. The N-hydroxysuccinimide ester form of the ORIGEN® label, ruthenium (II) Tris(bipyridine) (Rubpy). This label was used for the DNA ECL reactions.

The ECL label is a chelate of ruthenium and Tris(bipyridine) complex (Rubpy) (Fig. 1) which produces light through electrochemical interactions. Reactive species, in this highly sensitive assay system, are generated from stable precursors at the electrode surface. The ruthenium label is oxidized at the electrode, forming a strong oxidant. Tripropylamine (TPA), in the buffer, is also oxidized at the electrode. TPA becomes spontaneously deprotonated, then donates an electron to the ruthenium atom. The decay of this electron from its excited state emits a photon at a wavelength of 620 nm (Fig. 2). The cyclical reaction continues by the ruthenium label and more TPA being oxidized at the electrode. Each label can emit may photons during the measurement cycle.

We present here data on the detection and quantitation of two different nucleic acid targets using ECL. Probe assays included the sensitive and specific detection of HIV-1 gag gene DNA, developed to demonstrate the sensitivity of the ECL oligonucleotide probe system. In addition, a scheme was developed whereby the precise input copy number could be determined by competitive PCR amplification, using internal standards of JC virus (JCV) DNA from clinical samples.

Chemiluminescence of Electrogenerated Reactants

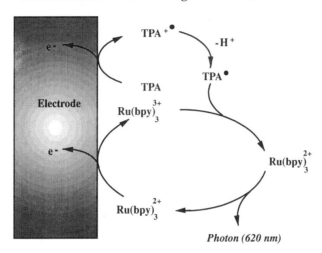

Figure 2. Proposed mechanism for the ECL reaction of Rubpy and tripropylamine (TPA). The Rubpy label is oxidized at the electrode surface forming a strong oxidant. Simultaneously, TPA, present in vast molar excess, is oxidized to form a cation radical which is spontaneously deprotonated to form a strong reductant (TPA•). This latter molecule reacts with the oxidized $Ru(bpy)_3{}^{3+}$ label to form the excited state of the ruthenium complex. The excited state ruthenium complex decays through a normal fluorescence mechanism, emitting a photon at 620 nm. This process regenerates the normal form of Rubpy.

IGEN, Inc. (Rockville, MD) has developed an ECL detection method and instrumentation (ORIGEN® Analyzer, Fig. 3) for use in immunoassays and DNA probe assays. Assays are performed on magnetic microspheres. This increases rate kinetics dramatically over other solid phase systems. Typical detection limits for immunoassays are 0.1 pg (T. Wu, personal communication). The instrument is automated allowing the run through of 50 samples per carousel at a rate of one sample reading in 30-60 seconds. Microspheres, in a sample tube, are drawn up through the fluidics of the instrument and are captured in a flow cell by a magnetic field. The microsphere capture sequence is followed by a wash of assay buffer. Only molecules immobilized on the microbeads, by interaction with a specific ligand, are counted by the system. Quantitation of the light produced by the ECL reaction is performed using a photomultiplier tube in the ORIGEN® Analyzer and the instrument's software.

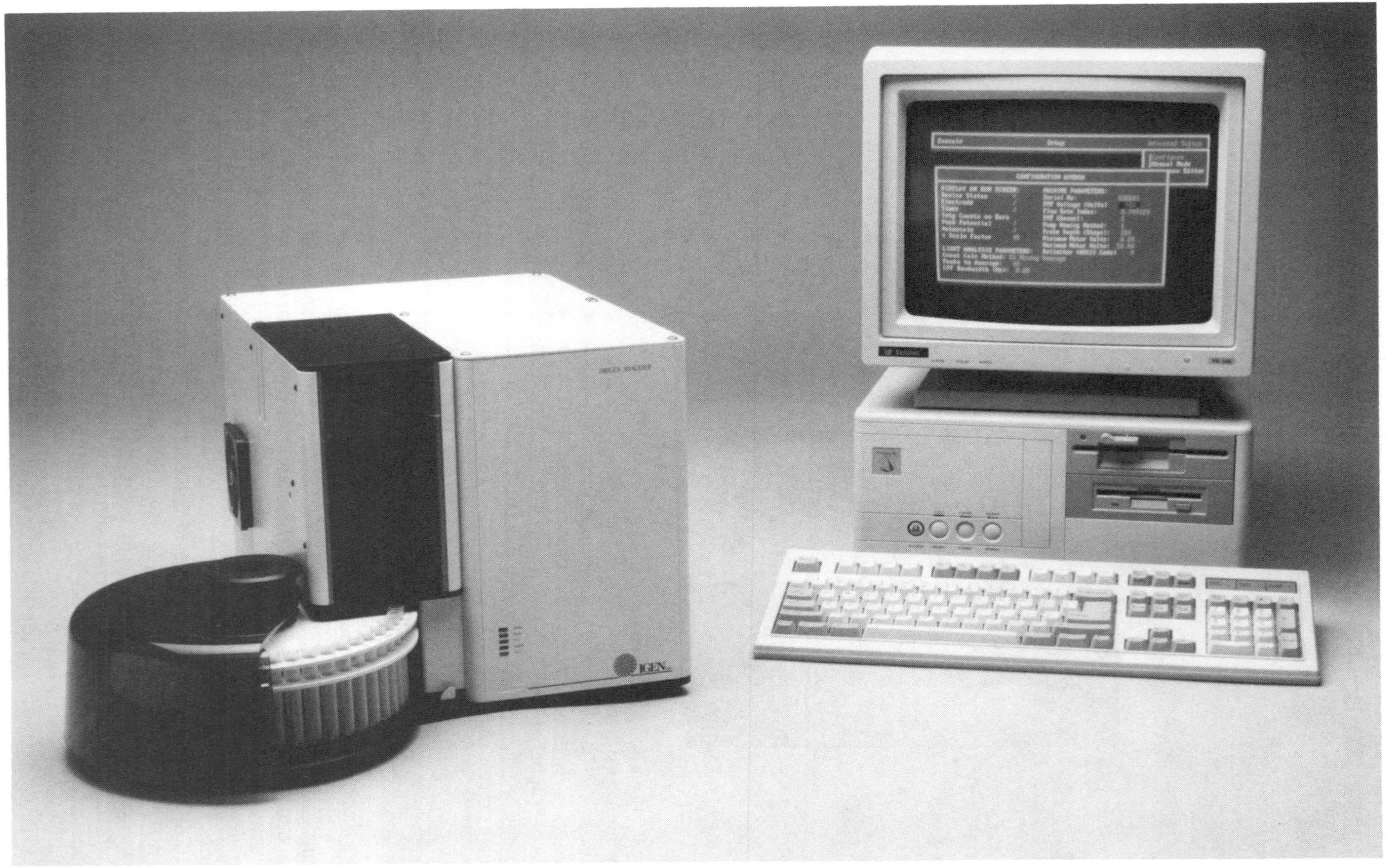

Figure 3. The IGEN ORIGEN® Analyzer with computer.

EXPERIMENTAL STUDIES

HIV-1 Gag Gene DNA Assay

A model sandwich hybridization/capture probe system was developed to characterize the ECL system. The assay consisted of a biotinylated oligonucleotide to immobilize analyte onto the magnetic beads and a Rubpy-labeled oligonucleotide probe for identification.

The following oligonucleotide probes and synthetic target DNA samples were used in the assays described. The target DNA (BA) was a 60-base fragment from the *gag* gene of HIV-1. Both DNA and RNA oligonucleotides were made for the BA target sequence. The A1 biotin probe was a 25-base oligonucleotide, biotinylated at the 5' end, homologous to a region near the 3' end of the BA sequence. The B2 (Rubpy) probe was a 28-base fragment, Rubpy labeled at both the 5' and 3' ends, homologous to a region at the 5' end of the BA target. All nucleic acid preparations were made up in hybridization buffer [1X SSPE/10X Denhardt's (1% Ficoll, 1% PVP, 1% BSA)/0.1% SDS)].

The oligonucleotides were biotinylated at the 5'-NH_2 site using a biotin NHS-ester and 5'3' Rubpy labeled by a Rubpy phosphoramidite or Rubpy-NHS ester. The labeled oligonucleotides were purified by denaturing polyacrylamide gel chromatography and high performance liquid chromatography.

Sandwich Hybridization/Capture Probe Assay. The oligonucleotide probe hybridization/magnetic bead capture was performed in one step. This was followed by the addition of assay buffer (essentially a phosphate buffer of neutral pH containing TPA and Triton X-100) to bring the reaction mixture to the required volume and concentration for reading in the ORIGEN® Analyzer. Streptavidin-coated, 208-micron magnetic beads were procured from Dynal, A.S. (Oslo,Norway). Beaded were suspended in ORIGEN assay buffer to give a concentration of 20.0 µg/50 µl prior to use. The value of 20.0 µg of beads per assay was determined empirically.

One-Step Assay Protocol:

1. Add the following:
   10 µl of test nucleic acid is aliquoted to the assay tube
   20 µl Abio probe/B2Rubpy probe (1.4 µg/ml each)
   50 µl streptavidin-coated magnetic beads (Dynal, 20 µg)
2. Mix on a rotary shaker, 15 minutes at 42°C
3. Add 200 µl assay buffer
4. Read sample

Assays were read using the IGEN ORIGEN® Analyzer (IGEN, Inc., Rockville, MD) fitted with platinum electrode cells. The instrument was set to an internal temperature of 35°C.

Time Course of Assay. A sample containing 10^9 molecules of target DNA was used for the study. Assays were performed at full volume and put on the instrument carousel in triplicate, alternating between control and positive samples. Time-course measurements were accomplished on the instrument according to cycle time and sample tube position in the carousel. Signal increased rapidly reaching a plateau at about 50 minutes. Background also leveled at about this point. These data indicated that a low volume hybridization should be performed followed by the addition of assay buffer in order to bring tube volume to the level accepted by the instrument. Positive results were obtained with a 15-minute low-volume incubation (data not shown).

One Step Test - Standard Curve. Under the standard assay conditions and buffers described above, BA DNA as well as RNA test samples were assayed in the ORIGEN system. Log concentrations of DNA range from 10^6 to 10^{13} molecules per 10 µl aliquot used in the assay. Probe concentration was 10^{12} per assay. Triplicate samples were assayed in three different instrument runs.

A standard curve was plotted (Fig. 4) on a log-log scale using these data. The dynamic range was shown to be five orders of magnitude. Signal at 10^{12} molecules approached the maximum of the system. There was a marked decrease in signal at 10^{13} molecules. This was due to excess unbound target nucleic acid molecules binding labeled probes. The slope of the plot approached 1.0 with excellent linearity. Results using the RNA target were equivalent (data not shown).

15 MIN ONE STEP ASSAY

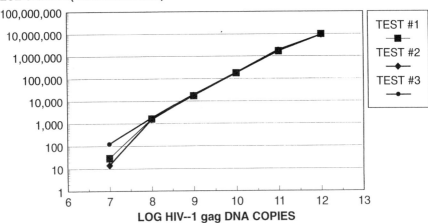

Figure 4. Sandwich hybridization assay for HIV-1 gag gene DNA. 10^{12} molecules each of biotinylated capture probe and Rubpy-labeled detection probe were incubated with target analyte per assay. Three separate tests were performed with triplicate samples. The plot indicates a sensitivity of 10^7 molecules with a dynamic range of five orders of magnitude. The ECL signal is calculated as the signal of the negative control plus two standard deviations, subtracted from the signal of the test sample.

In a related experiment investigating maximum sensitivity, the Abiotin/B2TAG probe set was made to 10^{11} each and magnetic beads used at a concentration of 2 µg per assay. Samples were run as above with a 45-minute incubation. Assay sensitivity was shown to be 10^5 with a range to 10^{11} (Fig. 5). The curve of the plot did not have a slope approaching 1 and was bimodal. This may have been due to the differing diffusion characteristics of the different concentrations of target.

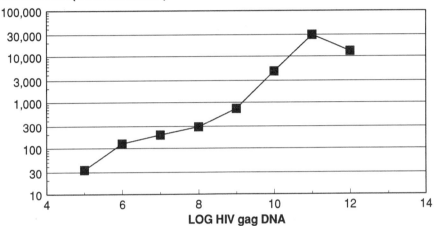

10¹¹ PROBES, 30 MIN

Figure 5. Sandwich hybridization assay for HIV-1 gag gene DNA, with incubation time extended to 30 minutes and 10^{11} molecules each of biotinylated capture probe and Rubpy labeled detection probe, incubated with target analyte per assay. These data indicate a sensitivity of 10^5 molecules with a dynamic range of six orders of magnitude, in a bimodal curve. ECL signal is calculated as the signal of the negative control plus 2 standard deviations, subtracted from the signal of the test sample.

Competitive PCR for the Quantitation of JC Virus

JC virus (JCV), a human polyoma virus, is the etiologic agent of progressive leukoencephalopathy (PML) (for review, see ref. 2). The existence of a large group of patients without PML but with JCV in their peripheral blood lymphocytes (PBLs) requires a more quantitative analysis of the levels of the virus to help determine their risk in acquiring PML.[3] In order to obtain a more quantitative evaluation of the presence of JCV, an assay was developed for the quantitative detection of JCV using a competitive PCR technique.

Several schemes have been developed to quantitate the input copy number of PCR-amplified analyte.[4-6] Quantitation can be done by methods such as densitometry of analyte on gels. The signal of the test sample is then compared by proportionality. This method, although widely used, has the disadvantage of having no internal standard for the amplification efficiency of the PCR process for the test sample, and quantitation is generally only accurate in the linear portion of the plot of the standard curve.

Competitive PCR (CPCR)[7,8] uses a control piece of DNA which has the same primer sites as the test sample and is included in the same PCR reaction, but is identified separately. Identification of the two species has been accomplished by having the control DNA be either a different size or having an unique internal restriction site, so that separation on gels can be achieved.[7,9] Quantitation is done by having a series of concentrations of the control DNA, coamplified as an internal standard, in PCR reactions with a set amount of sample DNA. These two targets use the same set of primers. At the point where the copy number of the test sample and control are equivalent, the two are amplified to the same level.

The accuracy of CPCR depends on the amplification of the control DNA and test sample being equal. Amplification can be influenced by DNA sequence and length. We determined the input copy number of JCV using CPCR. A control DNA piece was constructed to be of the same length and nucleotide pairing as the JCV but contained a 53-base region at the sample probe site which was a reversed sequence from the wild type. This created a novel site for the control probe and determination by ECL.

Construction of the pBRJCH3con Control Plasmid for CPCR Analysis. The recombinant JC plasmid pMad1 was obtained from Dr. Richard Frisque[10] (Pennsylvania State University, College Park, PA). PML DNA was obtained from Dr. Carlo Tornatore and prepared from a 0.5 cm^3 piece of brain autopsy tissue essentially as described previously.[3]

In order to construct the JCV CPCR control plasmid pBRJCH3con, a 416-bp HindIII-HindIII fragment was removed and isolated from the recombinant JCV plasmid pMad1. This fragment contains the coding region near the 5' end (nucleotides 4615 to 4668) of the JCV large T and small t antigens (Fig. 6). It was ligated into the HindIII site of pBR322 to give the plasmid pBRJCH3. Before insertion of the JCV fragment into pBR322, the SphI restriction site in the pBR322 vector was eliminated.

pBRJCH3 was further modified as shown in Figure 7 for use in CPCR analysis. pBRJCH3 was digested with BstXI (JCV nucleotide 4615) and SphI (JCV nucleotide 4668) to remove a 53-bp fragment. A 71-bp oligonucleotide which contained the reverse sequence of the JCR 53-bp BstXI-SphI fragment and flanked by BstXI and SphI restriction sites was prepared. After the 71-bp oligonucleotide was digested with BstXI and SphI to give a 53-bp fragment, the digested oligonucleotide was ligated into pBRJCH3, in which the original 53-bp BstXI-SphI fragment had been removed. The new plasmid pBRJCH3con was sequenced in the region of the new insertion to confirm the sequence and orientation of the replacement oligonucleotide.

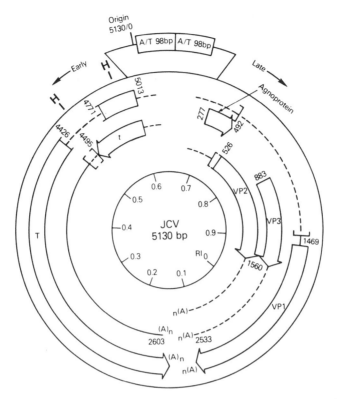

Figure 6. Schematic diagram of the JC virus genome adapted from Frisque et al.[10] The 416 bp
*Hind*III-*Hind*III fragment used to prepare the quantitative PCR control template is located near
the 5'-end of the T-antigen coding region in the early region. H represents *Hind*III restriction
sites.

Oligonucleotides and Primers. A pair of complimentary 71-base oligo-
nucleotides, with *Bst*XI and *Sph*I restriction sites, for construction of the JCV
CPCR control plasmid was obtained from Integrated DNA Technologies, Inc.
(Coralville, IA). A pair of 20-base oligonucleotide primers (JCPMER5 and
JCPMER3) used for PCR amplification were obtained from Synthecell/Vega Bio-
molecules Corp. (Columbia, MD). JCPMER5 was biotinylated for capture of the
PCR product onto streptavidin-coated magnetic beads.

Two probes (JCWT and JCCON) were synthesized by Synthecell/Vega Bio-
molecules for use in the ECL system to identify the PCR products. These oligonucleotides were amine-modified and labeled using the Rubpy NHS ester. Both
probes hybridize to the same map region of the amplified product; however, they
are reversed sequences and therefore unique.

PCR and CPCR Amplification. PCR and CPCR analyses were performed with reagents obtained from Perkin Elmer Cetus (Norwalk, CT) and used
as recommended by the manufacturer. One-hundred μl reaction mixtures with
2.5 units of AmpliTaq DNA polymerase were incubated in a Perkin Elmer Cetus
DNA ThermalCycler with a program of 95°C for 1 minute, 55°C for 1 minute, and
72°C for 2 minutes, for 30 cycles. Primers JCPMER5 and JCPMER3 were used
at 25 pmol each per reaction mix, and the amount of DNA template used as
stated in each figure for both PCR and CPCR analysis. PCR products (10 μl
aliquots) were analyzed on a 5% polyacrylamide gel after staining with ethidium
bromide.

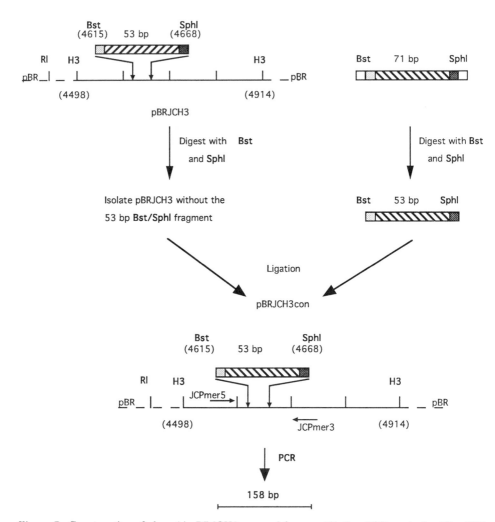

Figure 7. Construction of plasmid pBRJCH3con used for quantitative PCR analysis. The JCV 416-bp *Hin*III-*Hind*III fragment cloned into pBR322 (pBRJCH3) is shown on the upper left. The location of the 53-bp *Bst*XI-*Sph*I fragment which was removed from the 416-bp *Hin*III-*Hind*III fragment is shown above. On the upper right is the replacement oligonucleotide. Next to the bottom is the new construct (pBRJCH3con) with the location of the PCR primers. The JCPMER5 primer is biotinylated. RI and H3 represent *Eco*RI and *Hind*III, respectively.

Analysis of PCR Products with pBRJCH3con, pMad1, and PML DNA. PCR was used to generate specific products with the newly constructed pBRJCH3con plasmid and the recombinant JCV pMad1 plasmid. The PCR products were analyzed by polyacrylamide gel electrophoresis. Twenty-five pmol of each primer, JCPMER5 and JCPMER3, were used in each reaction. Figure 8A (lanes 1-6) shows that with an increasing amount of pMad1 DNA (0.0001-10 pg), there was an increasing amount of a 158-bp PCR product. The production of this

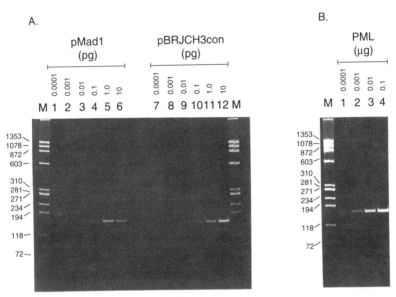

Figure 8. Electrophoretic analysis of PCR products using pMad1, pBRJCH3con, or PML DNA templates. A. PCR products with increasing amounts of either pMad1 (lanes 1-6) or pBRJCH3con (lanes 7-12) DNAs. B. PCR products with increasing amounts of DNA from a PML patient. Ten µl of each PCR reaction was examined by polyacrylamide gel electrophoresis. Twenty-five pmol of each primer was used in all PCR reactions. Lanes labeled M are φX174 HaeIII size markers.

specific product depended on both the DNA template and specific primers (data not shown). When the CPCR control plasmid pBRJCH3con was used at increasing concentrations (0.0001-10 pg), a similar size PCR product was produced as that with pMad1 DNA (Fig. 8A, lanes 7-12). In addition, when DNA extracted from brain tissue from a PML patient was used as the template at different concentrations (0.0001-0.1 µg) with the same primers as above, the same size PCR product was obtained as with the pMad1 and pBRJCH3con DNA templates (Fig. 8B). Therefore, the same expected size PCR product was obtained with the three different DNA templates with the same pair of primers.

Electrochemiluminescent Detection of PCR Products. For each competitive PCR amplification reaction, two hybridization reactions were set up: one using a Rubpy-labeled JCWT probe, and one using a Rubpy-labeled JCCON probe. 30 µl of the PCR product, 30 µl of ruthenium-labeled probe [10^{14} copies/ml in hybridization buffer (1X SSPE, 10X Denhardt's, 0.1% SDS)], and 30 µl of yeast tRNA (0.1 mg/ml in hybridization buffer) were mixed in a microfuge tube. The samples were incubated at 95°C for 5 minutes and then allowed to hybridize for 15 minutes at 42°C. Each sample was then divided into three assay tubes (30 µl per tube), mixed with 50 µl (20 µg) of Dynal M-280 streptavidin-coated beads (Fig. 9), and incubated for 15 minutes while vortexing at 88 r.p.m. on the Analyzer carousel. Finally, 200 µl of assay buffer was added to each tube, and the samples were read on the IGEN ORIGEN® Analyzer (internal temperature set to 35°C).

A series of control DNA samples at known, increasing concentrations were amplified by PCR, then assayed by ECL. At the same time, 1 µg (total DNA) of three known JCV/PML patient samples was also amplified and assayed using the same methods. A standard curve was derived from the control DNA and the signals of the patient samples plotted against this (Fig. 10). The input copy number of the patient samples was determined in this manner. In the following experiments, 100 ng (1/10 of these samples) were quantitated by CPCR.

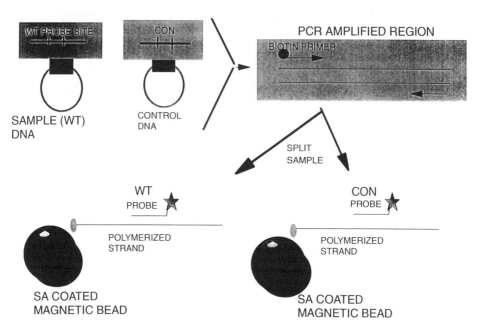

Figure 9. Scheme for competitive PCR/ECL assay. Sample DNA and control DNA are both mixed in the same PCR reaction, competing for the same set of primers. One primer was biotinylated so that this strand of the amplified product could be immobilized onto streptavidin-coated magnetic beads. After amplification, the PCR reaction mix is split into two aliquots and these used in two different Rubpy labeled oligonucleotide probe assays, in order to quantitate the amplified product.

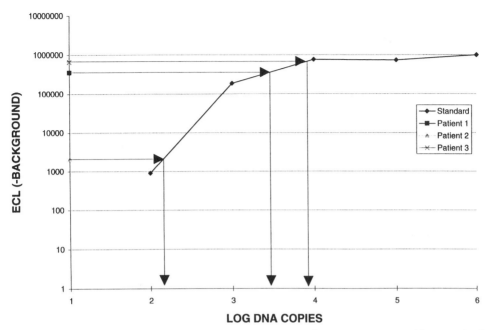

Figure 10. Quantitation of the input copy of JC virus, after PCR, by comparison with a standard curve. In a separate PCR reaction, a set of samples of known copy number were amplified. The signal of a 1 µg (total genomic) DNA sample, from three PML patients containing JC DNA, was then compared to this plot.

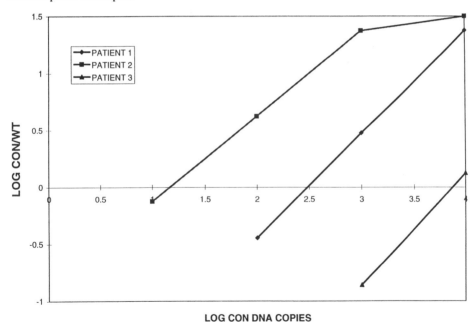

Figure 11. Calculation of the input copy number of JC virus in test patient DNA by competitive PCR. The logarithm of the ratio of the control to test sample ECL signal was plotted against the copy number of the control DNA. At log(con/wt) = 0, the input copy number of the control and the test sample is equivalent.

Competitive PCR Quantitation. In the competitive PCR reaction, the control DNA, pBRJCH3con, was added to the PCR reaction mixes in four ten-fold increasing concentrations; replicate samples of patient test DNA were added to each of the four tubes at a concentration of 0.1 µg per reaction (1/10 that of the amount used for ther standard curve experiment listed above). A competitive PCR reaction was then done on this set. After PCR, two aliquots of each reaction were prepared. A Rubpy-labeled JCWT probe, complementary to the test sample PML DNA, was added to one and a Rubpy-labeled control probe (JCCON) added to the other. An ECL assay was performed and hybridizations of the two markers were counted using the ORIGEN® Analyzer. The ECL signal from four increasing samples of pBRJCH3con DNA (CON) increased and intersected the plot of the PML DNA. At the point where the ECL signal from the WT and CON samples were equivalent, the copy number of the WT DNA is equal to the copy number of the CON DNA. Estimation of the input copy number was determined by taking the logarithm of the ratio of the CON to the WT ECL signal and plotting this value against the logarithm of the input copy number of the control DNA (Fig. 11). The input copy number of the PML sample DNA was calculated at the point where log(CON/WT) = 0. Calculation of this value indicated a copy number of 1.25, 2.5 and 3.8 logs for patients 2, 1 and 3, respectively. These data correlated very closely with that of the standard curve except for patient 3. This inaccuracy may have been due to the signal on the standard curve being in the plateau of the plot.

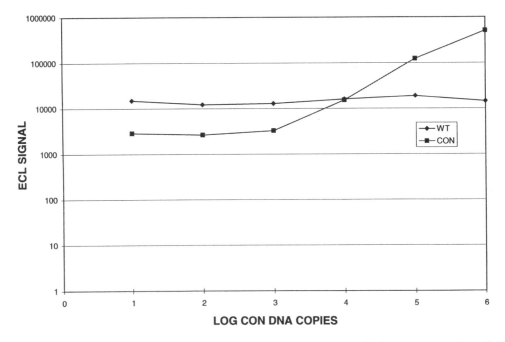

Figure 12. Competitive PCR of JCV DNA of known copy number. An input copy number of 10,000 copies returned the same value when determined by this method.

A series of samples of known copy number of test DNA (WT) were assayed using the methods described above. This was done to further determine the accuracy of the CPCR method using ECL as the detection system. A sample of 10,000 copy number DNA was diluted 1/10 (1,000 copies) and both tested by CPCR. The plot of the intersect of the WT and CON amplificates indicates the expected copy numbers of the input samples (Figs. 12 and 13).

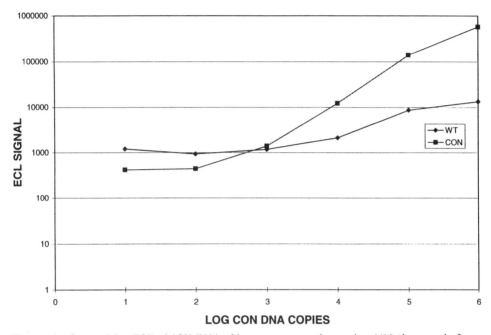

Figure 13. Competitive PCR of JCV DNA of known copy number, using 1/10 the sample from Figure 12. An input copy number of 1,000 copies returned a value of 850 copies when determined by this method.

CONCLUSIONS

Data presented here demonstrate the utility of ECL in the detection and quantitation of analytes such as nucleic acids. The Rubpy label is a nonisotopic, low molecular weight metal chelate, with a stable shelf life of longer than one year. Labeling can be achieved via a convenient NHS ester chemistry,[11] although phosphoramidite labels[12] are available for automated oligonucleotide synthesis (Perkin Elmer, Norwalk, CT). Due to the low molecular mass of the label and its hydrophobicity, proteins and nucleic acids can be labeled without affecting their solubility or binding kinetics. DNA probe hybridizations are similarly unaffected.

DNA probe assays were performed in a rapid, one step, no wash format. The HIV-1 gag gene assay illustrated the wide dynamic range of the ECL system. The dynamic range was five orders of magnitude with a sensitivity of 10^7 molecules, in an assay which used 10^{12} molecules of probe. The sensitivity/range window can be shifted downward by reducing the concentration of probe used and increasing incubation time. The sensitivity and specificity of the ECL DNA probe assay for HIV-1 was excellent, having a detection limit as low as 10^5 molecules using a probe set of 10^{11} molecules.

Probe formats other than a no wash, one-step, sandwich hybridization can be accomplished using the ECL system. Assays in which biotin was incorporated into a polymerized DNA strand have been performed. This format was used to

295

assay the amplified product in a competitive PCR reaction for the quantitation of JC virus.

Quantitation of input copy number in a PCR reaction can be performed by a comparison with a standard curve.[6,13] This method, however, has some limitations. Most significantly, there is no internal standard for the PCR reaction condition in the test sample and quantitation is most accurately done in the linear portion of the standard curve. This may result in a three-order of magnitude linear dynamic range; if the signal of the test sample lies outside this region, quantitation may be inaccurate. These problems are obviated in competitive PCR. Quantitation can be done over the entire range of control samples and these control samples are contained within the PCR reactions of the test samples.

The control DNA for the competitive PCR was constructed by altering the detection probe site of the wild type DNA (PML). This was done by excising a segment which included the probe site and replacing it with a synthesized sequence of the excised segment read in reverse. This eliminated the wild type probe site and replaced it with a unique control probe site while maintaining the size and base composition of the segment to be amplified. This has the advantage of mitigating any differential amplification due to sequence or size of the target.[4,14] This scheme also enabled splitting the PCR material into two aliquots and then using two different probes.

PCR of the PML DNA in the competitive reaction did not result in very high signals in the PML samples that were at a higher concentration than the competing control This was probably due to inefficient amplification or a PCR reaction which did not reach saturation. This was not an impediment, however, to calculating the input copy number of the test sample. Four internal control DNA concentrations were used in these experiments; it would have been possible to use a greater number of controls for quantitation across a wider range. The ECL signal of the controls increased exponentially and intersected the plot of the test samples.

A calculation of the input copy number of the PML DNA, using the competitive PCR technique, resulted in a very good correlation between the standard curve and CPCR. Comparison of the two methods while good was not exact in all samples. These results were not unexpected, since the standard curve method uses standards from a separate PCR reaction, not internal controls, and quantitation of the inordinate sample was done in the plateau portion of the standard curve. Testing the CPCR method using a known copy number of test samples resulted in an almost exact return of the input copy number.

ECL is a technology which can be used for conducting assays in a variety of formats. Simple labeling protocols facilitate the use of this system. Key features of the ECL system are its sensitivity and wide dynamic range. These characteristics were particularly advantageous in the quantitation of input copy number by competitive PCR.

Acknowledgement

The authors would like to thank Dr. Carlo Tornatore for the PML DNA. John Link, Guy Johnson, and Linda Durham provided excellent technical assistance.

REFERENCES

1. G.F. Blackburn, H.P. Shah, J.H. Kenten, et al. Electrochemiluminescence detection for development of immunoassays and DNA-probe assays for clinical diagnostics. *Clin. Chem.* 37:1534 (1991).
2. E.O. Major, K. Amemiya, C.S. Tornatore, S.A. Houff, and J.R. Berger. Pathogenesis and molecular biology of progressive multifocal leukoencephalopathy, the JC virus-induced demyelinating disease of the human brain. *Clin. Microbiol. Rev.* 5:49 (1992).

3. C.Tornatore, J.R. Berger, S.A. Houff, et al. Detection of JC virus DNA in peripheral lymphocytes from patients with and without progressive multifocal leukoencephalopathy. *Ann. Neurol.* 31:454 (1992).

4. A.M. Wang, M.V. Doyle, and D.F. Mark. Quantitation of mRNA by the polymerase chain reaction. *Proc. Natl. Acad. Sci. USA* 86:9717 (1989). [Erratum,. 87:2865 (1990)]

5. B. van Gemen, T. Kievits, R. Schukkink, et al. Quantification of HIV-1 RNA in plasma using NASBA™ during HIV-1 primary infection. *J.Virol. Meth.* 43:177 (1993).

6. J. DiCesare, B. Grossman, E. Katz, et al. A high-sensitivity electrochemiluminescence-based detection system for automated PCR product quantitation. *BioTechniques* 15:152 (1993).

7. G. Gilliland, S. Perrin, K. Blanchard, and H.F. Bunn. Analysis of cytokine mRNA and DNA: detection and quantitation by competitive polymerase chain reaction. *Proc. Natl. Acad. Sci. USA* 87:2725 (1990).

8. P.D. Siebert, and J.W. Larrick. PCR Minics: competitive DNA fragments for use as internal standards in quantitative PCR. *BioTechniques* 14:244 (1993).

9. M. Piatak, Jr., K-C. Luk, B. Williams, and J.D. Lifson. Quantitative competitive polymerase chain reaction for accurate quantitation of HIV DNA and RNA species. *BioTechniques* 14:70 (1993).

10. R. Frisque, G. Bream, and M. Canulla. Human polyomavirus JC virus genome. *J. Virol.* 51:458 (1984).

11. J.H. Kenten, J. Casadei, S. Link, et al. Rapid electrochemiluminescence assays for polymerase chain reaction products. *Clin. Chem.* 37:1626 (1991).

12. J.H. Kenten, S. Gudibande, J. Link, J. Willey, and E. Major. An improved electrochemiluminescent label for DNA probe assays: rapid quantitative assays for HIV-1 polymerase chain reaction products. *Clin. Chem.* 38: 873 (1992).

13. J.M. Wages, L. Dolenga, and A.K. Fowler. Electrochemiluminescence detection and quantitation of PCR-amplified DNA. *Amplifications* (Perkin Elmer) 10:1 (1993).

14. R.W. Cone, A.C. Hobson, M.-L. W. Huang. Coamplified positive control detects inhibition of polymerase chain reactions. *J. Clin. Microbiol.* 30:3185 (1992).

DEVELOPMENT OF NEW TECHNIQUES AND METHODS APPLIED TO AIDS

TECHNIQUES IN PCR AND PCR EVALUATION TECHNOLOGY AND ITS APPLICATION TO THE STUDY OF CEREBROSPINAL FLUID IN HIV DISEASE

Peter Schmid, Andrew Conrad, Karl Syndulko, Elyse J. Singer, Ximing Li, Gongming Tao, Daniel Handley, Bridget Fahy-Chandon, and Wallace W. Tourtellotte

Neurology and Research Services
VA Medical Center West Los Angeles
Los Angeles, California 90073
Department of Neurology
University of California School of Medicine
Los Angeles, California 90024

INTRODUCTION

An early and substantial involvement of the central nervous system (CNS) in human immunodeficiency virus (HIV) disease became obvious quite soon after the onset of the AIDS epidemic.[1] Clinical classifications have since emerged,[2] and the pathological correlates have been described.[3] The direct presence of HIV in the brain in spite of the inability of the virus to pass the blood-brain barrier (BBB) was found and explained by mechanisms in which the virus intracellularly traverses the barrier, in particular through its capacity to infect macrophages.[4]

The harmful effects of HIV on the CNS are well documented and range from subtle cognitive or motor neuropsychological findings to the full blown HIV-1 associated cognitive/motor complex. While numerous theories have emerged to account for these CNS effects, the precise pathogenetic pathways have not yet been elucidated. The rare availability of direct tissue material for the study of molecular pathogenesis in the early stages of HIV CNS involvement and the need to conduct longitudinal studies make the cerebrospinal fluid (CSF) a logical choice to investigate viral activity and status in terms of the presence of proviral forms, intensity of cellular lysis, and titer of infective virions both in cellular and noncellular compartments of the CSF. In addition, a comparison of these aspects of viral activity between blood and CSF evaluated directly by quantitative assay of the molecular species representing the genetic material of HIV as it progresses through its life cycle, is likely to provide insight into any special role that the CNS might play through its immunoprivileged position in the overall and intricate mechanisms of pathogenesis, persistence, and resilient adaptation of HIV to the body's natural defense systems. Similarly, a realistic account of the quantitative presence of HIV in the CNS will be necessary to assess the potential limits of efficacy or immunotherapy schemes if the drug in question does not penetrate the BBB. In addition, through the relative ease with which the CSF can be obtained, quantitative studies of the proviral and free virion forms might provide critical markers of actual CNS involvement in a

Technical Advances in AIDS Research in the Human Nervous System
Edited by E.O. Major and J.A. Levy, Plenum Press, New York, 1995

301

particular patient and is likely to serve as a prognostic tool for HIV CNS disease, if such a correlation can indeed be shown.

From the foregoing, the importance of a molecular technique for the reliable quantitative assessment of HIV RNA and DNA forms is obvious, as is the need to conduct longitudinal studies on well-classified cohorts of HIV-positive patients whose neurologic status is routinely examined. The relatively small quantities of HIV nucleic acid materials present in blood and CSF require using an extremely sensitive technique. The polymerase chain reaction (PCR), in principle, can detect such small quantities of nucleic acids, and several methods to perform PCR quantitatively have been reported.[5,6] However, PCR is not a specific technique, but rather a wide range of methods that share the principle of cyclic enzymatic replication using thermostable polymerases. A critical integrative analysis of the fundamental aspects of biochemistry, thermocycling, and post-amplification analysis was performed as well as a study of the limitations and hidden possibilities that reside in the hardware. The following will cover some of the concepts and inventive results that have emerged as the results of an optimization development of this important methodology over several years. The last section will present some of the result in the investigation of HIV in the CSF and blood using those techniques and how these findings relate to the clinical disturbances in CNS function.

IMPROVING THE RELIABILITY OF QUANTITATIVE PCR

The exponential amplification of PCR is also the Achilles heel of PCR quantitation. Inconsistencies in any of the factors that determine the amplification efficiency per individual cycle will lead to an exponential amplification of the resulting tube-to-tube variation as well. This severely limits the use of external quantitative standards in the reaction, and prompted the development of QC-PCR that employs an internal standard in the same reaction vessel. In its most elaborate form for the quantitation of HIV RNA, a competitive standard is already used in the reverse transcription reaction, and the standard has the same length and sequence as the unknown, except for a single restriction site that is later cut to distinguish sample RNA from standard. Perfect cutting efficiency is a prerequisite for this method and due to the need for several standard tubes per sample, the method is very labor-intensive and costly.

An alternate way to address the problem is to identify the sources of tube-to-tube inconsistency and find novel ways to reduce them as much as possible. While inconsistencies resulting from the variable background nucleic acid content of the sample are difficult to reduce (but note below that hot start dramatically reduces these inconsistencies), all the other factors can be increased in precision. The first strategy is to reduce the impact of factor variations by reducing the amplification of errors, which can be mostly directly accomplished by reducing the PCR cycle number to a minimum. However, a decrease in PCR cycle number must be accompanied by a corresponding increase in the sensitivity of post-PCR detection. To underscore this point, a system has been offered that uses such ultrahigh specific activity probes that no PCR is used at all.[7] In taking a middle ground position, we believe that "low cycle number low wobble" PCR should be combined with the highest sensitivity and specificity detection method for the amplicon produced.

In comparing the various post-PCR detection methods, it is necessary to consider a number of factors inherent in PCR. Nonspecific background synthesis always exists, even if little or no primer dimer is produced. Therefore, global labelling of all synthesized products through labelled precursors or of all products whose synthesis is initiated from a labelled primer will lead to a high background. While stringent annealing conditions can reduce this background, the price for such high compensatory annealing stringency will be a lower per cycle efficiency with resulting magnification of errors through the need for higher cycle numbers. Fundamentally, electrophoresis of PCR products will have the effect of cleaning the amplicon from masking false synthesis products. Still, if one uses a high-sensitivity detection system, weak bands from very low-copy number PCR or from low-cycle number PCR could still be masked inside a smear of unwanted background synthesis. Those effects become very apparent once one leaves the classic 10 ng limit sensitivity of ETBr detection, for example, by using an end-detection system such as digoxigenin binding AB linked to alkaline phosphatase, which can detect 0.01 picogram of DNA on a membrane.

One solution to the problem of background synthesis is the use of product-specific high-activity probes that will ignore all but the specific amplicon band. All these measures increase sensitivity beyond the simple limit of the detection system for the PCR product, since they dramatically reduce background and thereby allow reliable quantitative readings of very small amounts of specific DNA. In turn, the number of cycles used to produce such a signal can be reduced.

A related method, oligomer liquid hybridization followed by gel separation, produces bands consisting of partly double-, partly single-stranded DNA. These bands are less sharp than those obtained in Southern blots, and since there is no transfer to a membrane, radioactive probes are needed for detection. After careful consideration, we found that the most sensitive and specific detection method for the amplification product is a combination of Southern blotting with product-specific probe hybridization. This conclusion was supported by direct comparative studies, where the Southern blot method has been shown to be 10,000 times more sensitive than standard gel detection.[8]

Despite these inherent qualifications, the Southern blot-probe detection method of PCR evaluation is typically only used on very limited research samples where only a few PCR runs need to be evaluated. Large numbers of specimens simply cannot be conveniently processed using existing Southern blot technology,[9] since these procedures require many time-consuming steps and skilled personnel are needed to perform these techniques. If the procedure is not optimized, it is likely to fail catastrophically.

In response to this situation, one author (P.S.) has contributed long-term efforts to make the benefits of PCR and Southern blots available to process a very high number of specimens. This was possible through the development of several rather complex, robotic instruments that permit completely operator-independent performance of this procedure from gel electrophoresis to the visualization of bands on the membrane. The system whose technical details cannot be presented in the scope of this chapter, currently provides a maximum capacity of 840 PCR reactions per automated run and a total processing time of approximately 24 hours. One picogram of amplified PCR product can be clearly detected. A further important aspect of such an automatic system is the capacity to optimize several conditions; for example, the concentrations of the various reagents in a PCR reaction, electrophoresis, chemical gel treatment, transfer, hybridization and wash stringencies.

In addition, in any manual set-up for the pipetting, mixing, and incubation steps that need to be done in the pre-PCR phase of the procedure, it is almost impossible to avoid uneven treatment of the different samples. Therefore, the important aspect of uniformity in sample preparation and treatment is further enhanced through the use of automatic processing machines, where samples are placed in a circular fashion on a large centrifuge rotor and reagent addition is done by automatic pipetters that are built into these machines and controlled by a computerized program. The rotor arrangement allows for homogeneous mixing by rapid inversions of rotor direction and reliable collection of small amounts of added reagents or condensation after incubations at high temperatures. Incubations at the various temperatures for the reverse transcription reaction are also done in these computer-controlled processors.

Beyond the advantages of high sensitivity end-product detection that help to reduce the number of required amplification cycles, we also attempted to further improve the sample-to-sample precision that is so critical for the use of quantitative PCR by using external standard. After optimization of the biochemical aspect of the amplification reaction through proper primer selection, magnesium concentration, and determination of optimum annealing temperatures, sample-to-sample variation other than the one inherent to the starting material itself, is mainly caused by trivial factors like pipetting inaccuracy, incomplete evenness of master mixes and reaction assemblies, and most importantly, by variations in the thermoprofile between individual tubes as well as the precision of the thermoprofiles. The surprisingly short subcycle times required by "air cyclers" that use the low thermal conductance medium air, alerted us to the fact that heat transfer is not only dependent on latent heat of the transfer medium, but also on the local speed of the transfer medium to overcome the "skin effect" that tends to isolate a tube thermally. While encountering substantial technical difficulties, the logical answer to maximum speed plus uniformity in thermocycling is the rapid direct rotary dipping of thin-walled sample tubes into intensely stirred and precisely thermoregulated, segmentally arranged water baths. This arrangement virtually eliminates any differences in thermal exposure between samples. This uniformity is in marked contrast to thermocyclers which heat metal blocks.

Hot Start Procedure

The hot start procedure results in substantial improvement of amplification efficiency of low-copy number targets. It reduces the influence of varying amounts of background DNA on cycle efficiency that results from the initially occurring false binding of primers at temperatures below the annealing point. This enhances overall sensitivity, and sample-to-sample variation resulting from background DNA is reduced. Technically, it requires the initiation of amplification/polymerization at temperatures clearly above the annealing temperatures for the given primer pair. Traditionally, hot starting is done by adding a wax bead to each tube which, while still in the clean pre-PCR environment, is molten and solidifies as a septum above which further essential components of the polymerization reaction are placed. Inside the thermocycler, the wax septum melts again and floats to the top, thereby generating a synthesis-competent mix. Aside from being cumbersome, the biggest problem is the slow and unpredictable mixing of the two phases. In our system, the hot start procedure is performed in a special machine that becomes an integral part of the thermocycling system and allows the simultaneous heating of the lower part of the sealed tubes containing the PCR mix minus an essential component for the polymerization reaction, that is later introduced simultaneously from a reservoir inside the sealed tubes. This provides for even mixing at the high temperature (approximately 80°C) after all the reaction components are assembled and thermocycling starts immediately. This elimination of tube-to-tube variation in hot starting is essential to harness the strong potential of this method for quantitative PCR.

Densitometric Evaluation of Band Intensity Development Over Time

Probe-bound alkaline phosphatase catalyzes the formation of insoluble dye polymers from NPT/X-phosphate precursors at the locations of bands on the membrane. For a given set of standards, some are below and some are above an intensity that it useful for quantitation. Therefore, to use each standard in its optimum range, the Southern blot membrane is scanned at intervals during colorimetric dye development to help ascertain the time point at which the derived standard curve is most linear. Each membrane contains quantity standards of post-PCR material generated from serial dilutions of a known copy number (1, 10, 100, 1,000 and sometimes 10,000 copies) of cloned pBR322 containing the HIV-1 *gag* sequence (Perkin-Elmer). The blots are scanned at 300 dpi, 256-level gray scale, 100% size using a Microtek 300 GZ flatbed scanner in conjunction with Adobe Photoshop™ software. An image processing program (Image version 1.47 written by Wayne Rasband, N.I.H.) is then used to manually identify and outline bands (image particles) and quantify band area and mean band density. The product of band area and mean density provides a reliable indication of the amount of "blackness" present in a band, and is used in conjunction with the derived standard curve on the same membrane to obtain a numerical value of RNA or DNA viral copy number for each band.

Application of Automated Quantitative PCR for the Study of HIV Neurologic Disease

Several recent papers have attempted using quantitative PCR to measure proviral load in blood, brain tissue, and CSF with relatively small numbers of subjects.[10-13] The methods for PCR quantitation vary in these papers from simple visual comparisons to the complex and labor-intensive quantitative competitive PCR.[14-16] We initially attempted to quantify the number of HIV-1 proviral copies per 1,000 CD4+ cells in CSF and blood in relationship to the stage of infection and HIV-1 neurologic disease (HND) in order to find prognostic indicators of HIV disease progression. A related purpose was to provide direct evidence of the presence of HIV-1 in the CNS *in vivo*, as suggested by recent findings.[17-19]

Cohort Study Subjects

Eighty-seven HIV-1 seropositive males without CNS opportunistic infections, tumors or neurosyphilis, and 9 high-risk seronegative controls underwent a structured interview, as well as physical and neurologic examination followed by blood and CSF collection. Laboratory tests confirmed that the subjects were free of CNS opportunistic infections, tumors, and neurosyphilis; blood and CSF were collected in a standardized fashion and nucleic acids were extracted immediately. The blood and/or CSF of 14 (DNA studies) and 18(RNA studies) not-at-risk seronegative controls were obtained from the National Neurological Research Specimen Bank (NNRSB).[20]

At the time of the examination, seropositive subjects were classified into three groups based on the infectious disease questionnaire and the physical examination. Asymptomatic seropositive (ASP) subjects were defined as HIV-1 antibody seropositive patients (with or without lymphadenopathy) with no opportunistic infections or other systemic manifestations of HIV-1. The category corresponds roughly to the Centers for Disease Control (CDC) Groups II and III,[21] which was in effect at the time this study was initiated. AIDS-related complex (ARC) was defined by the presence of one or more of the following: oral candida; oral hairy leukoplakia; herpes zoster in the past 3 years; chronic intermittent diarrhea of at least one-month duration with at least 3 liquid stools/day by work-up without definable cause; weight loss in the past 3 years of at least 10 pounds or 10% of the body weight, without a definable cause; drenching whole-body night sweats on at least 3 occasions in the previous 3 months; recorded temperatures of at least 100°F for at least one month; chronic fatigue which interferred with normal activity at least twice weekly for the past 6 months; and recurrent seborrheic dermatitis or tropical pruritic folliculitis. This category is more inclusive than the CDC groups IVa and IVc2.[21] AIDS was defined as follows: medically documented episodes of *Pneumocystis carinii* pneumonia, extraintestinal strongyloidosis, isopsoriasis, esophageal or bronchial candidiasis; *Mycobacterium avium intracellulaire* or *M. kansasii* infection; chronic, mucocutaneous herpes simplex or disseminated herpes simplex; cytomegalovirus infection (nonneurologic); or other infections listed by the CDC as AIDS-defining infections, but not involving the CNS; biopsy-documented Kaposi's sarcoma, lymphoma or other syndromes such as chronic lymphoid interstitial pneumonitis, or wasting syndrome. We did not use CD4 cell counts or "HIV-1 encephalopathy" as an AIDS-defining diagnosis. This category corresponded roughly to the CDC group IV, except it does not include CDC groups IVa or IVb.[21]

On the basis of history and neurologic examination subjects were categorized neurologically as follows: neurologically negative (NeuroNeg), which was defined as the absence of HIV-1-related neurologic signs and symptoms; and neurologically positive (NeuroPos), which was defined as the documented presence of HIV-1-related neurologic signs and symptoms. Neurologic disease unrelated to HIV-1 was not used to define either of these categories. HIV-1-related HND was subclassified as cognitive, CNS motor (weakness, spasticity, incoordination, movement disorder) or peripheral neuropathy. Behavioral abnormalities (e.g., depression) were evaluated, but did not contribute to a diagnosis of NeuroPos. The severity grading system (mild, moderate and severe) for HND was adapted from the AIDS Treatment Evaluation Unit clinical trial number 005 protocol.[22]

Lumbar puncture (LP) was performed in a standardized fashion and CSF (25 cc) was collected into a 30-ml syringe. An aliquot was taken for cell counts, and the remaining fluid was centrifuged to concentrate the cells. Routine clinical CSF testing included white and red blood cell (RBC) counts, glucose, total protein ,and VDRL. Cultures, cytology and serologies were ordered when clinically indicated. Because of the sensitivity of the PCR reaction, any blood introduced into the CSF specimen because of LP-induced trauma could falsely promote positive HIV findings in the CSF. Therefore, only LPs with RBC counts less than 30 cells/mm3 were used for PCR analyses.

Negative controls for blood and CSF consisted of 9 seronegatives at high risk for HIV-1 infection, of whom 5 had concurrent CSF and blood collections, and 14 paired blood/CSF seronegative control specimens with no known risk for HIV infection were obtained from the NNRSB.

Proviral DNA Load Calculations

Proviral loads were calculated using the following formulae that were based on the findings of many investigators that the overwhelming cell type infected in the blood is the CD4+ cell.[23-26] Flow cytometric analysis was also used on selected CSF samples to confirm the notion that the percentage of CD4+ cells in the CSF cells is close to the CD4+ percentage of peripheral blood mononuclear cells.

Number of blood CD4+ cells added to each PCR reaction =
(CD4+ cells in blood[a]/mm3) (ml whole blood[b]) (1,000 mm3/ml) (0.68[c])
(0.05 fraction added)[d]

Number of CSF CD4+ cells added to each PCR reaction =
(CD4+ cells in CSF[e]/mm3) (ml CSF[f]) (1,000 mm3/ml) (0.125 fraction added[d])

where:

[a]Determined by flow cytometry.[27]
[b]Blood used ranged from 4-7 ml, mean ± 1 SD = 4.5 ± 0.3 ml.
[c]Peripheral blood mononuclear cell recovery is on average $68 \pm 13\%$ with the Ficoll-Hypaque kit (Sigma) used.
[d]Volume fraction of nucleic acid preparation used for each PCR reaction.
[e]Since we did not determine directly the number of CD4+ cells in the CSF, this number was estimated by multiplying the measured number of CSF mononuclear cells by the CD4+ cell concentration in the blood, i.e.:

(CSF mononuclear cells/mm3) $\left(\dfrac{CD4+ \text{ cells in blood/mm3}}{\text{blood lymphocytes/mm3}}\right)$ based on the finding

that the CD4+ cell concentrations in blood and CSF were essentially the same.[28,29]
[f]CSF used ranged from 8-22 ml, mean ± 1 SD = 18.0 ± 4.0 ml.

The number of HIV-1 proviral DNA copies determined by band image analysis for the respective blood or CSF specimen were then divided by the numbers of CD4+ cells calculated from these formulae. This ratio was then multiplied by 1,000 to yield the number of copies per 1,000 CD4+ cells.

RESULTS

All seropositive subjects were ambulatory and living in the community. The demographic, functional and laboratory profiles are presented in Tables 1-3.

Table 1. Demographic profile of HIV-1 high-risk seronegative and seropositive individuals.

	HIV-1 Seronegative (n=9)	HIV-1 Seropositive (n=87)	P-VALUE
Age (years)	41.1 ± 8.6†	38.7 ± 8.6	.4452*
Risk Factor (percent of cases)			
Homosexual or Bisexual	89%	90%	
Homosexual or Bisexual & IV Drug Use	11%	10%	
Source (percent of cases)			
Clinic or Physician Referrals	0	20%	
Community self-referrals through advertisements	100%	80%	

† mean ± one standard deviation
* p-value, probability level from t-test comparing HIV-1 seropositive and seronegative subjects

Table 2. Disability status of seropositive individuals.

Disability Variable	HIV-1 Systemic Disease Stage			HIV-1 Neurologic Disease	
	ASP	ARC	AIDS	Neuro Neg	Neuro Pos
Functional	n=34	n=46	n=7	n=60	n=27
Work Status - % of cases (#)					
Working full time	97% (33)	61% (28)	14% (7)	88% (53)	33% (9)
Working part time	0%	9% (4)	14% (1)	2% (1)	15% (4)
Unemployed / Unable to Work	3% (1)	30% (14)	71% (5)	10% (6)	52% (14)
Karnofsky Index of Performance % of cases (#)					
100% of Normal Functioning	82% (28)	35% (16)	14% (1)	68% (41)	15% (4)
90%	12% (4)	20% (9)	0% (0)	15% (9)	15% (4)
80%	6% (2)	24% (11)	14% (1)	12% (7)	26% (7)
50, 60 or 70%	0% (0)	22% (10)	71% (5)	5% (3)	44% (12)
Neurologic Disease % of cases (number)					
None	91% (31)	61% (28)	14% (1)	100% (60)	0% (0)
Mild	6% (2)	15% (7)	14% (1)	0% (0)	37% (10)
Moderate	3% (1)	24% (17)	71% (5)	0% (0)	63% (17)
Severe	0% (0)	0% (0)	0% (0)	0% (0)	0% (0)
Anti-retroviral Treatment % of cases (#)					
None	62% (21)	20% (9)	0% (0)	47% (28)	22% (6)
Treated at time of examination	38% (13)	80% (37)	100% (9)	53% (32)	78% (21)

Table 3. Laboratory parameters in HIV-1 seropositive individuals.

Lab Parameter	HIV-1 Systemic Disease Stage			HIV-1 Neurologic Disease	
	ASP	ARC	AIDS	Neuro Neg	Neuro Pos
BLOOD	n=34	n=46	n=7	n=60	n=27
$CD4^+$ cell count (cells/mm^3)	637±260	428 ±275	137 ±139	581 ± 268	275 ± 244
% (#) <200 $CD4^+$ cells/mm^3	6% (2)	17% (8)	57% (4)	7% (4)	37% (10)
200-499 $CD4^+$ cells/mm^3	21% (7)	43% (20)	43% (3)	33% (20)	37% (10)
≥ 500 $CD4^+$ cells/mm^3	73% (25)	39% (18)	0 %	60% (36)	26% (7)
$CD4^+ : CD8^+$ ratio	.65 ± .34	.4 ± .27	.15 ± .1	.59 ± .32	.24 ± .16
CSF	n=28	n=33	n=6	n=47	n=20
Leukocyte count (cells/mm^3)	4.1 ± 5.6	2.8 ± 3.0	2.5 ± 4.7	3.7 ± 4.7	2.5 ± 3.3
% leukocytes ≥ 5 cells/mm^3	18% (5)	15% (5)	17% (1)	19% (9)	10% (2)
Trans-Blood-Brain-Barrier Albumin Leakage (AL) Rate (mg/day)	21.2 ± 31.8	44.8 ± 52.5	26.7 ± 31.6	21.4 ± 28.5	61.2 ± 60.7
% (#) abnormal AL Rate≥75 mg/day	7% (2)	21% (7)	0%	2% (1)	40% (8)
Intrathecal IgG Synthesis					
By Rate Formula (mg/day)	10.2 ±12	22.8 ± 27	12.4 ±9.3	13.6±16.4	23.6±29.2
By Oligoclonal Bands (OB,#)	1.9 ± 2.8	2.2 ± 2.2	2.5 ± 1.8	2.0 ± 2.6	2.2 ± 2.0
% (#) abnormal by rate formula ≥ 3.3 mg/day	50% (14)	70% (23)	67% (4)	60% (28)	65% (13)
% (#) abnormal by OB ≥ 1 band	50% (14)	67% (22)	83% (5)	55% (26)	75% (15)
% (#) abnormal by rate formula ≥ 6 mg/day or OB ≥ 1 band	68% (19)	85% (28)	100% (6)	74% (35)	90% (18)

◊ Mean±1 standard deviation

Table 4 shows results for the detection of HIV-1 provirus in blood CD4+ cells. Ninety-three percent of the HIV-1 seropositives had positive PCRs for HIV-1 provirus detection (Table 4A). There were no significant differences in frequency of positive PCRs among either the systemic or neurologic subgroups (Table 4B). A single HIV-1 seronegative high-risk control showed a positive PCR, and this result was confirmed on a subsequent sample, although the subject's ELISA and Western blot remained negative. None of the 14 no known risk controls showed a positive PCR.

Table 5 indicates the detection rate of HIV-1 provirus in CSF cells. Ninety percent of the HIV-1 seropositives were PCR-positive (Table 5A). Two high-risk seronegative controls showed a positive PCR and one of these cases also showed PCR-positive blood. These findings were confirmed on the next CSF sample for each subject. There were no significant differences in frequency of positive PCRs among either the systemic or neurologic subgroups (Table 5B). None of the 14 no known risk controls were PCR positive.

Table 4A. Frequency of HIV-1 proviral detection by PCR in blood CD4+ cells in HIV-1 seronegative and seropositive individuals.

| PCR Result | HIV-1 Seronegative | | HIV-1 Seropositive n=87 |
	No-known risk factors n=14	High Risk n=9	
Negative	100% (14/14)	89% (8/9)	7% (6/87)
Positive	0% (0/14)	11% (1/9)	93% (81/87)

Table 4B. Frequency of HIV-1 provirus detected by PCR in blood CD4+ cells in clinically classified HIV-1 seropositive individuals.

| PCR Results | HIV-1 Systemic Disease Stage | | | HIV-1 Neurologic Disease | |
	ASP	ARC	AIDS	NeuroNeg	NeuroPos
Negative	12% (4/34)	4% (2/46)	0% (0/7)	10% (6/60)	0% (0/27)
Positive	88% (30/34)	96% (44/46)	100% (7/7)	90% (54/60)	100% (27/27)
	p=0.3265, Chi-Square=2.24			p=.2129, Chi-Square=1.55	

Table 5A. Frequency of HIV-1 provirus detection by PCR in CSF CD4+ cells in HIV-1 seronegative and seropositive individuals.

| PCR Result | HIV-1 Seronegative | | HIV-1 Seropositive |
	No-known risk factors	High Risk	
Negative	100% (14/14)	60% (3/5)	10% (6/63)
Positive	0% (0/14)	40% (2/5)	90% (57/63)

Table 5B. Frequency of HIV-1 provirus detection by PCR in CSF CD4+ cells in clinically classified HIV-1 seropositive individuals.

| PCR Results | HIV-1 Systemic Disease Stage | | | HIV-1 Neurologic Disease | |
	ASP	ARC	AIDS	NeuroNeg	NeuroPos
Negative	15% (4/26)	3% (1/31)	17% (1/6)	10% (4/42)	10% (2/21)
Positive	85% (22/26)	97% (30/31)	83% (5/6)	90% (38/42)	90% (19/21)
	p=0.2423, Chi-Square=2.82			p=.6489, Chi-Square=0.21	

The proviral DNA loads for blood and CSF cells from subjects who had both CSF and blood specimens at the same visit are presented in Table 6. In blood CD4+ cells, the median number of proviral copies/1,000 cells for all seropositive subjects was 0.6; whereas, in CSF the median number was 25. The CSF proviral load was significantly greater than that for blood over all seropositive subjects (p = 0.0001). Proviral load also varied as a function of HIV-1 disease status. For blood CD4+ cells, the number of proviral copies/1,000 cells was significantly different among ASP, ARC and AIDS subgroups, with proviral load lowest for ASP (0.09 copies/1,000 cells), higher for ARC (1.4 copies/1,000 cells) and highest for AIDS (10.7 copies/1,000 cells). Similarly, the proviral load in blood CD4+ cells was significantly greater in NeuroPos than in NeuroNeg individuals. For CSF cells, there was a trend for proviral load to be greater in NeuroPos (43.5 copies/1,000 cells) than in NeuroNeg (17.6 copies/1,000 cells) individuals. In addition, CSF proviral load differed significantly as a function of HIV-1 systemic disease status, against lowest in ASP and highest in AIDS (p = 0.0316). The effects of anti-retroviral therapy could not be adequately evaluated because this comparison was confounded by the fact that the subjects on treatment had significantly lower mean CD4+ cell counts than those not on treatment (p = 0.0001); that is, subjects on treatment generally had more advanced HIV-1 disease than those not on treatment.

Table 6. HIV-1 proviral DNA load[†] in blood and CSF CD4+ cells from HIV-1 seropositive individuals with concurrent CSF and blood samples.

GROUP		Blood	CSF	P-Value
All Seropositives (n=63)	median	0.6	25	.0001*
	inter-quartile range	0.04 - 4.0	2.4 - 144	
Asymptomatic seropositive (ASP)(n=26)				
	median	0.09	10.5	
	inter-quartile range	0.01 - 1.1	0.32 - 53	
ARC (n=31)	median	1.4	54	
	inter-quartile range	0.17 - 11.5	12.5 - 206	
AIDS (n=6)	median	10.7	155	
	inter-quartile range	0.04 - 54	5.6 - 1160	
ASP vs. ARC vs. AIDS		p=0.0281**	p=0.0316**	
NeuroNegative (n=42)	median	0.4	17.6	
	inter-quartile range	0.02 - 2.5	1.2 - 95	
NeuroPositive (n=21)	median	1.6	43.5	
	inter-quartile range	0.1 - 21.2	12.2 - 747	
NeuroNegative vs. NeuroPositive		p=0.0357***	p=0.0614***	

* Wilcoxon Signed-Rank Test; **Kruskal-Wallis H corrected for ties;
***Mann-Whitney U

[†] copies per 1000 CD4+ cells

The frequency of HIV-1 RNA detection in serum (at 40 cycles of PCR amplification) was 93% (62/67) for al seropositive subjects (Table 7A) and did not vary significantly with HIV-1 disease status or the presence of neurologic disease (Table 7B). Table 8 shows that HIV-1 RNA was significantly related to CD4+ cell count. The RNA values were highest in seropositive subjects with counts less than 200 cells/mm3 and lowest in those with counts at or above 500 cells/mm3. The RNA detection frequency was less in CSF than in serum, but the CSF data are still being evaluated. Preliminary quantitative evaluation of CSF RNA suggests lower amounts than in the serum.

Table 7A. Frequency of HIV-1 RNA detection by PCR in serum of HIV-1 seronegative and seropositive individuals.

PCR Result	HIV-1 Seronegative Low Risk n=18	HIV-1 Seronegative High Risk n=6	HIV-1 Seropositive All Stages n=67
Negative	100% (18/18)	83% (5/6)	7% (5/67)
Positive	0% (0/18)	17% (1/6)	93% (62/67)

Table 7B. Frequency of HIV-1 RNA detection in serum of clinically classified HIV-1 seropositive individuals.

PCR Results	HIV-1 Systemic Disease Stage			HIV-1 Neurologic Disease	
	ASP	ARC	AIDS	NeuroNeg	NeuroPos
Negative	8% (2/25)	8% (3/36)	0% (0/0)	10% (5/44)	0% (0/18)
Positive	92% (23/25)	92% (33/36)	100% (6/6)	90% (44/49)	100%(18/18)
	p=0.766, Chi-Square=0.53			p=3.35, Chi-Square=0.341	

Table 8. HIV-1 RNA in serum from HIV-1 seropositive individuals: relationship to CD4+ cell counts.

GROUP	Serum RNA*
CD4+ cell count 0-199 cells/mm3 (n=11)	100,000
200-499 cells/mm3 (n=23)	53,000
≥ 500 cells/mm3 (n=31)	12,000

Comparison among CD4+ cell groups, p=0.0041

* Median copies per ml

DISCUSSION

PCR Blood Results

We found that 94% of the HIV-1 seropositive blood specimens were PCR-positive using two HIV-1 *gag* region primers and that the detection frequency was not related to either systemic or neurologic disease status. The overall detection frequency is similar to that reported for peripheral blood mononuclear cells in other HIV studies.[30-35]

The quantified proviral DNA data suggest that the level of HIV-1 infection in blood CD4+ cells is highly variable, but related to disease status. The absolute proviral load values reported here are similar to those reported elsewhere, and also confirm that the highest levels of infection occur in subjects with more advanced HIV-1 disease.[10,26,33,36] These data indicate that in the later stages of HIV-1 infection, the relative proviral load in blood CD4+ cells increases substantially and may be the basis for the rapid decline of CD4+ cells seen in these patients.[35]

PCR CSF Findings

A few investigators have extended PCR detection of HIV to the CSF and compared directly the results in blood and CSF.[17,18,37] If we discount the patients with opportunistic infections and CNS lymphoma, Shaunak and colleagues[17] had a positive HIV-1 PCR detection rate of only 60% (9/15). In contrast, we report here a detection rate of 90% (19/21) in the subgroup who were NeuroPos and without opportunistic infection, tumor, or neurosyphilis. Likewise, we also report a higher detection rate in subjects without neurologic findings (38/42, or 90%) than did Shaunak et al. (1/7, or 14%).[17] The differences in detec-tion rates between our CSF findings and those of Shaunak and colleagues may stem from methodologic or sensitivity issues. Further support for this explanation and our results can be found in a paper by Sönnerberg and colleagues[18] who performed a series of experiments which most closely parallel our work on PCR detection of HIV in CSF; however, they did not quantitate the PCR results. They performed PCR on 28 seropositive patients, 24 of whom showed no neurologic signs, and reported a PCR detection rate of 86% in the CSF.

In the only other paper dealing with proviral load in CSF, Steuler et al. report amounts of virus in the CSF similar to those we report here.[37] In contrast to our results, they reported that the HIV-1 proviral load in CSF cells did not correlate with CDC disease stage. However, 7 of their 13 patients had a CNS opportunistic infection. Additionally, Steuler and colleagues used a different form of proviral quantitation than we employed so results are not directly comparable. However, their results provide some corroborating evidence that the level of HIV-1 provirus in the CSF cells is higher per cell than that reported in peripheral blood.

What Is the Source of HIV-1 Proviral DNA in CSF Cells?

There is sparse knowledge regarding the source and migration of lymphocytes and monocytes in the brain and CSF. While it is generally accepted that HIV is initially introduced into the CNS intracellularly aboard infected monocytes, its further mode of propagation inside the CNS is unknown. Although others have not observed virus-expressing lymphocytes within the HIV-infected brain, our data indicate that at least a substantial portion of the cells in the CSF are indeed carrying the HIV proviral genome.

We find a frequency of infection of CSF cells almost equal to that in blood. Autopsy studies have shown the presence of HIV DNA determined by PCR in all cases with evidence of encephalitis and similarly, Pang and colleagues[12] found HIV proviral DNA in 90% of all cases with postmortem evidence of HIV encephalitis. In a case of severe accidental inoculation with HIV, the virus was detectable in the brain after 15 days with no signs of encephalitis. Additionally, Masliah and colleagues found that although only 16% of the cases they examined showed histologic signs of HIV-1 encephalitis, up to 50% had moderate to severe HIV-1 infection.[38] Golswami and colleagues using HIV RNA PCR found 23 of 24 patients with neurodisease were HIV RNA positive in the CSF, but not 4 of 20 asymptomatic patients. These conflicting results are likely to be caused by a variation in the sensitivity of the PCR assay that was actually used.

In an attempt to explain the surprisingly high frequency of proviral DNA per CSF cell, it seems likely that of the variety of mechanisms that have been shown or are suspected to reduce the number of infected (and uninfected) CD4+ cells in peripheral blood via immunoreactive means most will be less rigorously effective in eliminating cells in the CSF, where the infection can spread more readily among the few available CD4+ cells. In addition, the brain might act as a continuous extravascular source of HIV. More esoteric possibilities include that there is some unknown selection method that concentrates infected cells from blood in the CSF, and that this mechanism accounts for the disproportionate level of proviral infected cells in the CSF. Another notion is that there is some permissive factor which allows HIV-1 to replicate more readily in the CSF than in blood.

The studies of Gendelman et al.[4], as well as others, localize HIV-1 in brain microglia and macrophages, where they appear to thrive as suggested by electron micrographs that show budding virions. Pathologic studies indicate that deep brain regions are frequently the site of intense HIV encephalitis, and that these regions are in turn characterized by the presence of multinucleated giant cells.[39,40] Accordingly, it is possible that there may be exfoliation of HIV-1 laden monocytes (histiocytes) into the ventricular CSF,[41] an extension of the extracellular space of the brain, from deep brain regions. This hypothesized movement from infected brain to CSF may account for the higher CSF proviral load when compared to blood. This concept is supported by our data that higher levels of HIV-1 provirus in the CSF were associated with the presence of clinical neurologic disease. Another hypothesis is that there may be an unknown selection method in the choroid plexus, the main source of CSF. In this view, the choroid plexus preferentially sequesters HIV-1-infected blood CD4+ cells and passes them into the CSF. To our knowledge, nobody has done a systematic histopathological study of the choroid plexus in HIV-1 brain to check for pathology.

Another notion is that infected CSF cells release virions which in turn infect over CD4+ cells. This reinfection may be facilitated in the CSF because of a higher concentration to activate T cells[42] and less rigorous immune surveillance.

SIGNIFICANCE

Determinations of proviral DNA load and replicative activity by HIV RNA PCR could serve as useful prognostic tools for CNS involvement of HIV disease in individual patients. Our findings further support the theory that an important aspect of HIV chronicity could be the continuous shedding of virus from the immunoprivileged CNS/CSF into the main circulation. A related notion is that the virus uses the CNS/CSF as a breeding ground for variants that are resistant against the body's natural defenses. Under this hypothesis, these variants would not have had the necessary time to develop in the immunoactive area of the body. It is known that the initial immune response against HIV is strong and effective. If a significant amount of virus is produced in the CNS/CSF then the continuous backflow through the natural exit of the CSF, the arachnoid villus, at 500 ml per day, could amount to a very substantial source of reinfection from an unattackable reservoir. Similar considerations apply to the use of initially effective drugs that are excluded from the CNS.

CSF is an easily obtainable fluid. In ongoing and future clinical therapeutic trials, where direct measurement of level of free virions in blood using quantitative HIV RNA PCR will soon be used widely, it might be important to determine the CSF viral load in collateral measurements. This will likely be a good indicator of the response of the brain infection to the therapy. If a tested drug does not pass the blood-brain barrier or is not effective inside the CNS, resistant variants will have a chance to form within this protected space and eventually reinfect the body.

ACKNOWLEDGMENTS

We express special appreciation to Peter Ruane, M.D. and Paul Singer, M.D. for assistance in recruitment and clinical classification of subjects; Carol Silbar, R.N., John Zhang, Ph.D., and Julie Kim, B.A., for their efforts in coordinating the HIV-1 project; Dan Stokes and Eugene Chiang, B.A., for laboratory analyses of CSF; Iris Rosario, R.N., for her coordination of the staff and activities of the NNRSB; and Giane Guntrip, Deborah Kovac, Diane Varnas, and Gerald Synder for admnistrative assistance.

REFERENCES

1. B.A. Navia, B.D. Jordan, and R.W. Price. The AIDS dementia complex. I. Clinical features. *Ann. Neurol.* 19:517 (1986).
2. American Academy of Neurology: Nomenclature and research case definitions for neurologic manifestations of human immunodeficiency virus type 1 (HIV-1) infection. Report of a Working Group of the American Academy of Neurology AIDS Task Force. *Neurology* 41:778 (1991).
3. L.R. Sharer. Pathology of HIV-1 infection of the central nervous system. A review. *J. Neuropath. Exp. Neurol.* 51:3 (1992).
4. H.E. Gendelman, J.M. Orenstein, L.M. Baca, et al. The macrophage in the persistence and pathogenesis of HIV infection. *AIDS* 3:375 (1989).
5. A. Rolfs, I. Schuller, U. Finckh, and I. Weber-Rolfs. PCR: Clinical Diagnostics and Research. Springer-Verlag, New York (1992).
6. F. Ferre. Quantitative or semiquantitative PCR: reality versus myth. *PCR Methods and Applications* 1:21 (1992).
7. J.G. Wetmur. DNA probes, applications of the principles of nucleic acid hybridization. *Crit. Rev. Biochem. Mol. Biol.* 26:227 (1991).
8. S. Kaneko, R.H. Miller, S.M. Feinstone, et al. Detection of serum hepatitis B virus DNA in patients with chronic hepatitis using the polymerase chain reaction assay. *Proc. Natl. Acad. Sci. USA* 86:312 (1989).
9. S. Kaneko, M.S. Feinstone, and r.h. Miller. Rapid and sensitive method for the detection of serum hepatitis B virus using the polymerase chain reaction technique. *J. Clin. Microbiol.* 27:1933 (1989).
10. M.T. Schechter, P.W. Neumann, M.S. Weaver, et al. Low HIV-1 proviral DNA burden detected by negative polymerase chain reaction in seropositive individuals correlates with slower disease progression. *AIDS* 5:373 (1991).
11. E. Stoeckl, N. Barrett, F.X. Heinz, et al. Efficiency of the polymerase chain reaction for the detection of human immunodeficiency virus type 1 (HIV-1) DNA in the lymphocytes of infected persons: comparison of antigen-enzyme-linked immunosorbent assay and virus isolation. *J. Med. Virol.* 29:249 (1989).
12. S. Pang, Y. Koyangi, S. Miles, et al. High levels of unintegrated HIV-1 DNA in brain tissue of AIDS dementia patients. *Nature* 343:85 (1990).
13. L.E. Davis, B.L. Hjelle, V.E. Miller, et al. Early viral brain invasion in iatrogenic human immunodeficiency virus infection. *Neurology* 42:1736 (1992).
14. M. Stieger, C. Démollière, L. Ahlborn-Laake, and J. Mous. Competitive polymerase chain reaction assay for quantitation of HIV-1 DNA and RNA. *J. Virol. Meth.* 34:149 (1991).
15. A. Teleni, P. Imboden, and D. Germann. Competitive polymerase chain reaction using an internal standard: application to the quantitation of viral DNA. *J. Virol. Meth.* 39:259 (1992).
16. M.J. Piatak, K.C. Luk, B. Williams, and J.D. Lifson. Quantitative competi-

tive polymerase chain reaction for accurate quantitation of HIV DNA and RNA species. *Biotechniques* 14:70 (1993).

17. S. Shaunak, R.E. Albright, M.E. Klotman, et al. Amplification of HIV-1 provirus form cerebrospinal fluid and its correlation with neurologic disease. *J. Infect. Dis.* 161:1068 (1990).

18. A.B. Sönnerborg, B. Johansson, and O,. Strannegard. Detection of HIV-1 DNA and infectious virus in cerebrospinal fluid. *AIDS Res. Human Retroviruses* 7:369 (1991).

19. H. Steuler, B. Storch-Haglenlocher, and B.Wildemann., Distinct populations of human immunodeficiency virus type 1 in blood and cerebrospinal fluid. *AIDS Res. Human Retroviruses* 8'53 (1992).

20. W.W. Tourtellotte and K. Bermann. Brain Banking. Birkhauser, Boston (1987).

21. Centers for Disease Control: Revision of the CDC surveillance case definition for acquired immunodeficiency syndrome. *Morbid. Mortal. Wkly. Rep.* 36 (Suppl. 15):1s (1987).

22. National Institute of Allergy and Infectious Diseases ATEU: A multicenter placebo-controlled, double-blind trial to evaluate treatment of the AIDS dementia complex and central nervous system in HIV infection (ATEU 005) (1987).

23. D. Klatzman, F. Brun-Vezinet, C. Rouzioux, et al. Selective tropism of lymphadenopathy-associated virus (LAV) for helper-inducer T lymphocytes. *Science* 225:59 (1984).

24. S. Gartner, P. Markovits, D.M. Markovits, et al. The role of mononuclear phagocytes in HTLV-III/LAV infection. *Science* 233:215 (1986).

25. D.D. Ho, T.R. Rota, and M.S. Hirsch. Infection of monocyte/macrophages by human T lymphotropic virus type III. *J. Clin. Invest.* 77:1712 (1986).

26. S.M. Schnittman, M.C. Psallidopoulos, H,.C. Lane, et al. The reservoir for HIV-1 in human peripheral blood is a T cell that maintains expression of CD4. *Science* 245:305 (1989).

27. J.L. Fahey, H. Prince, M. Weaver, et al. Quantitative changes in TR helper or T suppressor/cytotoxic lymphocyte subsets that distinguish ADS from other immune subset disorders. *Am. J. Med.* 76:95 (1984).

28. J.B. Margolick, J.C. McCarthur, E.R. Scott, et al. Flow cytometric quantitation of cell phenotypes in cerebrospinal fluid and peripheral blood of homosexual men with and without antibodies to human immunodeficiency virus type I. *J. Neuroimmunol.* 20:73 (1988).

29. J.C. McCarthur, E. Sipos, D.R. Cornblath, et al. Identification of mononuclear cells in CSF of patients with HIV infection. *Neurology* 39:66 (1989).

30. K.Y. Young, J.B. Peter, and R.E. Winters. Detection of HIV DNA in peripheral blood by the polymerase chain reaction: A study of clinical applicability and performance. *AIDS* 4:389 (1990).

31. L. Ratner. Measurement of human immunodeficiency virus load and is relation to disease progression. *AIDS Res. Human Retroviruses* 5:115 (1989).

32. F.T. Hufert, D. von Laer, C. Schramm, A. Tärnok, and H. Schmitz. Detection of HIV-1 DNA in different subsets of human peripheral blood mononuclear cells using the polymerase chain reaction. *Arch. Virol.* 106:341 (1989).

33. F.T. Hufert, D. von Laer, T.E. Fenner, et al. Progression of HIV-1 infection. Monitoring of HIV-1 DNA in peripheral blood mononuclear cells by PCR. *Arch. Virol.* 120:233 (1991).

34. S. Oka, K. Urayama, Y. Hirabayashi, et al. Quantitative analysis of human immunodeficiency virus type 1 DNA in asymptomatic carriers using the polymerase chain reaction. *Biochem. Biophys. Res. Commun.* 167:1 (1990).

35. S.M. Schnittman, J.J. Greenhouse, H.C. Lane, P.F. Pierce, and A.S. Fauci. Frequent detection of HIV-1-specific mRNAs in infected individuals suggests ongoing active viral expression in all stages of disease. *AIDS Res. Human Retroviruses* 7:361 (1991).

36. N.L. Michael, M. Vahey, D.S. Burke, and R.R. Redfield. Viral DNA and

mRNA expression correlate with the stage of human immunodeficiency virus (HIV) type 1 infection in humans: evidence for viral replication in all stages of HIV disease. *J. Virol.* 66:310 (1992).

37. H. Steuler, S. Munzinger, B., Wildemann, and B. Strock-Hagenlocher. Quantitation of HIV-1 proviral DNA in cells from cerebrospinal fluid. *J. AIDS Syndr.* 5:405 (1992).

38. E. Masliah, C.L. Achim, N. Ge, et al. Spectrum of human immunodeficiency virus-associated neocortical damage. *Ann. Neurol.* 32:321 (1992).

39. H. Budka. Human immunodeficiency virus (HIV)-induced disease of the central nervous system: pathology and implications for pathogenesis. *Acta Neuropathol.* 77:225 (1989).

40. H.V. Vinters, and K.H. Anders. Neuropathology of AIDS. Boca Raton, CRC Press, Inc., 1990.

41. R.L. Katz, C. Alappattu, J.P.Glass, and J.M. Bruner. Cerebrospinal fluid manifestations of the neurologic complications of human immunodeficiency virus infection. *Acta Cytol.* 33:233 (1989).

42. D.G. Walker, S. Itagaki, K. Berry, and P.L.McGeer. Examination of brains of AIDS cases for human immunodeficiency virus and human cytomegalovirus nucleic acids. *J. Neurol. Neurosurg. Psychiatry* 52:583 (1989).

QUANTIFICATION OF QUINOLINIC ACID METABOLISM BY MACROPHAGES AND ASTROCYTES

Melvyn P. Heyes,[1] Eugene O. Major,[2] Kuniaki Sato,[1] and Sanford M. Markey[1]

[1]Section on Analytical Biochemistry
Laboratory of Clinical Science
National Institute of Mental Health
[2]Laboratory of Molecular Medicine and Neuroscience
National Institute of Neurological Disorders and Stroke
National Institutes of Health
Bethesda, Maryland 20892

INTRODUCTION

Neurologic abnormalities, brain atrophy, neurodegeneration and encephalitis may accompany infection with the human immunodeficiency virus (HIV).[1,12] Some neurologic symptoms can be attributed to opportunistic central nervous system (CNS) conditions such as toxoplasmosis, progressive multifocal leukoencephalopathy (PML) and lymphoma. However, because neurologic deficits can occur independent of opportunistic CNS infections, and because HIV appears to be preferentially localized in macrophages, monocyte infiltrates and microglia rather than the functional elements of the brain, there is considerable interest in whether host- or virus-coded mediators secreted by macrophages are involved in the neuropathogenic processes. Potential host-coded mediators include quinolinic acid (QUIN),[3-5] cytokines,[6,7] prostaglandin metabolites,[8,9] nitric oxide,[10] as well as several unidentified factors.[11-15] Virus-coded factors include gp120[13,16-18] and *tat*.[19] Other investigators have implicated the involvement of astrocytes.[8,9,18]

QUINOLINIC ACID ASSAY

Quinolinic acid (QUIN) is a neurotoxic agonist of N-methyl-D-aspartate (NMDA) receptors,[20] and a metabolite of the L-tryptophan-kynurenine pathway (Fig. 1), with a history of consideration as an etiologic agent in neurologic diseases. During 1986-1988, we developed a highly sensitive, specific and accurate assay for QUIN.[21,22] Samples of cerebrospinal fluid (CSF) (100 µl), plasma (20 µl) and QUIN standards (0-150 pmol) are mixed with [^{18}O]-QUIN (6-30 pmol) as internal standard and freeze-dried overnight. Samples of tissue are homogenized in either buffer or hydrochloric acid containing [^{18}O]-QUIN (6-30 pmol) and washed with chloroform. Samples are then frozen at -70°C overnight, then thawed and centrifuged. The aqueous supernatant containing the QUIN and [^{18}O]-QUIN is collected and freeze-dried. QUIN and [^{18}O]-QUIN are then esteri-

Technical Advances in AIDS Research in the Human Nervous System
Edited by E.O. Major and J.A. Levy, Plenum Press, New York, 1995

317

fied to their dihexafluoroisopropanol esters by heating with 50 µl of 1,1,1,3,3,3-hexafluoroisopropanol and 50 µl of trifluoroacetylimidazole at 80°C. After cooling, samples are washed with 250 µl of water and extracted into 250 - 1000 µl of heptane. One or two microliter-injections of the heptane extract are made on a column (80°C) onto a 1 m x 0.35 mm deactivated silica precolumn that was connected to a 15 m x 0.25 mm DB-5 chromatography column at 111°C, with helium as a carrier (head pressure 10 Torr).

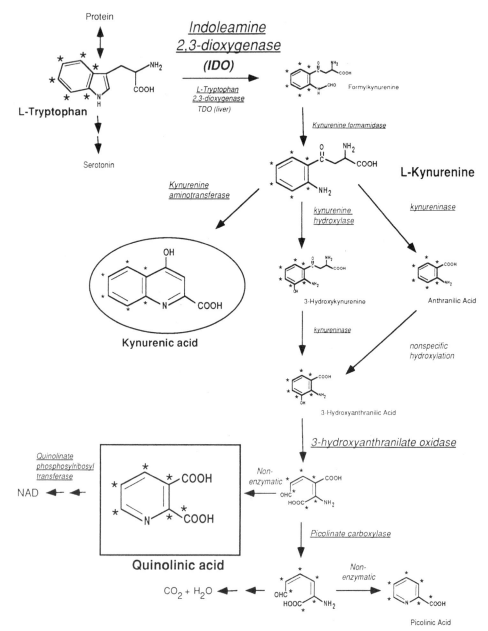

Figure 1. Overview of the kynurenine pathway. Enzymes are underlined. The [13C] atoms in [13C6]-L-tryptophan are indicated by an asterisk (*).

Samples were passed directly into the ion source of a Hewlett-Packard 5988 mass spectrometer (transfer line and ion source at 175°C) with methane (0.5 Torr) as reagent gas. QUIN and [^{18}O]-QUIN are then monitored as the molecular ions (m/z 467, 471 and 473), respectively, and quantified as the peak at the appropriate retention time (minimum sensitivity 500 amol injected). The minimum sensitivity of the assay is 80 fg (479 amol). Accuracy was obtained by using an isotopomer of QUIN, rather than structural isomers or chemical analogs. The use of negative chemical ionization, rather than electron impact ionization, reduced the degree of fragmentation of QUIN and thereby enhanced the specificity of the assay.

CLINICAL FINDINGS

The assay has been applied to a number of clinical and experimental conditions. The concentrations of QUIN are increased in cerebrospinal fluid (CSF), brain tissue and blood of patients infected with HIV, as well as in macaques infected with the simian immunodeficiency virus (SIV).[3,23-26] Increases in CSF QUIN were associated with motor deficits in early-stage HIV-infected patients and SIV-infected macaques.[25-27] CSF QUIN levels also correlated with quantitative measures of neuropsychologic deficits in later-stage adult and pediatric patients.[3,25,26,28] The highest QUIN levels were found in HIV-infected patients with dementia, aseptic meningitis or opportunistic CNS conditions.[23,27,28] Increases in QUIN also occurred in other inflammatory conditions associated with infection or injury,[3,5,23,29-32] but were not found to be elevated in noninflammatory conditions such as Huntington's disease, Alzheimer's disease or complex partial seizures.[5,33-35] Consequently, QUIN was implicated in the etiology of neurologic deficits associated with immune activation.

Several animal models of immune activation have since been used to develop the following model of the sources of QUIN accumulations in brain (Fig. 2). In conditions of CNS-restricted inflammation, QUIN originates from macrophages and perhaps constitutive brain cells such as astrocytes. In conditions of systemic immune activation, QUIN is synthesized within several tissues, and some QUIN may enter the brain from the blood. In both conditions, the increase in QUIN production following immune activation is related to increased activity of indoleamine-2,3-dioxygenase, the first enzyme of the kynurenine pathway.[5,30,37-41] Additional studies have suggested that kynurenine-3-hydroxylase is also a modulatory enzyme.[30-32,43,44]

An important issue regarding our model (Fig. 2) is whether macrophages and astrocytes can be a source of QUIN.[30-32,43,44] We have used the QUIN assay system to evaluate the capacity of these cell types to synthesize QUIN.

MEASUREMENT OF L-TRYPTOPHAN CONVERSION TO QUINOLINIC ACID

Macrophages and astrocytes were incubated with media containing [^{13}C$_6$]-L-tryptophan, and stimulated with interferon-γ or infected with HIV or unchallenged. The amounts of [^{13}C$_6$]-QUIN are then quantified in the incubation media. [^{13}C$_6$]-QUIN (mass 473 when esterified) can readily be distinguished from QUIN (mass 467) and [^{18}O]-QUIN (mass 471). The concentrations of L-kynurenine were also quantified as an index of indoleamine-2,3-dioxygenase activity.

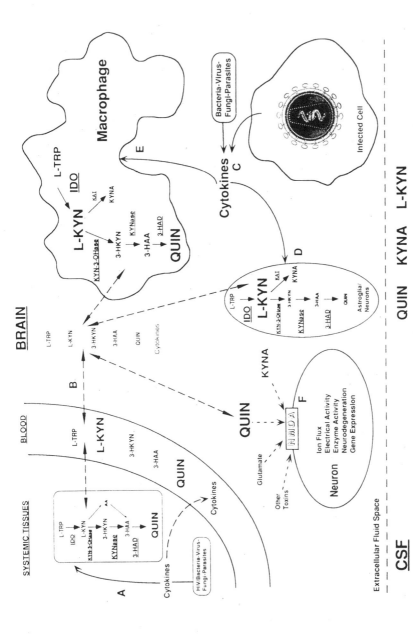

Figure 2. Model of the sources of quinolinic acid (QUIN) in HIV infection. Some QUIN may originate from systemic tissues (A) following induction of indoleamine-2, 3-dioxygenase (IDO) by interferon-γ, tumor necrosis factor-α, and other cytokines. QUIN may then enter the blood and cross the blood-brain barrier, particularly if the permeability is increased (B). Cytokines released from HIV-infected cells or in response to opportunistic infections (C) increase IDO activity in macrophages, astrocytes, and other CNS cells. L-kynurenine is the major product in astrocytes, and very little QUIN is produced (D). In macrophages, and perhaps microglia, there is high activity of IDO, kynurenine-3-hydroxylase, kynureninase and 3-hydroxyanthranilate-3,4-dioxygenase and QUIN is synthesized in large quantities (E). If QUIN accumulates in brain regions containing N-methyl-D-aspartate receptors, neuronal activity may be altered and neurodegeneration may also occur.

Cell cultures of human brain[45] were incubated in Eagle's MEM medium supplemented with 10% fetal bovine serum (FBS) (containing approximately 20 µM nonlabeled L-tryptophan), 25 µg/ml gentamicin at 37°C under humidified air containing 5% CO_2. Cultures consisted of a heterogeneous population of cells identified as astrocytes (approximately 65%) and neurons (approximately 25%) by using a monoclonal antibody to either the intermediate filaments of GFAP (Lab Systems, Amsterdam) or neurofilament (Boeringer-Mannheim, Germany). While neither myelin nor myelin basic protein was detected in these cultures, a few cells ($< 1\%$) were gal/C positive, and have been referred to as oligodendrocyte progenitor cells. Cells were expanded in cultured into 25 cm^3 flasks and used at the third passage. Each flask contained approximately 2.3 x 10^6 cells. At this generation period, there is no evidence of microglial cells[46] when tested for Fc receptors and reactivity to macrophage markers, including Mac 1. THP-1 cells and U373MG cells (an astrocyte cell line) were obtained from the American Type Culture Collection (Rockville, MD) and incubated in a 75 cm^3 plastic culture flask (approximately 10^5 to 10^6 cells/ml in 20 ml of tissue culture medium) at 37°C under humidified air containing 5% CO_2. The medium consisted of RPMI-1640 supplemented with 10% heat-inactivated FBS, 2 mM of L-glutamine, and 20 µM mercaptoethanol. Cocultures of THP-1 cells and human brain were made by attachment of 10^6 THP-1 cells onto a confluent layer of brain cells in a culture medium that consisted of RPMI-1640 supplemented with 10% heat-inactivated FBS and gentamicin at 37°C under humidified air containing 5% CO_2.

The concentrations of L-kynurenine and [$^{13}C_6$]-QUIN after 168 hours of incubation are presented in Figs. 3A and B, respectively. In THP-1 cells, both interferon-γ and infection with HIV-1 increased both L-kynurenine and [$^{13}C_6$]-QUIN accumulation compared to controls. In the human brain cultures, L-kynurenine release was increased by interferon-γ stimulation. However, only small quantities of [$^{13}C_6$]-QUIN were detected. It should be noted that the amounts of QUIN formed by the human brain cultures were more than 87-fold less than from the THP-1 cultures, even though the concentration of L-kynurenine was higher in the human brain cultures compared to the THP-1 cells. Transfection of human brain cultures with HIV-1 was not associated with production of either L-kynurenine and [$^{13}C_6$]-QUIN. In the combined cultures of THP-1 cells and human brain cells stimulated with interferon-γ, both L-kynurenine and [$^{13}C_6$]-QUIN were detected. The small counts of L-kynurenine and QUIN that were produced in the human fetal brain and THP-1 cell cultures, may be secondary to the release of cytokines, and QUIN synthesis within the THP-1 cells. In the astrocytoma cell line, interferon-γ produced large increases in L-kynurenine accumulation to concentrations greater than 50 µM, but no [$^{13}C_6$]-QUIN was detected. U373 MG cells were also found to produce large quantities of L-kynurenine in response to 24 and 48 hours of interferon-γ stimulation. However, no [$^{13}C_6$]-QUIN was detected.

CONCLUSIONS

These results demonstrate that activated macrophages have a high capacity to synthesize QUIN. While astrocytes have a high capacity to convert L-tryptophan to L-kynurenine in response to interferon-γ or HIV-1 infection, the capacity of astrocytes to synthesize QUIN is limited. The present results support the hypothesis that macrophages are a major source of QUIN in conditions of brain inflammation.

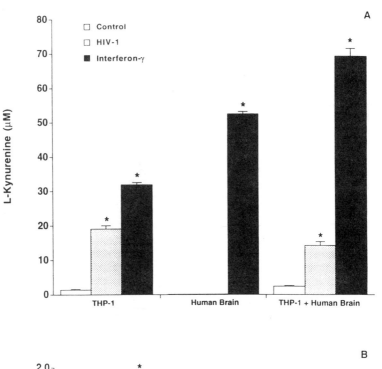

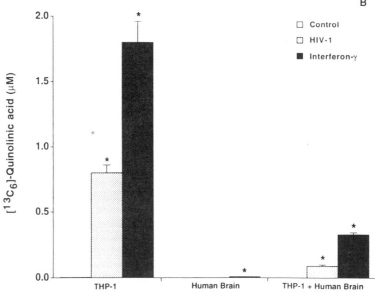

Figure 3. L-kynurenine (A) and [13C6]-QUIN (B) production by cultures of human fetal brain and THP-1 cells *in vitro*.

REFERENCES

1. E. Masliah, N. Ge, M. Morey, et al. Cortical dendritic pathology in human immunodeficiency virus encephalitis. *Lab. Investig.* 66:285 (1992).
2. D.C. Spencer and R.W. Price. Human immunodeficiency virus and the central nervous system. *Annu. Rev. Microbiol.* 46:655 (1993).
3. M.P. Heyes, B.J. Brew, A. Martin, et al. Quinolinic acid in cerebrospinal fluid and serum in HIV-1 infection: Relationship to clinical and neurologic status. *Ann. Neurol.* 29:202 (1991).
4. M.P. Heyes, D. Rubinow, C. Lane, et al. Cerebrospinal fluid quinolinic acid concentrations are increased in acquired immune deficiency syndrome. *Ann., Neurol.* 26:275 (1989).
5. M.P. Heyes, K. Saito, J. Crowley, et al. Quinolinic acid and kynurenine pathway metabolism in inflammatory and noninflammatory neurologic disease. *Brain* 115:1249 (1992).
6. C.L.Achim, M.P. Heyes and C.A. Wiley. Quantitation of human immunodeficiency virus, immune activation factors and quinolinic acid in AIDS brains. *J. Clin. Invest.* 91:2769 (1993).
7. W.R. Tyor, J.D.Glass, and J.W. Griffin. Cytokine expression in the brain during AIDS. *Ann. Neurol.* 31:249 (1992).
8. L.G. Epstein and H.E. Gendelman. Human immunodeficiency virus type 1 infection of the nervous system: pathogenic mechanisms. *Ann. Neurol.* 33:429 (1993).
9. P. Genis, M. Jett, E.W. Bernton, et al. Cytokines and arachidonic acid metabolites produced during human immunodeficiency virus (HIV)-infected macropahge-astrocyte interactions: Implications for the neuropathogenesis of HIV disease. *J. Exp. Med.* 176:1703 (1992).
10. V. Mollace, M. Colasanti, T. Persichini, et al. HIV gp120 glycoprotein stimulates the inducible isoform of NO synthetase in human cultured astrocytoma cells. *Biochem. Biophys. Res. Comm.* 194:439 (1993).
11. E.W. Bernton, H.U. Bryant, m.A. Decoster, et al. No direct neuronotoxicity by HIV-1 virions or culture fluids from HIV-1-infected T cells or monocytes. *AIDS Res. Human Retroviruses* 8:495 (1992).
12. D. Giulian, K. Vaca and C.A. Noonan. Secretion of neurotoxins by mononuclear phagocytes infected with HIV-1. *Science* 250:1593 (1990).
13. D. Giulian, E. Wendt, K. Vaca, et al. The envelope glycoprotein of human immunodeficiency virus type 1 stimulated the release of neurotoxins from monocytes. *Proc. Natl. Acad. Sci. USA* 90:2769 (1993).
14. L. Pulliam, B.G. Herndier, N.M. Tang, et al. Human immunodeficiency virus-infected macrophages produce soluble factors that cause histological and neurochemical alteration in cultured human brains. *J. Clin. Invest.* 87:503 (1991).
15. M. Tarieu, C. Henry, S. Peudenier, et al. Human immunodeficiency virus type 1-infected monocytic cells can destroy human neural cells after cell-to-cell adhesion. *Ann. Neurol.* 32:11 (1992).
16. D.E. Brenneman, G.L. Westbrook, S.P. Fitzgerald, et al. Neuronal cell killing by the envelope protein of HIV and its prevention by vasoactive intestinal peptide. *Nature* 335:639 (1988).
17. S.A. Lipton, N.J. Sucher and P.K. Kaiser. Synergistic effects of HIV coat protein and NMDA receptor-mediated neurotoxicity. *Neuron* 7:111 (1991).
18. L. Pulliam, D. West, N. Haigwood, et al. HIV-1 envelope gp120 alters astrocytes in human brain cultures. *AIDS Res. Hum. Retroviruses* 9:439 (1993).
19. J-M. Sabatier, E. Vives, K. Mabrouk, et al. Evidence for neurotoxic activity of *tat* from human immunodeficiency virus type-1. *J. Virol.* 65:961 (1991).
20. T.W. Stone. Neuropharmacology of quinolinic and kynurenic acids. *Pharmacol. Rev.* 45:309 (1993).
21. M.P. Heyes and S.P. Markey. [^{18}O]-quinolinic acid: Its esterification with-

out back exchange for use as internal standard in the quantification of brain and CSF quinolinic acid. *Biomed. Environ. Mass. Spectrom.* 15:291 (1988).

22. M.P. Heyes and S.P. Markey. Quantification of quinolinic acid in rat brain, whole blood and plasma by gas chromatography and negative chemical ionization mass spectrometry: Effects of systemic L-tryptophan administration on brain and blood quinolinic acid concentrations. *Anal. Biochem.* 174:349 (1988).

23. M.P. Heyes, E.K. Jordan, K. Lee, et al. Relationship of neurologic status in macaques infected with the simian immunodeficiency virus to cerebrospinal fluid and serum quinolinic acid and kynurenic acid. *Brain Res.* 570:237 (1992).

24. E.K. Jordan and M.P. Heyes. Virus isolation and quinolinic acid in primary and chronic SIV infection. *AIDS* 7:1173 (1993).

25. A. Martin, M.P. Heyes, A.M. Salazar, et al. Progressive slowing of reaction time and increasing cerebrospinal fluid concentrations of quinolinic acid in HIV-infected individuals. *J. Neuropsych. Clin. Neurosci.* 4:270 (1992).

26. A. Martin, M.P. Heyes, A.M. Salazar, et al. Impaired motor-skill learning, slowed reaction time, and elevated cerebrospinal fluid quinolinic acid in a subgroup of HIV-infected individuals. *Neuropsychology* 7:149 (1993).

27. D.M. Rausch, M.P. Heyes, E.A. Murray, et al. Cytopathologic and neurochemical correlates to motor/.cognitive impairments in SIV-infected rhesus monkeys., *J. Neuropathol. Exp. Neurol.* 1994 (in press).

28. P. Brouwers, M.P. Heyes, H. Moss, et al. Quinolinic acid in the cerebrospinal fluid of children with symptomatic human immunodeficiency virus type-1 disease: relationships to clinical status and therapeutic response. *J. Infect. Dis.* 168:1380 (1993).

29. A.R. Blight, K. Saito, and M.P. Heyes. Increased levels of the excitotoxin quinolinic acid in spinal cord following contusion injury. *Brain Res.* 632:314 (1993).

30. M.P. Heyes, K. Saito, D. Jacobowitz, et al. Poliovirus induces indoleamine-2,3-dioxygenase and quinolinic acid synthesis in macaque brain. *FASEB J.* 6:2977 (1992).

31. M.P. Heyes, K. Saito, E.O. Major, et al. A mechanism of quinolinic acid formation by brain in inflammatory neurologic disease: Attenuation of synthesis from L-tryptophan in inflammatory neurologic disease: Attenuation of synthesis from L-tryptophan by 6-chloro-tryptophan and 4-chloro-3-hydroxyanthranilate. *Brain* 116:1425 (1993).

32. K. Saito, T.S. Nowak, K. Suyama, et al. Kynurenine pathway enzymes in brain: responses to ischemic brain injury versus systemic immune activation. *J. Neurochem.* 61:2061 (1993).

33. M.P. Heyes, K. Saito, O. Devinsky, et al. Kynurenine pathway metabolites in cerebrospinal fluid and serum in complex partial seizures. *Epilepsia* 35:251 (1994).

34. M.P. Heyes, A.R. Wyler, O. Devinsky, et al. Brain and cerebrospinal fluid quinolinic acid concentrations in patients with intractable complex partial seizures. *Sixth International Study Group for Tryptophan Research*; Kynurenine and serotonin pathways, 683 (1991).

35. M.P. Heyes, K.J. Swartz, S.P. Markey, et al. Regional brain and cerebrospinal fluid quinolinic acid concentrations in Huntington's disease. *Neurosci. Lett.* 122:265 (1991).

36. M.M. Mouradian, M.P. Heyes, J-B Pan, et al. No changes in central quinolinic acid levels in Alzheimer's disease. *Neurosci. Lett.* 105:233 (1989).

37. K. Saito, J.S. Crowley, S.P. Markey, et al. A mechanism for increased quinolinic acid formation following acute systemic immune stimulation. *J. Biol. Chem.* 268:15496 (1993).

38. K. Saito, A. Lackner, S.P. Markey, et al. Cerebral cortex and lung indoleamine-2,3-dioxygenase activity is increased in type D retrovirus-infected macaques. *Brain Res.* 540:353 (1991).

39. K. Saito, S.P. Markey, and M.P. Heyes. Chronic effects of gamma-inter-

feron on quinolinic acid and indoleamine-2,3-dioxygenase in brain of C57BL6 mice. *Brain Res.* 546:151 (1991).

40. K. Saito, S.P. Markey, and M.P. Heyes. Effects of immune activation on quinolinic acid and kynurenine pathway metabolism in the mouse. *Neuroscience* 51:25 (1992).

41. K. Saito, T.S. Nowak Jr., K., S.P. Markey, et al. Mechanism of delayed increases in kynurenine pathway metabolism in damaged brain regions following transient cerebral ischemia. *J. Neurochem,* 60:180 (1993).

42. K. Saito, B.J. Quearry, M. Saito, et al. Kynurenine-3-hydroxylase in brain: species activity differences and effect of gerbil cerebra ischemia. *Arch. Biochem. Biophys.* 307:104 (1993).

43. M.P. Heyes, K. Saito and S.P. Markey. Human macrophages convert L-tryptophan to the neurotoxin quinolinic acid. *Biochem. J.* 283:633 (1992).

44. K. Saito, C.Y. Chen, M. Masana, et al. 4-Chloro-3-hydroxyanthranilic acid, 6-chlorotryptophan and norharmane attenuate quinolinic acid formation by interferon-γ-stimulated monocytes (THP-1) cells. *Biochem. J.* 291:11 (1993).

45. E.O. Major and D. Vacante. Human fetal astrocytes in culture support the growth of the neurotropic human polyomavirus. *J. Neuropathol Exp. Neurol.* 48:425 (1989).

46. G. Elder and E.O. Major. Early appearance of type II astrocytes in developing human fetal brain. *Dev. Brain Res.* 42:146 (1988).

TARGETED DEFECTIVE INTERFERING HIV-1 PARTICLES AS RENEWABLE ANTIVIRALS?

Manfred Schubert, Akhil C. Banerjea, Soon-Young Paik,
George G. Harmison, Chang-Jie Chen

Laboratory of Molecular Medicine and Neuroscience
National Institute of Neurological Disorders and Stroke
National Institutes of Health
Bethesda, Maryland 20892

INTRODUCTION

Defective viruses are viral mutants which are incapable of replication because they lack essential regions of the viral genome. They are ubiquitous and can be detected within all DNA and RNA virus families.[1] The replication of the defective virus requires functions which are carried out by gene products encoded in the missing regions. These functions must be provided in trans by a helper virus, which is usually the virus from which the defective virus originated. Many defective viral genomes contain all essential cis-acting nucleotide sequences, such as the origin of replication and the packaging signal necessary for viral assembly.[2] With defective proviruses, some of these cis elements may also be deleted and replaced by host sequences. In such cases, the defective virus cannot be transmitted by virus particle formation. Initial observations with acute trans-forming retroviruses led to the discoveries of oncogenes and the roles of defective proviruses and their regulatory sequences in neoplastic transformation.[3] Most defective proviruses, however, do not give rise to a recognizable cellular phenotype. Replication of these defective proviruses only occurs by cell division which the provirus itself can promote in some cases.

This contrasts with the replication of most nonretroviruses and/or viruses which do not integrate into the host genome and which replicate independently of the cell cycle. The replication of defective viruses from this large virus group is strictly dependent on coinfection with the parental virus. The life span of the host cell and the intracellular half-life of the defective genome itself determine their survival. Most critically, however, their survival depends on their ability to coinfect cells with parental helper virus. This ability is often limited by the low probability of such a coinfection.

Some defective viruses exhibit new biological properties which were first described in detail for influenza virus.[4,5] In fact, it was the ability to interfere with the replication of parental virus which led to their discovery. The replication of the defective virus depends on the presence of helper virus, but these coinfections often result in a dramatic and disproportionate reduction in the total number of virus progeny. This exciting new property initiated many studies on the origins of defective and interfering particles, their genomic organization, and their mechanisms of interference.[6-13] Their potential use as antivirals was considered but their primary use is as vaccines. Antigenetically, defective interfering particles are indistinguishable from their parental virus, but unlike their

Technical Advances in AIDS Research in the Human Nervous System
Edited by E.O. Major and J.A. Levy, Plenum Press, New York, 1995

parent, they are usually not pathogenic. It has recently been shown that some attenuated vaccine strains of measles virus, for example, do in fact contain defective and possibly even defective interfering virus particles.[14] It is uncertain whether their presence contributed to the total attenuation of the measles virus vaccine itself.

Many nonretroviral defective viruses which interfere with the replication of their parental virus in tissue culture have been described. Their general structural and biological characteristics were summarized by Huang and Baltimore,[15] who referred to them as DI (defective interfering) particles. There are only a few examples of defective interfering retroviruses, although defective proviruses are relatively abundant in retroviral infections. The presence of some defective proviruses has even been 'blamed' for the increased pathogenesis during a feline leukemia and a murine immunodeficiency viral infections.[16,17] These studies demonstrated that defective viruses can also perform complementary, helper functions in parental virus replication, and even modulate the disease process.

During coinfections of nonretroviral DI particles with wild type virus *in vitro*, cytopathogenesis is usually reduced and the infections may occasionally become persistent. Evidence for a widespread role of DI particles in establishing and maintaining persistent infections *in vivo*, however, is missing. Only a few persistent infections have been identified which involve DI particles,[7] suggesting that DI particles may be products of a selection process during repeated virus passages carried out at high multiplicity of infection in tissue culture, conditions which rarely exist *in vivo*. In addition, the sometimes rapid cell killing by some lytic viruses *in vivo* and the antiviral mechanisms of the host as well as the host's immune response are also unfavorable for DI particle replication.

When the virus distracts or weakens the immune system, as with the human immunodeficiency virus (HIV-1),[18] conditions may exist which are more suitable for generating DI particles and their survival. Until now, however, there has been no evidence for the presence of HIV-1 DI particles in patients. Increased numbers of defective HIV-1 proviruses have been observed during disease progression.[19,20] This of course, neither includes nor excludes a role for defective HIV-1 proviruses in viral replication or pathogenesis. Their increased abundance in later stages of the disease may simply be the result of higher viral burden. PCR methods now allow more sensitive studies on the presence of DI particle genomes in other persistent viral infections, for example, during the rare persistent measles virus infection of the brain. This infection causes a slow and fatal disease, subacute sclerosing panencephalitis (SSPE).[21] It will be interesting to see whether, in addition to the accumulation of large number of mutations in the measles virus genomic RNA,[22] defective and interfering particles also contribute to establishing and/or maintaining this persistent brain infection.

In the following sections of the chapter, we extrapolate this basic knowledge about defective particles and DI particles, and propose an antiviral strategy against HIV-1 which focuses on a novel type of recombinant DI particle, a targeted, defective interfering HIV-1 particle. Although the proposed particle functionally and structurally fits the general definition of DI particles,[15] its newly encoded biological features would place it into a new designer category of DI particles which are not found in nature. The proposed DI virus would, if all elements of the strategy are functional and optimized, be nonpathogenic but parasitic for another virus, HIV-1. As will be discussed in detail below, the genetically engineered DI virus genomes are reduced to only the cis-acting elements necessary for gene expression and replication. In addition, they encode gene products which may enable them to selectively interfere with HIV-1 replication without affecting their own replication. This may provide a selective advantage for these DI particles over their HIV-1 helper virus. It is the goal of this study, to develop DI particles which may overcome some of the replicative disadvantages of naturally occurring DI particles described above. The strategy, therefore, promotes coinfections of HIV-1-infected cells with DI particles, so these DI particles could ultimately function as renewable antivirals.

Recent findings that HIV-1 replicates efficiently at all times during the 8-10 years of the asymptomatic phase of the infection[23,24] provides an unique opportunity for intervention. The proposed antiviral strategy is especially adapted to HIV-1 infections. In this chapter, we introduce the first candidate designs of defective interfering HIV-1 particle genomes which may encode all the biological elements required for this antiviral strategy. The functionality of some of these elements is still hypothetical and needs to be further developed. Viral vectors similar to those proposed here could in the future also become valuable analytic as well as therapeutic agents for the targeted gene delivery to both dividing and nondividing cells. This will be of particular importance for cells of the central nervous system (CNS).

ANTIVIRAL STRATEGY: REVIEW AND DISCUSSION

Intracellular Immunization vs. Targeted Defective Interfering HIV-1 Particles

The genetic manipulation of cells which renders them resistant to a particular viral infection has previously been defined as intracellular immunization.[25] For this antiviral strategy to be effective, a substantial fraction of all potential target cells must become resistant to the virus to result in an overall decrease in viral pathogenesis and disease progression. Intracellular immunization, therefore requires a selected and resistant stem cell which confers resistance to all its progeny. With HIV-1 as the challenging virus, this stem cell should be of the hematopoietic cell lineage from which the majority of HIV-1-infected cells in the patient are derived. This includes T4 lymphocytes as well as monocytes and macrophages (Fig. 1, A-E).

The intracellular immunization of cells from HIV-1-infected patients appears to have some distinct disadvantages. Even if it were effective and safe, it would be extremely difficult at this time to treat millions of patients. It certainly would be a major, if not impossible task to genetically manipulate progenitor cells *ex vivo* (Fig. 1B) and then reintroduce the cells safely into such a large number of infected patients. A therapy with an *in vivo* delivery of the resistant gene by a DI particle would have significant advantages (Fig. 1, F-I). With an intracellular immunization gene therapy, it is still uncertain whether a large enough fraction of HIV-1 host cells can be made resistant, and whether the resistance gene product can be stably expressed. The size of the resistant cell fraction which is necessary to cause a delay, or ultimately prevent the onset of AIDS, is currently unknown. The possibility nevertheless exists, that the immune system could be partially protected and/or restored through gene therapy, and the accessibility of hematopoietic cells lends itself to genetic manipulation.

Cells which do not belong to the hematopoietic cell lineage, however, such as endothelial cells or astrocytes, would remain susceptible to HIV-1. The same may apply to cells present in the CNS, such as microglial cells[26-28] and astrocytes[29,30] which are inaccessible to genetic manipulation. The severe problem of HIV-1 neuropathogenesis is not addressed by intracellular immunization of hematopoietic stem cells. HIV-1 infection of the brain can cause neuronal loss and dementia, even in the absence of neuronal infections.[27,30] Several indirect mechanisms for HIV-1 neuropathogenesis have been proposed.[26,31] While restoration of the patient's immune function is of central importance, it may not be sufficient to reduce HIV-1 neuropathogenesis. The enormous plasticity of the HIV-1 genomic sequence together with the diversity of HIV-1-infected cells clearly indicate that a combination of several antiviral therapies may be needed against HIV-1.

For a gene therapy, retroviruses such as Moloney murine leukemia virus, the first virus to be approved for human gene therapy,[32] and other defective nonpathogenic viruses, which integrate into the chromosomal DNA, like adeno-associated virus, have been considered as vectors for gene therapy as well as for the delivery of antiviral gene(s) against HIV-1.[33] Defective viral vectors or HIV-1 vectors, which encode mutant negative trans-dominant HIV-1 gene products

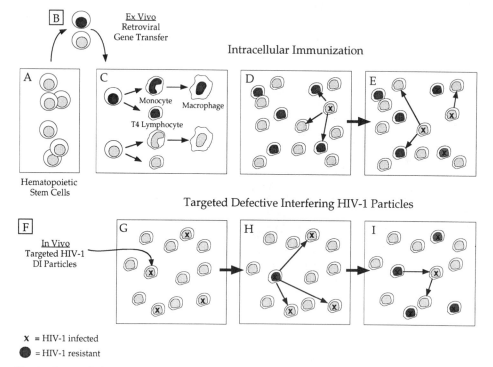

Intracellular Immunization

Targeted Defective Interfering HIV-1 Particles

x = HIV-1 infected

● = HIV-1 resistant

Fig. 1. Intracellular immunization/gene therapy (A-E): Hematopoietic stem cells are isolated from the bone marrow of HIV-1-infected patients and the HIV-1 resistant gene is inserted into these cells *ex vivo* by retroviral gene transfer.[25,32] Resistant stem cells are selected, enriched, and subsequently returned to the patient. Cells derived from these progenitor cells, such as T4 lymphocytes, monocytes, and macrophages, remain HIV-1 resistant and do not permit HIV-1 replication. Antiviral strategy involving targeted defective interfering HIV-1 particles (F-I): Recombinant defective HIV-1 particles are prepared in tissue culture in the absence of infectious HIV-1 and are introduced into HIV-1-infected patients. These targeted virus particles specifically adsorb to and infect any cell expressing the HIV-1 Env protein on the surface. After integration and expression, its gene products specifically interfere with the replication of IIIV-1, but they allow replication of the defective virus. New defective interfering virus particles are released which repeat this cycle in other HIV-1-infected cells.

that interfere with viral replication have been proposed as antiviral agents.[34-39] The ultimate goal of these strategies is to completely block HIV-1 gene expression or replication and thereby dramatically reduce the levels of infectious virus released from the resistant cells.

The antiviral strategy, which we propose here, is conceptually quite different from intracellular immunization (Fig. 1, F-I). Unlike intracellular immunization and the complete inhibition of HIV-1 replication, the strategy proposed here focuses on a selective inhibition of some, but not all, HIV-1 functions. The strategy involves an uniquely designed, targeted, defective interfering HIV-1 particle, which would be able to spread the antiviral genes and products of HIV-1 infected cells. These DI particles should have the following structural and biological properties:

(a) The defective interfering HIV-1 genome contains all cis-acting elements for gene expression and replication.

(b) The defective genome is only expressed, replicated, and assembled in the presence of wild type HIV-1, which provides all structural and regulatory proteins.

(c) The gene products encoded by the defective genome interfere selectively with the replication of infectious wild type HIV-1, but not with the replication of the defective genome.

(d) Defective interfering HIV-1 particles are assembled which specifically target and infect other HIV-1 expressing cells to complete and repeat the cycle.

The complete inhibition of HIV-1 gene expression and viral assembly is clearly not the goal of this strategy. In fact, a complete inhibition of all HIV-1 functions would be detrimental to this approach. A therapy which employs these particles could potentially be carried out *in vivo* and it would not require gene transfer to isolated stem cells. Different from an intracellular immunization, this strategy involves a mobile element, the targeted, defective interfering HIV-1 particle. Such an unique HIV-1 DI particle would replicate at the expense of wild type HIV-1 and be able to target and repeat this cycle in other HIV-1-infected cells. As is characteristic for DI particles, their replication would totally depend on the presence of wild type HIV-1, which would provide all helper virus functions.

Some of the key features for such a putative HIV-1 DI particle are shown in Figure 2. The ability and efficiency of the DI particles to target and infect cells which express the HIV-1 envelope protein Env on their surface is essential for this approach. The effectiveness will in part depend on the ability to insert, for example, a functional HIV-1 receptor, CD4 or a chimeric receptor molecule into its envelope. Different from the intracellular immunization of progenitor cells, such targeted defective viruses may be able to infect all HIV-1-infected cells, independent of their origin, if they express HIV-1 Env on the cell surface. This may enable the DI particle to reach any location HIV-1 is able to reach, and thereby deliver the interfering genes to different cell types, including, but not limited to, cells of the hematopoietic cell lineage. Similar to a gene therapy, over time, increasingly more HIV-1-expressing cells would be included. The potential kinetics of such an infection are addressed below.

Targeting HIV-1-Infected Cells by Defective Pseudotype HIV-1 Viruses

Targeting and delivering genetic information to specific cells through either viral vectors, liposomes or other transfer mechanisms, are desirable tools for many areas in the life sciences, which would allow one to genetically manipulate cells for analytic and/or therapeutic purposes. Many viruses already demonstrate a high degree of target cell specificity, which can be as specific as high-affinity antigen/antibody interactions. For example, HIV-1 primarily infects a subset of T lymphocytes as well as monocytes/macrophages,[40] which express the HIV-1 receptor, the CD4 membrane protein.[41-43] This highly efficient and specific interaction of the viral envelope protein with its receptor has been the focus of several antiviral strategies. For example, the use of a truncated, soluble

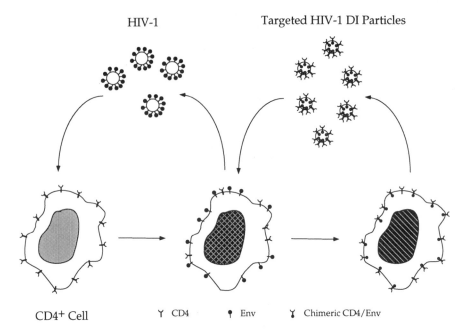

HIV-1   Targeted HIV-1 DI Particles

CD4⁺ Cell   Y CD4   Env   Chimeric CD4/Env

Fig. 2. HIV-1 primarily infects CD4⁺ cells by binding Env to its receptor, followed by the fusion of viral and cellular membranes which initiates the infection process. After proviral integration, HIV-1 down-regulates the surface expression of CD4, and high levels of the viral glycoprotein Env are expressed on the cell surface. HIV-1 particles are released from these cells which reinfect other CD4⁺ cells. The proposed targeted HIV-1 DI particles would carry a functional viral receptor in their envelope. They would be able to adsorb to and infect HIV-1-infected cells which express Env on their surface. The gene products encoded by the DI particle would reverse the down-regulation of CD4 and down-regulate the viral Env protein instead. One of the gene products of the DI genome would encode a chimeric CD4 protein, which is expressed on the cell surface, where it would be inserted into the envelope of the newly released DI particles. These new particles may again carry the chimeric receptor which allows us to target and infect other HIV-1 Env-expressing cells.

form of the CD4 protein has been used to physically block HIV-1 cell entry.[44] Chimeric CD4-toxin molecules were developed to selectively target and kill HIV-1-expressing cells in tissue culture with an exceptionally high degree of specificity.[45] *In vivo*, the use of the targeted toxin may have the disadvantage that it must be supplied continuously, which could trigger an undesired immune response. In addition, it would also be unable to cross the blood-brain barrier.

Changing the host range of a virus experimentally has been achieved with several enveloped viruses. Coinfections of cells with two unrelated enveloped viruses can result in a mixing of the viral glycoproteins in the cell membrane, and it can subsequently lead to the insertion of functional glycoprotein(s) of one virus into the envelope of the other virus and *vice versa*. This can broaden the host range of these phenotypically mixed viruses. Neutralizing antibodies against its own envelope proteins can be used to restrict the host range of these virus particles to the host range of the second virus only. The resultant virus is called a pseudotype virus. Genomic sequences are not exchanged during this phenotypic mixing, and pseudotype viruses loose the foreign envelope protein by membrane fusion at the time of infection. Coinfections of vesicular stomatitis virus (VSV) with other enveloped viruses, can, for example yield pseudotype VSV fractions of 30%; other combinations only yield 0.01% or less.[43,46-48] HIV-1 pseudotype viruses with VSV and herpes virus envelopes, HTLV-1 or with an envelope of an endogenous murine retrovirus have been described.[49-52] HIV-1 pseudotype particles with a widened host range could conceivably play an important role during the initial infection step, especially when the foreign envelope protein is more stable and efficient than HIV-1 Env, resulting in a more infectious virus.

The specific interactions between membrane glycoproteins, membrane lipids and other cytoplasmic viral proteins at the site of virus assembly are still poorly understood for most viruses and in particular for HIV-1. It is still unclear which protein domains determine the efficiency and specificity of glycoprotein insertion during HIV-1 assembly. Glycoprotein levels are important, but they are not considered the primary determining factor for insertion. The low level insertion of cellular membrane proteins into viral envelopes has also been described.[53] A specific exclusion of cellular proteins at the site of viral assembly was initially suggested, and an intrinsic structural difference between viral and cellular glycoproteins was postulated to explain the sometimes high efficiency of pseudotype virus formation ("pseudotypic paradox").[48] Such a distinction may possibly occur during specific interactions of the cytoplasmic tail region of the envelope protein with other membrane-associated or cytoplasmic viral proteins, such as the viral matrix protein.[54]

To study the requirements of pseudotype formation and to be able to target HIV-1 Env-expressing cells, we initially inserted the HIV-1 receptor, the CD4 protein, into the envelope of a rhabdovirus, VSV. Since the ectodomain of CD4 is sufficient for receptor function,[55,56] we also constructed a chimeric CD4 molecule, which consists of the ectodomain of CD4 precisely fused to the transmembrane and cytoplasmic portions of the VSV glycoprotein G, to increase the efficiency of membrane insertion. When either one of the proteins, CD4 or CD4/G was expressed in a coinfection with VSV using vaccinia virus recombinants, about 42% of the phenotypically mixed VSV could be specifically immunoprecipitated using a monoclonal antibody to CD4 without neutralizing the virus.[56] In addition, there was surprisingly no significant difference in the efficiency of CD4 or CD4/G insertion into the viral envelope, which resulted in a relatively large fraction of phenotypically mixed virus as shown for CD4/G in Table 1.

Other investigators have successfully inserted the CD4 or a chimeric CD4 molecule into the envelopes of avian leukosis virus[57] and herpes simplex virus,[58] respectively. Attempts with any of these phenoytpically mixed viruses, however, to specifically target and infect cells which express the HIV-1 Env protein on their surface have been unsuccessful to date. In contrast, it has recently been demonstrated that cellular membrane vesicles, which anchor CD4, and which were generated from HeLa cells, can fuse with HIV-1 Env-expressing cells.[59] Thus, the absence of a selective infection of HIV-1 Env-expressing cells by either avian leukosis virus or herpes simplex virus pseudotypes, which carry CD4 on their surface cannot be explained at this time.

Surface expression of CD4 promotes HIV-1 adsorption, but its expression alone is insufficient for infection. CD4 protein expressed in mouse cells allows HIV-1 adsorption onto the cells, but not viral infection, although the cells are permissive for HIV-1 replication, as was demonstrated by transfection with a complete HIV-1 DNA clone.[43] The presence of CD4 on the surface of a nonhuman or even a human cell, does not assure viral entry and/or cell fusion.[60,61] Additional factor(s), besides the primary receptor, seem to be required, which have not been identified as yet. These putative factors (galactosyl ceramide[62,63] and CD26 have recently[64] been proposed as alternate or as coreceptors, respectively) could also be membrane-associated and located in close proximity to CD4. Or they could be copackaged into a pseudotype virus envelope together with CD4. Consequently, the cellular source of a CD4-carrying pseudotype virus may not only affect its binding to HIV-1 Env-expressing cells, it could also affect its infectivity.

Table 1. Immunoprecipitations of phenotypically mixed vesicular stomatitis virus carrying a chimeric CD4/G protein.*

Total virus titer (PFU/ml)	Anti-CD4 antibody	Virus titer (PFU/ml)		% Phenotypically mixed virus in pellet
		Supernatant	Pellet	
VSV (CD4/G)	OKT4	7×10^5	5×10^5	42
6×10^6	Leu3a-Leu3b	7×10^5	5×10^5	42
	No 1st Ab	3×10^6	5×10^3	0.2
VSV				
5×10^6	OKT4	3×10^6	4×10^3	0.1
	Leu3a-Leu3b	3×10^6	4×10^3	0.1
	No 1st Ab	4×10^6	4×10^3	0.1

*Vesicular stomatitis virus (VSV) was coinfected with a recombinant vaccinia virus expressing a chimeric CD4/G protein. CD4/G consisted of the ectodomain of CD4 precisely fused to the transmembrane and cytoplasmic domains of the VSV glycoprotein G.[56]

Placing the receptor into the viral envelope and the fusogenic envelope protein of the virus into the cell membrane represents a functional role reversal of cellular and viral membranes. It may allow viral adsorption but it may not be permissive for membrane fusion and infection. The relative densities of viral Env and CD4 at the adsorption site may also be critical for membrane fusion. As compared to membrane vesicles, smaller virus particles may only package a limited number of CD4 molecules, which could be insufficient for membrane fusion. Alternatively, intracellular events past membrane fusion could also be critically affected and block infection.

For the proposed antiviral strategy, it is important to develop HIV-1 DI particles, which are able to target and infect other HIV-1-infected cells. This is a very important element of the strategy, which still requires a more detailed study. Transfer of the viral genomic RNA could also occur through CD4-Env-dependent cell fusions in the absence of particle formation. In fact, this mode of genome transfer occurs during cocultivations of susceptible cells and is most efficient.[65] Cell fusions, however, generally result in a shortened half-life of the participating cells. Therefore, a mobile, targeted HIV-1 DI particle will ultimately be required for a more effective spread of the interfering genes.

The Target Cells

Most HIV-1-infected cells are differentiated, nondividing cells. The ability of HIV-1 to infect and replicate in these cells is a characteristic of lentiviruses.[66] Unlike most other retroviruses, lentiviruses can transport the preintegration complex through nuclear pores prior to the integration into chromosomal DNA.[67] Quiescent host cells have a limited half-life of approximately 6 weeks. HIV-1 must, therefore, replicate and reinfect other cells in order to continue the infection process. Consequently, the infection cannot remain latent. Without reinfections, the virus would be lost entirely from the population unless stem cells were infected. There is, however, no evidence for an HIV-1 infection of stems cells which do not express CD4. On the other hand, HIV-1 also does not rapidly kill every infected host cell. The low level and the quasilatent state of the HIV-1 infection in the peripheral blood could possibly explain the very low level of HIV-1 expression and the long asymptomatic phase of the infection. Initially it did not easily explain how the virus was maintained, and particularly how this low number of infected cells could lead to AIDS.

An HIV-1-infected cell reservoir which bridges this gap has recently been discovered in two separate laboratories.[23,24] Large numbers of HIV-1-infected

CD4+ cells have been detected in lymph nodes, which are actively expressing HIV-1. These observations led to a new and important view on HIV-1 infection kinetics and disease progression. Different from the earlier perspective, high numbers of persistently infected, HIV-1-expressing cells are present at all times. There is no latency with respect to the viral population, although many individual cells can be latently infected. It is unknown how the less symptomatic phase of the infection progresses to AIDS. Virus load, integrated as well as free virus, most likely plays an important role and includes the overall size and heterogeneity of the replicating and continuously evolving virus population.[20,68,69]

Any antiviral strategy must be designed to down-regulate this virus load. Since proviruses cannot be removed from cells, the total number of infected cells as well as the state of viral expression and replication, become important parameters. Any decrease in these levels, even if they may seem very small, could over time, have a significant impact on the size of the infected cell population and possibly even delay the onset of AIDS. The antiviral strategy discussed here requires that the cells, which are infected with HIV-1 and which express HIV-1 Env protein on their surface, can be targeted and infected by the proposed HIV-1 DI particles. The highest density of HIV-1-infected cells has been found in lymph nodes, where they are immobile in contrast to the peripheral blood. These conditions are clearly more permissive for viral adsorption and infection, and consequently more favorable for an antiviral strategy that depends on superinfections.[65]

Different from most other retroviruses, the HIV-1 infection itself is cytopathic. T4 helper cells are often killed within a few days after infection, whereas monocytes and macrophages usually survive for a longer time. They are also infected through the CD4 receptor, but often replicate HIV-1 less efficiently than T4 helper cells and accumulate virions in cytoplasmic inclusions.[27,70] Thus, monocytes/macrophages are an important fraction of the virus reservoir. These cells continuously produce HIV-1 particles at low levels and are able to survive for a longer time. They thereby become stable targets for DI particle infection within the proposed antiviral strategy. Presumably because of lower HIV-1 expression levels, they can express both the CD4 protein as well as the HIV-1 Env protein on their surface. HIV-1-infected cells do not appear to generally exclude other HIV-1 particles from superinfection, which is essential for the proposed use of the DI particles.[71-74] Viral exclusion of superinfection, however, has been reported in some cases. Such an exclusion was caused either by receptor down-regulation after infection or possibly by events past viral entry.[75,76]

Mechanisms of Interference

All antiviral gene therapies proposed so far focus on the complete inhibition of HIV-1 replication. Antiviral gene products, which can be either constitutively expressed or upon induction in the presence of HIV-1, should be highly efficient in interrupting critical elements in the HIV-1 replication cycle, resulting in reduced levels of infectious virus released from these cells. Candidate antiviral products and their targets are presented in Table 2, which also includes an evaluation for their potential use for HIV-1 DI particles. Although each antiviral mechanism may be very effective in tissue culture, the efficiency of most of them *in vivo* will be limited to the cell type and size of the cell fraction which can be made nonpermissive by gene therapy. Survival of the infected cells itself depends on the antiviral gene product and its mechanism of action.

Table 2. Antiviral genes for gene therapy and HIV-1 DI particles.*

Gene Product	Antiviral mechanism	Particle release	Infectivity of released virus	Suitability for DIs
Mutant viral proteins:				
Tat	transcription	+	+ + + +	−
Rev	mRNA proces.	+	+ + + +	−
Gag	viral assembly	+	+/−	−
Env	infectivity	+ + + +	−	+/−
RNA transcripts:				
Tar decoys	transcription	+ +	+ + + +	−
antisense	translation	+ +	+/−	+/−
ribozymes	translation	+ +	+/−	+ +
Recombinant cellular proteins:				
CD4-derivatives	infectivity	+ + + +	−	+ + + +
linear Env-antibody	infectivity	+ + + +	−	+ + + +

*For references see text.

For example, cells which express a recombinant, transdominant mutant HIV-1 Gag protein that interferes with virus maturation, may still be killed by high levels of viral expression. Some antiviral strategies have been proposed to involve gene products which inactivate the cell upon induction after HIV-1 infection, for example, through the cytopathic effect caused by the VSV matrix protein.[77] This type of approach also contributes to limiting virus spread and virus load within the cell population. Although this strategy initially appears to worsen viral pathogenesis for the infected cell, it could protect the population of all HIV-1 susceptible cells by limiting virus spread.

Many proposed interfering gene products are of viral origin, including several negative transdominant mutant proteins such as for Gag, Rev, and Tat.[37-39] Regulatory proteins such as Tat and Rev affect either the level, posttranscriptional processing, transport, or stability of HIV-1 RNAs. All these proteins could subsequently affect viral replication by inhibiting HIV-1 gene expression or by disrupting the multimerization of Gag during the formation of the viral core structure. The expression of RNA fragments has been proposed, which could act as decoys for the viral Tat protein.[78] This approach requires high levels of RNA decoy expression, and relies upon depletion of viral regulatory proteins. Since these RNAs may also attract cellular factors, they may also deplete factors which are potentially needed for cellular functions.

The expression of ribozymes or antisense RNA molecules targeted against HIV-1 RNA has been shown to specifically inhibit viral replication.[79-85] Their antiviral effects depend on hybrid formation between the HIV-1 and the antisense transcript. Excess molar amounts of the antiviral RNA are required at the same subcellular location. Since ribozymes are believed to cleave target RNA catalytically *in vivo*, they can in contrast to antisense RNA be used repeatedly. This differs from antisense RNAs which form stable hybrids with their target RNAs.

Several types of ribozyme motifs have been described which can be very efficient in RNA cleavage reactions *in vitro*.[86-88] Their effectiveness *in vivo* cannot be predicted as yet, and has to be determined empirically. Ribozymes are not antigenic and there is no evidence for cell toxicity, and as will be shown below, they can be encoded by the DI genome. In fact, the genomic RNA of the proposed HIV-1 DI itself can function as a catalytic RNA, and it can cleave wild type HIV-1 RNAs without self destruction. Because of the potential selection of ribozyme-resistant viral mutants, it can be anticipated that single ribozymes, as the only antiviral component of a strategy, will not be effective over a long period of time.

We have developed the first multitarget ribozymes - ribozymes which are directed to cleave HIV-1 RNA at up to nine different sites. All selected target sites are located within the ectodomain region of Env mRNA which does not contain any other open-reading frames (Fig. 3A).[80] The selected target sequences (Fig. 3B) are highly conserved among more than 30 HIV-1 isolates sequenced so far. All individually targeted monoribozymes contain the hammerhead ribozyme motif (Fig. 3C), and they were combined into an approximately 500-nucleotide long, completely synthetic nonaribozyme (Fig. 3D), targeted to cleave at nine of the ten selected target sites. At the same molar concentration, multitarget ribozymes were much more effective in cleaving the same substrate than single ribozymes. This may explain why in contrast to single ribozymes, multitarget ribozymes also remain highly active even when they are part of a larger RNA transcript, such as the HIV-1 D1 genomic RNA.

Multiple cleavages of HIV-1 Env mRNA by the nonaribozyme *in vitro* and *in vivo* are shown in Figure 4. *In vitro* incubation of a 1,335-nucleotide substrate RNA, which contains all the ribozyme target sites listed in Figure 3B, with the nonaribozyme Rz636 (Fig. 3D) resulted in a complete degradation of Env RNA (Fig. 4A). The multiple RNA fragments were of the predicted sizes, which indicated that they were the result of multiple cleavages of the same RNA molecule. The nonaribozyme RNA itself was not cleaved under these conditions (data not shown). Since both RNAs were combined at equal molar ratios, the multiple cleavages are strong evidence that the cleavage reactions were catalytic.

The result of a coexpression of the approximately 3.5 kb prototype HD3 and HD4 DI DNAs (Fig. 5) with HIV-1 Env RNA in HeLa-Tat 3 cells is shown in Figure 4B. In the presence of the DI DNA HD3, which did not contain the nonaribozyme, there was only a partial reduction in the amounts of expressed Env RNA (compare lanes 1 and 2). Insertion of the nonaribozyme DNA into HD3 DNA created HD4. Coexpression of the large HD4 transcript resulted in a dramatic reduction of Env transcripts. Rehybridization of the same blot with a nonaribozyme probe, demonstrated the presence of the uncleaved HD4 transcript in the same RNA sample (lane 3'). This strongly suggested that the large RNA transcript encoded by HD4 DNA also functioned as a multitarget ribozyme *in vivo*.

We conclude from these results that ribozymes, and in particular, multitarget ribozymes, could be effective in modulating HIV-1 gene expression and viral infectivity. Ribozymes could potentially be used to favor the packaging of the DI genomic RNA at the expense of the wild type virus. In contrast to antisense RNA, ribozymes could be used to alter the genomic makeup of released virus particles. Depending on the position of the target sequences within HIV-1 RNA, there may also be a differential effect on the cleavage and stability of the individual mRNA species in the presence of ribozymes. There are many different viral mRNA species in HIV-1-infected cells which do not contain the target sequence(s) and would not be cleaved. For a strategy which, in part, relies on the selective down-regulation of the HIV-1 Env protein in the viral envelope, a partially selective inhibition of Env protein expression would be an advantage.

There are other antiviral strategies that also change the infectivity of released virus particles without reducing the number of released virus particles.[89] To target HIV-1 Env-expressing cells, the makeup of the envelope of the HIV-1 DI particles needs to be altered to specifically limit its host range. We hope to be able to achieve this by expressing a chimeric CD4/Env protein on the particle's surface. In HIV-1-infected cells, however, in which the virus is expressed, a down-regulation of the HIV-1 receptor on the cell surface is usually observed, which in the extreme case, can be complete and possibly even lead to

A   Multitarget-Ribozyme Cleavage Sites in HIV-1 RNA

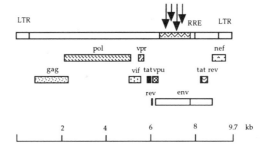

B   Specific Target Sites within the HIV-1 env Region

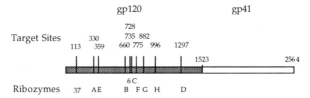

C   Monoribozyme Structure/Catalytic Center

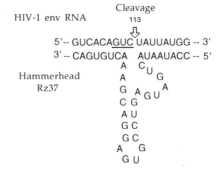

D   Structure of Multitarget-Ribozyme Rz636

Rz37-RzE-RzF-RzG-RzH-RzA-RzB-RzC-RzD

Figure 3. Multitarget ribozyme construct and its target sites in HIV-1 RNA.[80] A, all cleavage sites in the env region were selected so they do not overlap with any other open-reading frames within HIV-1 RNA. B, the chosen sites are located within highly conserved regions of the Env ectodomain. C, the target sites were 17 nucleotides in length and contained the conserved GUC cleavage site.[87] D, nine different monoribozymes were linked to an approximately 400-nucleotide nonaribozyme, targeted to cleave at up to nine sites (B).

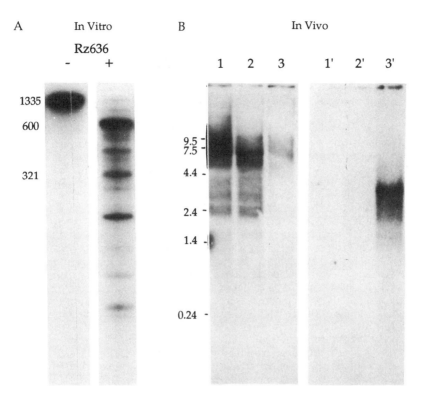

Figure 4. *In vitro* and *in vivo* multitarget ribozyme cleavages of HIV-1 Env RNA. A, isotopically labeled *in vitro* transcripts of HIV-1 Env RNA, which contain all the ribozyme target sites shown in Figure 3B, were incubated with the same molar amount of the approximately 400-nucleotide long nonaribozyme transcript Rz636 for 30 minutes at 55°C. B, equal amounts of pHenv DNA encoding HIV-1 Env mRNA were cotransfected with an unrelated control DNA (1), HD3 DNA (2), and HD4 DNA which encodes the nonaribozyme Rz636 (3), respectively, into HeLa-Tat-3 cells. Total RNAs were isolated 48 hours after transfection, separated on an agarose gel, blotted on nitrocellulose, and hybridized with an isotopically labeled DNA to detect env transcripts (1,2,3) or nonaribozyme sequences (1', 2', 3'). Indicated sizes are in either nucleotides (A) or kilobases (B), respectively.

an exclusion of superinfection by other HIV-1 particles. Three different mechanisms have been described which are involved in this CD4 down-regulation: (a) the complex formation between CD4 and Env proteins in the endoplasmic reticulum;[90-93] (b) degradation of the receptor in the presence of Env and the viral protein Vpu;[94] and (c) the down-regulation by the viral Nef protein.[95]

In the context of the proposed strategy, receptor down-regulation must be prevented. Therefore, these three mechanisms must be addressed, potentially circumvented or inactivated. Functionality of the CD4 protein as the receptor for HIV-1 depended only on the ectodomain of CD4. The cytoplasmic domain of CD4 can be replaced, as was done during the development of the chimeric receptor described earlier (Fig. 2). On the other hand, the down-regulation of CD4 by Vpu and/or Nef requires the cytoplasmic domain of CD4 which is missing the chimeric receptor.[96-98] We, therefore, anticipate that the chimeric receptor will not be down-regulated by either Nef or Vpu.

Trapping CD4/Env by complex formation with Env in the endoplasmic reticulum, however, can still occur. To further down-regulate Env expression, the multitarget ribozyme was also directed against the ectodomain region of Env. This region does not overlap with any open-reading frames. For HIV-1 DI particle assembly, these mRNAs are needed for the continued expression of the structural and regulatory proteins of the virus. Engaging all Env protein molecules in an intracellular complex formation with CD4/Env, possibly by excess CD4/Env expression, would result in virus particles which are less infectious, simply because they carry fewer Env molecules. The transport of HIV-1 Env as well as CD4 or CD4/Env to the cell surface are hindered by complex formation, but also by the poor transport of Env itself.[99] Coexpression of a nonmembrane-bound CD4 protein or a protein which specifically binds to the CD4 binding site on Env, may help to achieve both: the neutralization of Env protein and a more efficient transport of the chimeric CD4/Env protein to the cell surface.

A soluble CD4 molecule which lacks the transmembrane and cytoplasmic domains but contains a KDEL retention signal at its carboxyl terminus, may be able to carry out such a function. This protein can inhibit Env protein transport to the cell surface.[90,100] The specificity of this interaction is very high, and most, if not all HIV-1 isolates could be affected. Similarly, the intracellular expression of a designer antibody, which consists of covalently linked variable regions of the heavy and light chains with a functional binding domain directed against the CD4 binding site of Env, also very effectively inhibited HIV-1 replication.[89] This antibody fragment specifically bound to Env intracellularly, inhibited its transport to the cell surface, and thereby, decreased the infectivity of the released virus without reducing the total number of released virus particles. This small antibody fragment could help generate the proposed DI particles by promoting the transport and thereby the insertion of CD4/Env into their envelope.

As indicated in Table 2, the suitability of an antiviral gene product for the proposed HIV-1 DI particle depends on its ability to decrease the infectivity of released virus by reducing the amount of functional HIV-1 Env protein, while keeping the total number of virus particles released from the cells high. These noninfectious virus particles represent the potential pool from which DI particles could be formed by altering the makeup of the envelope proteins and the genome. A select combination of these interfering mechanisms and their corresponding gene products have in part been encoded in the DI genomic RNAs as described in the following section.

Defective Interfering HIV-1 Proviral Genomes

We have assembled several defective prototype HIV-1 particle genomes (Fig. 5), starting with the infectious HIV-1 DNA clone pNL4-3.[101] A DNA region was deleted from the clone, starting with the translational start codon for the Gag polyprotein and including the last amino acid of the ectodomain region of the Env protein. This large deletion removes all the Gag and Pol sequences as well as the smaller genes Vpu and Vif, the first exons of Tat and Rev. It leaves the 5' LTR region and the leader sequence intact as well as the transmembrane and cytoplasmic regions of Env, the entire Nef coding regions, and the 3' LTR (compare with Figure 3A). This deleted region was precisely replaced by the coding region for the ectodomain of the human CD4 protein,[102] so that the translational start codon for CD4 substituted for the start codon of Gag. The DNA fusions resulted in an initial construct with two open-reading frames encoding a chimeric CD4 Env and Nef protein. In each subsequent DNA construct, the 5' portion of Nef was replaced stepwise by sequences of a monoribozyme, a Rev responsive element[103] and a multitarget ribozyme.[80] Expression of each of these DNAs depended on the transactivation in the presence of the HIV-1 Tat protein provided in trans for example by HIV-1 itself (data not shown).

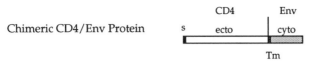

Chimeric CD4/Env Protein

Defective Interfering Proviral DNAs

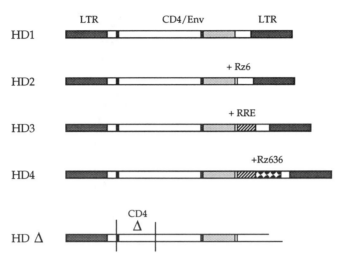

Fig. 5. Defective interfering HIV-1 proviral DNAs. The DNAs were assembled starting with the infectious HIV-1 clone pNL4-3,[101] and cDNA clone encoding the HIV-1 receptor, the human CD4 protein.[102] A chimeric CD4/Env encoding DNA was assembled by gene fusion, resulting in the ectodomain of CD4 including the signal peptide(s) precisely fused to the transmembrane (Tm) and the cytoplasmic domains (cyto) of Env. The chimeric gene was inserted into the pNL4-3 DNA, replacing the entire region from the translational start of Gag to the end of the ectodomain of Env (compare with Fig. 3A). With subsequent constructs, the Nef region was stepwise replaced by the monoribozyme Rz6,[80] a 240-nucleotide rev responsive element from pNL4-3 DNA,[103] and the nonaribozyme Rz636.[80] In the HD Δ constructs, the amino terminal portion of CD4/Env including the translational start codon were removed to yield HD1Δ, HD3Δ, and HD4Δ DNAs, respectively, preventing a functional CD4/Env protein expression.

Coexpression of any of these DNAs with HIV-1 proviral DNA in cotransfection assays results in an inhibition of HIV-1 replication in HIV-1 permissive cells, such as HeLa T4 cells (Fig. 6). A decrease in cell fusions as well as a decrease in infectious virus in cell supernatants was detected as measured by p24 Gag antigen release as well as by the total infectious virus titer release. In this assay, inhibition of virus spread was primarily caused by the expression of the chimeric receptor CD4/Env, since deletions within CD4/Env of HD1, HD3, and HD4 which abolish CD4/Env expression, partially restored HIV-1 replication (Fig. 6). The data also suggest that in cotransfection assays, HIV-1 DI vector DNA itself can also partially inhibit HIV-1 replication, possibly by competing for limited amounts of cellular or viral proteins needed for efficient expression.

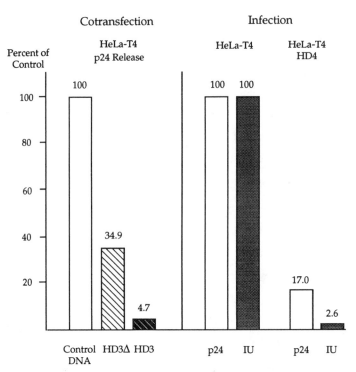

Fig. 6. Inhibition of HIV-1 replication by defective interfering HIV-1 provirus/DNA. Cotransfections of HIV-1 permissive HeLa T4 cells were carried out using lipofectin and a 1:20 ratio between pNL4-3 and an unrelated control DNA, HD3Δ or HD3 DNAs, respectively. Cell supernatants were collected daily for 5 days, combined, and the amount of released p24 antigen was determined by ELISA. HeLa-T4-HD4 cells were selected in the presence of hygromycin. The insertion of HD4 DNA was confirmed. HeLa-T4-HD4 cells and the parental HeLa-T4 cells were infected with HIV-1 stock from the supernatants of pNL4-3-transfected HeLa-T4 cells. Cell supernatants harvested 4 days postinfection were combined and the amounts of released p24 antigen were determined by ELISA. The infectivity of released virus (IU) was determined in parallel using a HeLa CD4-β-gal indicator cell line.[104]

An HIV-1 permissive HeLa-T4 cell line was selected which harbors one of the defective interfering HIV-1 proviruses (HD4). Upon challenge, HIV-1 was able to infect the cell as efficiently as the parental HeLa-T4 cell. After reverse transcription, the HIV-1 provirus also integrated into the cellular genome with approximately the same efficiency (data not shown). Despite this fact, the cell line with the HD4 provirus was dramatically less permissive for HIV-1 replication than without the HD4 provirus. Typical syncytia formation which was seen with control cells was absent or drastically reduced (data not shown). The amounts of released virus particles were reduced by 80% as measured by p24 antigen release (Fig. 6). In contrast, the amounts of infectious virus (IU) were reduced even greater, by more than 95%. This difference indicated that not only was the overall amount of released HIV-1 progeny decreased, the released virus also appeared to be less infectious. This strongly suggests that the makeup of released particles was altered possibly by the combined effects of both the coexpression of CD4/Env and the cleavage by the multitarget ribozyme. In addition, these results also indicated that HIV-1 DI proviruses can be transactivated upon HIV-1 infection, which in turn resulted in efficient interference with wild type virus replication.

This change in the makeup of the virus particles released from the HD4 cell line is promising for the generation of the proposed DI particles; however, two additional elements must still be functional with the DI proviruses: (a) their genomic RNAs must be efficiently packaged into infections particles; and (b) the DI particles must be able to target other HIV-1 Env-expressing cells. We have preliminary evidence that polyadenylated genomic DI RNA can indeed be packaged into virus particles, using either HIV-1 or a defective packaging helper virus construct, which we have developed (data not shown). The efficiency of packaging, however, is lower than with wild type virus. Currently, the packaging sequences for HIV-1 are not well defined. A picture of more complex sequence requirements appears to be emerging and more studies are needed to precisely define the cis-acting sequences.[105,106] CD4/Env has also not been detected on HIV-1 particles as yet but will be needed for targeting. The anticipated formation of complexes between CD4/Env and Env in the endoplasmic reticulum may be detrimental to CD4/Env transport to the cell surface. Co-expression of a nonmembrane-bound, chimeric antibody fragment, which specifically interacts with the CD4 binding site of Env may in the future help to totally inactivate Env and support the insertion of CD4/Env and/or another targeting protein into the viral envelope. The development of DNA constructs which include these additional elements are in progress.

There are several elements which must still be worked out and optimized to be able to assemble a defective interfering HIV-1 particle with the desired biologic properties. The complexity as well as safety require a high level of specificity on all levels. Expression levels of the different interfering gene products may need adjustment, and the coordinated used of alternate internal promoters or internal ribosome entry sites[107] will have to be employed to carry out all these functions from a single DI RNA transcript. In addition, a marker gene would be helpful to be able to follow the gene transfer quantitatively. The available rapid gene fusion procedures using synthetic oligonucleotides should allow a rearrangement of the sequences without serious technical limitations in the future. The final assembly of functional DI particles requires a detailed understanding of all processes of viral replication and pathogenesis. Thus, the basic understanding of the molecular biology of virus/DI virus and virus/host interactions becomes equally important to the ultimate goal of generating such HIV-1 DI particles.

Quantitating Infection Kinetics

Mathematical modeling of the kinetics of HIV-1 infection and disease progression have been carried out by Perelson et al.[108] Initially, they developed models to describe the long asymptomatic phase of HIV-1 infections. Since many parameters of the infection are still unknown, any mathematical model cannot with absolute certainty describe both the quantitative and qualitative effects of each parameter. Nevertheless, mathematical models can, despite these limitations, provide a better evaluation of the potential effects of some parameters, especially those values which can be estimated more realistically, such as infectivity, virus yield, cell killing, natural lifespan of uninfected and infected target cells, etc. Such evaluations were carried out by Perelson et al.,[108] initially focusing only on the population of T4 helper cells in the peripheral blood. Many other compartments in which the virus also replicates in the infected patients were not considered by the simplified model at the time.

Starting from these models, Perelson and Nelson subsequently developed a model which included coinfections with our hypothetical HIV-1 DI particles.[109] A model for its coinfection with HIV-1 was formulated and various numerical values were assigned to several parameters. In summary, their study suggested that only with highly optimistic values and only under the most favorable conditions, would the DI particle have a chance to down-regulate the HIV-1 load. This would take several years. Under less favorable conditions, however, which are more realistic, the DI particles would be lost from the cell population, as it would occur with most naturally occurring DI particles. This was not unexpected, since the model only describes T4 lymphocyte infections in the peripheral blood, where there is a low density of HIV-1-expressing cells as well as a high fluidity, which are not favorable for superinfections even by a targeted virus.

Infection kinetics in lymph nodes, however, can be expected to be quite different and much more favorable for DI particle replication, because of the high density of HIV-1-expressing cells and the decreased mobility of the cells. Under these conditions, the DI particles will have a much better chance to replicate in HIV-1-expressing cells and thereby have a chance to survive within this compartment, which appears to be the main reservoir of persistently infected cells. We anticipate that any potential HIV-1 DI particle therapy would take several years to be effective, especially since the wild type virus is already established before the addition of the DI particles. If the DI particles, however are able to deliver the inhibitory elements to HIV-1-infected cells, we anticipate that after a certain time, an equilibrium between wild type virus and DI particles may form, which could limit the total number of HIV-1-infected cells. Thus, the selective disadvantage of many naturally occurring DI particles would be offset by the cell targeting and the specifically adapted interference mechanisms encoded by the DI genome itself, mechanisms which would cooperate to promote DI particle replication at the expense of HIV-1. This could potentially limit or decrease virus load which could lead to a significant delay in the onset of AIDS.

Safety

Over a long period of time, the effectiveness of this strategy will depend on the rate at which HIV-1 generates escape mutants and how quickly they are selected. The targets for interference have specifically been chosen to involve highly conserved interactions between virus and cells, such as the interaction between CD4 and Env, which at the same time do not inhibit virus particle formation. The dependency of the virus on the functionality of these interactions will greatly determine the length of the therapy's effectiveness.

The continuous mutational changes of the HIV-1 genome during the many years of the asymptomatic phase of the infection is a characteristic not only for HIV-1 but for all viruses and in particular RNA viruses, which leads to the generation of a quasispecies.[69,110,111] Some genomic changes are subsequently selected if they promote viral replication. Dramatic changes may arise more quickly through recombinational events. Moreover, the presence of a defective virus can increase pathogenesis in the case of feline and murine immuno-deficiency viruses.[16,17] These examples demonstrate that during coinfections, complementation and/or recombinational events can take place which could undesirably lead to a more pathogenic virus. With the defective HIV-1 genomes proposed here, no complete viral genes are encoded. All sequences which are present in the DI particle are either of cellular origin or completely synthetic, such as the ribozymes. This drastically reduces the possibility of homologous recombinations. Future experiments will have to indicate whether the 5' and 3' LTRs of the DI virus genome itself are sufficient to complement other endogenous defective HIV-1 proviruses, and if they could have an effect on disease progression. Alternatively, the gene products themselves could elicit an immune response which may eliminate the DI-infected cell altogether. Since the DI particle infected cell would also contain HIV-1, it is not possible to evaluate whether this would be beneficial or detrimental to the strategy.

With HIV-1 infections, the induction of neoplastic transformation of cells does not appear to play a significant role if at all. This will most likely also apply to DI particles. The presence and potential biological roles of defective HIV-1 particles have not been studied in detail as yet. With the related simian immunodeficiency virus (SIV), defective SIV proviral genomes increase with disease progression; this probably reflects the increased virus load in later stages of the infection rather than the cause of the increased pathogenesis. Currently, there is no evidence that these defective proviruses or the proposed DI particles would help disease progression or cause any other undesirable side effects.

Until now, there has been no animal model which could be used to study the effectiveness and safety of HIV-1 DI particles *in vivo*. This complicates the potential initial evaluation of these particles as antiviral agents. HIV-1-infected chimpanzees may present the only animal model to study the safety and possibly the spread of the interfering genes as well as their effect on virus load. In fact, the infection of chimpanzees with the high prevalence of HIV-1 in lymph nodes may be an adequate model for the asymptomatic phase of the human HIV-1 infection.[112] Since none of the infected chimpanzees have become immuno-deficient until now, use of this model will be limited as can be expected for any other model. The proposed antiviral strategy would most likely require several years of the asymptomatic phase of the infection to reach the anticipated equilibrium with wild type virus. The infection of nonhuman primates with SIV-1 usually spreads very rapidly.[113] Although functionally equivalent defective interfering SIV-1 particles could be developed, the disease progression may not allow sufficient time for the SIV-1 DI particle to become established in the animal. The use of the SIV-1 model may, therefore, be limited.

Finally, to be able to employ DI particles in any antiviral trials, they will have to amplified to high numbers, in the absence of wild type HIV-1. This should be possible by generating helper virus cell lines which can constitutively supply all the structural proteins for the DI particle without the formation of infectious virus through recombinational events. We have evidence (data not shown) that this could be achieved by coexpressing the structural and regulatory proteins of the virus in the same cell from several template sources.

Note

Multitarget ribozymes and CD4/Env encoding defective interfering HIV-1 genomes were first presented by M.S. in 1991 at the International AIDS Meeting of the Laboratory of Tumor Cell Virology, National Cancer Institute, National Institutes of Health, Bethesda, Maryland.

REFERENCES

1. J.J. Holland. Defective viral genomes, *in:* "Virology," B.N. Fields, D.M. Knipe, eds., Raven Press, New York (1990).
2. J.M. Coffin. Retroviridae and their replication, *in:* "Virology," B.N. Fields, D.M. Knipe, eds., Raven Press, New York (1990).
3. T. Benjamin, and P.K. Vogt. Cell transformation by viruses, *in:* "Virology," B.N. Fields, D.M. Knipe, eds., Raven Press, New York (1990).
4. P. von Magnus. Studies on interference in experimental influenza. I. Biological observations. *Mineral. Geol.* 24:1 (1947).
5. P. von Magnus. Incomplete forms of influenza virus. *Adv. Virus Res.* 2:59 (1954).
6. A.D.T. Barrett, and N.J. Dimmock. Defective interfering viruses and infections of animals. *Curr. Topics Microbiol. Immun.* 128:55 (1986).
7. A.S. Huang, and D. Baltimore. Defective interfering animal viruses, *in:* "Comprehensive Virology," H. Fraenkel-Conrat, R.P. Wagner, eds., Plenum Press, New York (1977).
8. R.A. Lazzarini, J.D. Keene, and M. Schubert. The origins of defective interfering particles of the negative-strand RNA viruses. *Cell* 26:1456 (1981).
9. D. Nayak, T. Chambers, and R. Akkina. Defective interfering (DI) RNAs of influenza viruses: origin, structure, expression and interference. *Curr. Topics Microbiol. Immunol.* 114:103 (1985).
10. M. Nonoyama, and A.F. Graham. Appearance of defective virions in clones of reovirus. *J. Virol.* 6:693 (1970).
11. J. Perrault. Origin and replication of defective interfering particles. *Curr. Topics Microbiol. Immunol.* 93:151 (1981).
12. L. Roux, A.E. Simon, and J.J. Holland. Effects of defective interfering virus

on virus replication and pathogenesis. *Adv. Virus Res.* 40:181 (1991).

13. S. Schlesinger. The generation and amplification of defective interfering RNAs, *in:* "RNA Genetics," E. Domingo, J.J. Holland, P. Ahlquist, eds. CRC Press, Boca Raton, Florida (1988).

14. P. Calain, and L.Roux. Generation of measles virus defective interfering particles and their presence in a preparation of attenuated live-virus vaccine. *J. Virol.* 62:2859 (1988).

15. A.S. Huang, and D. Baltimore. Defective viral particles and viral disease processes. *Nature* 226:325 (1970).

16. H.C. Dhattopadhyay, H.C. Morse III, M. Makino, S.K. Ruscetti, and J.W. Hartley. Defective virus is associated with induction of murine retrovirus-induced immunodeficiency syndrome. *Proc. Natl. Acad. Sci. USA* 86:3862 (1989).

17. J. Oberbraugh, P.R. Donahue, E.A. Quackenbush, E.A. Hoover, and J.I. Mullins. Molecular cloning of a feline leukemia virus that induces fatal immunodeficiency disease in cats. *Science* 239:906 (1988).

18. A.S. Fauci. The human immunodeficiency virus: infectivity and mechanisms of pathogenesis. *Science* 239:617 (1988).

19. R.I. Connor, I. Mohri, Y. Cao, and D.D. Ho. Increased viral burden and cytopathicity correlate temporally with CD4+ T-lymphocyte decline and clinical progression in human immunodeficiency virus type 1-infected individuals. *J.Virol.* 67:1772 (1993).

20. A. Meyerhans, R. Cheynier, J. Albert, et al. Temporal fluctuations in HIV quasispecies *in vivo* are not reflected by sequential HIV isolates. *Cell* 58:901 (1989).

21. E. Norby, and M.N. Oxman. Measles virus, *in:* "Virology," B.N. Fields, D.M. Knipe, eds., Raven Press, New York (1990).

22. R. Cattaneo, A. Schmid, D. Eschle, et al. Biased hypermutation and other genetic changes in defective measles viruses in human brain infections. *Cell* 55:255 (1988).

23. J. Embretson, M. Zupancic, J.L. Ribas, et al. Massive covert infection of helper T lymphocytes and macrophages by HIV during the incubation period of AIDS. *Nature* 362:359 (1993).

24. G. Pantaleo, C. Graziosi, J.F. Demarest, et al. HIV infection is active and progressive in lymphoid tissue during the clinically latent stage of disease. *Nature* 362:355 (1993).

25. D. Baltimore. Intracellular immunization. *Nature* 335:395 (1988).

26. M. Dubois-Dalcq, C.A. Jordan, W.B. Kelly, and B.A. Watkins. Understanding HIV-1 infection of the brain: a challenge for neurobiologists. *AIDS* 5:567 (1991).

27. S. Koenig, H.E. Gendelman, M.J. Orenstein, et al. Detection of AIDS virus in macrophages in brain tissue from AIDS patients with encephalopathy. *Science* 233:1089 (1986).

28. B.A. Watkins, H.H. Dorn, W.B. Kelly, et al. Specific tropism of HIV-1 for microglial cells in primary human brain cultures. *Science* 249:549 (1990).

29. C. Tornatore, A. Nath, K. Amemiya, and E.O. Major. Persistent human immunodeficiency virus type 1 infection in human fetal glial cells reactivated by T-cell factors or by the cytokines tumor factor alpha and interleukin-1 beta. *J. Virol.* 65:6094 (1991).

30. C.A. Wiley, R.D. Schrier, J.A. Nelson, P.W. Lampert, and M. Oldstone. Cellular localization of human immunodeficiency virus infection within the brains of acquired immune deficiency syndrome patients. *Proc. Natl. Acad. Sci. USA* 83:7089 (1986).

31. R.T. Johnson, J.C. McArthur, and O. Narayan. The neurobiology of human immunodeficiency virus infections. *FASEB J.* 2:2970 (1988).

32. R.J. McLachlin, K. Cornetta, M.A. Eglitis, and F.W. Anderson. Retroviralmediated gene transfer. *Progr. Nucleic Acid Res. and Mol. Biol.* 38:91 (1990).

33. R.C. Mulligan. The basic science of gene therapy. *Science* 260:926 (1993).

34. I. Bahner, C.Zhou, X.-J. Yu, et al. Comparison of trans-dominant inhibitory

mutant immunodeficiency virus type 1 genes expressed by retroviral vectors in human T lymphocytes. *J. Virol.* 67:3199 (1993).

35. D. Bevec, M. Dobrovnik, J. Hauber, and E. Boehnlein. Inhibition of human immunodeficiency virus type 1 replication in human T cells by retroviral-mediated gene transfer of a dominant-negative Rev trans-activator. *Proc. Natl. Acad. Sci. USA* 89:9870 (1992).

36. E.O. Freed, E.L. Delwart, G.L. Buchschacher, and A.T. Panganiban. A mutation in the human immunodeficiency virus type 1 transmembrane glycoprotein gp41 dominantly interferes with fusion and infectivity. *Proc. Natl. Acad. Sci. USA* 89:70 (1992).

37. M. Green, M. Ishino, and P.M. Loewenstein. Mutational analysis of HIV-1 Tat minimal domain peptides: identification of trans-dominant mutants that suppress HIV-LTR-driven gene expression. *Cell* 58:215 (1989).

38. M.H. Malim, S. Bohnlein, J,. Hauber, and B.R. Cullen. Functional dissection of the HIV-1 rev transactivator - derivation of a trans-dominant repressor of rev function. *Cell* 58:205 (1989).

39. D. Trono, M.B. Feinberg, and D. Baltimore. HIV-1 gag mutants can dominantly interfere with the replication of the wild type virus. *Cell* 59:113 (1989).

40. M.S. Hirsch, and J. Curran. Human immunodeficiency viruses, *in:* "Virology," B.N. Fields, D.M. Knipe, eds., Raven Press, New York (1990).

41. A.G. Dalgleish, P.C.L. Beverly, P.R. Clapham, et al. The CD4 (T4) antigen is an essential component of the receptor for the AIDS retrovirus. *Nature* 312:763 (1984).

42. D. Klatzman, E. Champagne, S. Chamaret, et al. T lymphocyte T4 molecule behaves as the receptor for human retrovirus LAV. *Nature* 312:767 (1984).

43. P.J. Maddon, A.G. Dalgleish, J.S. McDougal, et al. The T4 gene encodes the AIDS virus receptor and is expressed in the immune system and the brain. *Cell* 47:333 (1986).

44. P. Clapham, J.N. Weber, D. Whitby, et al. Soluble CD4 blocks the infectivity of diverse strains of HIV and SIV for T cells and monocytes but not for brain and muscle cells. *Nature (Lond.)* 337:268 (1989).

45. V.K. Chaudhary, T. Mizukami, T.R. Fuerst, et al. Selective killing of HIV-infected cells by recombinant human CD4-Pseudomonas exotoxin hybrid protein. *Nature* 335:369 (1988).

46. J.C. Burns, T. Friedmann, W. Driever, M. Burrascano, and J.-K. Yee. Vesicular stomatitis virus G glycoprotein pseudotyped retroviral vectors: concentration to very high titer and efficient gene transfer into mammalian and nonmammalian cells. *Proc. Natl. Acad. Sci. USA* 90:8033 (1993).

47. R.A. Weiss. Rhabdovirus pseudotypes, *in:* "Rhabdoviruses," D.H.L. Bishop, ed. CRC Press, Boca Raton, Florida (1980).

48. J. Zavada. The pseudotypic paradox. *J. Gen.Virol.* 63:15 (1982).

49. N.R. Landau, K.A. Page, and D.R. Littman. Pseudotyping with human T-cell leukemia virus type 1 broadens the human immunodeficiency virus host range. *J.Virol.* 65:162 (1991).

50. P. Lusso, F. Veronese, B. Ensoli, et al. Expanded HIV-1 cellular tropism by phenotypic mixing with murine endogenous retroviruses. *Science* 247:848 (1990).

51. D.H. Spector, E. Wafde, D.A. Wright, et al. Human immunodeficiency virus pseudotypes with expanded cellular and species tropism. *J. Virol.* 64:2298 (1990).

52. Z. Zhu, S. Chen, and A.S. Huang. Pseudotypes of human immunodeficiency virus (HIV) with the envelope antigens of vesicular stomatitis virus (VSV) or herpes simplex virus (HSV), *in:* "Vth International Conference on AIDS," Montreal, Canada (1989).

53. L.M. Little, G. Lanman, and A.S. Huang. Immunoprecipitating human antigens associated with vesicular stomatitis virus grown in HeLa cells. *Virology* 129:127 (1983).

54. X. Yu, X. Yuan, Z. Matsuda, T.-H. Lee, and M. Essex. The matrix protein of

human immunodeficiency virus type 1 is required for incorporation of viral envelope protein into mature virions. *J. Virol.* 66:4966 (1992).

55. M. Jasin, K.A. Page, and D.R. Littman. Glycosylphosphatidylinositol-anchored CD4/Thy-1 chimeric molecules serve as human immunodeficiency virus receptors in human,but not mouse, cells and are modulated by gangliosides. *J. Virol.* 65:440 (1991).

56. M. Schubert, B. Joshi, D. Blondel, and G.G. Harmison. Insertion of the human immunodeficiency virus CD4 receptor into the envelope of vesicular stomatitis virus. *J. Virol.* 66:1579 (1992).

57. J.A.T. Young, P. Bates, K. Willert, and H.E. Varmus. Efficient incorporation of human CD4 protein into avian leukosis virus particles. *Science* 250:1421 (1990).

58. K.E. Dolter, S.R. King, and T.C. Holland. Incorporation of CD4 into virions by a recombinant herpes simplex virus. *J. Virol.* 67:189 (1993).

59. A. Puri, D.S. Dimitrov, H. Golding, and R. Blumenthal. Interactions of CD4 + plasma membrane vesicles with HIV-1 and HIV-1 envelope glycoprotein-expressing cells. *J. AIDS* 5:915 (1992).

60. P.A. Ashorn, E.A. Berger, and B. Moss. Human immunodeficiency virus envelope glycoprotein/CD4-mediated fusion of nonprimate cells with human cells. *J. Virol.* 64:2149 (1990).

61. R.D. Harrington, and A.P. Geballe. Cofactor requirement for human immunodeficiency virus type 1 entry into a CD4-expressing human cell line. *J. Virol.* 67:5939 (1993).

62. S. Bhat, S.L. Spitalnik, F. Gonzalez-Scarano, and D. H. Silberberg. Galactosyl ceramide or a derivative is an essential component of the neural receptor for human immunodeficiency virus type 1 envelope glycoprotein gp120. *Proc. Natl. Acad. Sci. USA* 88:7131 (1991).

63. J. Fantini, D.G. Cook, N. Nathanson, S.L. Spitalnik, and F. Gonzalez-Scarano. Infection of colonic epithelial cell lines by type 1 human immunodeficiency virus is associated with cell surface expression of galactosylceramide, a potential alternative gp120 receptor. *Proc. Natl. Acad. Sci. USA* 90:2700 (1993).

64. C. Callebaut, B. Krust, E. Jacotot, and A.G. Hovanessian. T cell activation antigen, CD26, as a cofactor for entry of HIV in CD4 + cells. *Science* 262:2045 (1993).

65. H. Sato, J. Orenstein, D. Dimitrov, and M. Martin. Cell-to-cell spread of HIV-1 occurs within minutes and may not involve the participation of virus particles. *Virology* 186:712 (1992).

66. O. Naryan, and J.E. Clements. Lentiviruses, *in*: "Virology," B.N. Fields, D.M. Knipe, eds. Raven Press, New York (1990).

67. M.I. Bukrinsky, N. Sharova, M.P. Dempsey, et al. Active nuclear import of human immunodeficiency virus type 1 preintegration complexes. *Proc. Natl. Acad. Sci.* 89:6580 (1992).

68. K. Cichutek, H. Merget, S. Norley, et al. Development of a quasispecies of human immunodeficiency virus type 1 *in vivo*. *Proc. Natl. Acad. Sci. USA* 89:7365 (1992).

69. J.M. Coffin. Genetic variation in AIDS viruses. *Cell* 46:1 (1986).

70. S. Gartner, P. Markovitz, M.D. Markovitz, et al. The role of mononuclear phagocytes in HLTV III/LAV infection. *Science* 233:215 (1986).

71. J.H. Kim, M.T. Vahey, R.J. McLinden, et al. Consequences of HIV-1 superinfection of chronically infected cells. *J. Cell. Biochem.* Suppl.17E:50 (1993).

72. M. LaGuern, and J.A. Levy. Human immunodeficiency virus (HIV) type 1 can superinfect HIV-2-infected cells: pseudotype virions produced with expanded cellular host range. *Proc. Natl. Acad. Sci., USA* 89:363 (1992).

73. K. Ohki, M. Kishi, K. Ohmura, et al. Human immunodeficiency virus type 1 (HIV-1) superinfection of a cell clone converting it from production of defective to infectious HIV-1 is mediated predominantly by CD4 regions other than the major binding site for HIV-1 glycoproteins. *J. Gen. Virol.* 73:1761 (1992).

74. M. Yunoki, K. Maotani-Imai, H. Kusuda, et al. Production of infectious par-

ticles from defective human immunodeficiency virus type 1 (HIV-1)-pro-
ducing cell clones by superinfection with infectious HIV-1. *Arch. Virol.*
116:143 (1991).
75. B. Taddeo, M. Federico, F. Titti, G.B. Rossi, and P. Verani. Homologous
superinfection of both producer and nonproducer HIV-infected cells is
blocked at a late retrotranscription step. *Virology* 194:441 (1993).
76. G.K. von Dalnok, A. Kleinschmidt, M. Neumann, et al. Productive
expression state confers resistance of human immunodeficiency virus
(HIV)-2-infected lymphoma cells against superinfection by HIV-1. *Arch.
Virol.* 131:419 (1993).
77. S.-Y. Paik, A.C. Banerjea, and M. Schubert. Transactivation of the vesicular
stomatitis virus matrix protein expression inhibits HIV-1 replication. *J.
Cell. Biochem.* Suppl.17E:35 (1993).
78. J. Lisziewicz, D. Sun, J. Smythe, et al. Inhibition of human immunodeficiency virus type 1 replication by regulated expression of a polymeric Tat
activation response RNA decoy as a strategy for gene therapy in AIDS.
Proc. Natl. Acad. Sci. USA 90:8000 (1993).
79. S. Chatterjee, P.R. Johnson, and K.K. Wong. Dual-target inhibition of HIV-
1 *in vitro* by means of an adeno-associated virus antisense vector. *Science*
258:1485 (1992).
80. C.-J. Chen, A.C. Banerjea, G.G. Harmison, K. Haglund, and M. Schubert.
Multitarget ribozyme directed to cleave at up to nine highly conserved
HIV-1 env RNA regions inhibits HIV-1 replication: potential effectiveness against most presently sequenced HIV-1 isolates. *Nucleic Acid Res.*
17:4581 (1992).
81. B. Dropulic, N.H. Lin, M.A. Martin, and K.-T. Jeang. Functional characterization of a U5 ribozyme: intracellular suppression of human immunodeficiency virus type 1 expression. *J. Virol.* 66:1432 (1992).
82. S. Joshi, A. Van Brunschot, S. Asad, et al. Inhibition of human immunodeficiency virus type 1 multiplication by antisense and sense RNA
expression. *J. Virol.* 65:5524 (1991).
83. K.M.S. Lo, M.A. Biasolo, G. Dehni, G. Palue, and W.A. Haseltine. Inhibition
of replication of HIV-1 by retroviral vectors expressing tat-antisense and
anti-tat ribozyme RNA. *Virology* 190:176 (1992).
84. N. Sarver, E.M. Cantin, P.S. Chang, et al. Ribozymes as potential anti-HIV-
1 therapeutic agents. *Science* 247:1222 (1990).
85. M. Weerasinghe, S.E. Liem, S. Asad, S.E. Read, and S. Joshi. Resistance to
human immunodeficiency virus type 1 (HIV-1) infection in human
CD4 + lymphocyte-derived cell lines conferred by using retroviral vectors
expressing an HIV-1 RNA-specific ribozyme. *J.Virol.* 65:5531 (1991).
86. T.R. Cech. The chemistry of self-splicing RNA and RNA enzymes. *Science*
236:1532 (1987).
87. J. Haselhoff, and W.L. Gerlach. Simple RNA enzymes with new and highly
specific endoribonuclease activities. *Nature* 334:585 (1988).
88. O.C. Uhlenbeck. A small catalytic oligoribonucleotide. *Nature* 328:596
(1987).
89. W.A. Marasco, W.A. Haseltine, and S.-Y. Chen. Design, intracellular expression, and activity of a human anti-human immunodeficiency virus
type 1 gp120 single-chain antibody. *Proc. Natl. Acad. Sci. USA* 90:7889
(1993).
90. B. Crise, L. Buonocore, and J.K. Rose. CD4 is retained in the endoplasmic
reticulum by the human immunodeficiency virus type 1 glycoprotein precursor. *J. Virol.* 64:5585 (1990).
91. M.A. Jabbar, and D.P. Nayak. Intracellular interaction of human immunodeficiency virus type 1 (ARV-2) envelope glycoprotein gp160 with CD4
blocks the movement and maturation of CD4 to the plasma membrane.
J. Virol. 64:6297 (1990).
92. I. Kawamura, Y. Koga, N. Oh-Nori, et al. Depletion of surface CD4 molecule
by the envelope protein of human immunodeficiency virus expressed in a
human CD4 + monocytoid cell line. *J. Virol.* 63:3748 (1989).
93. W.L. Marshall, D.C. Diamond, M.M. Kowalski, and R.W. Finberg. High

level of surface CD4 prevents stable human immunodeficiency virus infection in T-cell transformants. *J. Virol.* 66:5492 (1992).

94. R.L. Wiley, F. Maldarelli, M.A. Martin, and K. Strebel. Human immuno-deficiency virus type 1 vpu protein regulates the formation of intra-cellular gp160-CD4 complexes. *J. Virol.* 66:226 (1992).

95. J.V. Garcia, and A.D. Miller. Serine phosphorylation-independent down regulation of cell surface CD4 by nef. *Nature* 350:508 (1991).

96. M.-Y. Chen, F. Maldarelli, M.K. Karczewski, et al. Human immunode-ficiency virus type 1 vpu protein induces degradation of CD4 *in vitro*: the cytoplasmic domain of CD4 contributes to vpu sensitivity. *J. Virol.* 67:3877 (1993).

97. J.V. Garcia, J. Alfano, and A.D. Miller. The negative effect of human immunodeficiency virus type 1 nef on cell surface CD4 expression is not species specific and requires the cytoplasmic domain of CD4. *J. Virol.* 67:1511 (1993).

98. M.J. Vincent, N.U. Raja, and M. Jabbar. Human immunodeficiency virus type 1 vpu protein induces degradation of chimeric envelope glycopro-teins bearing the cytoplasmic and anchor domains of CD4: role of the cytoplasmic domain in vpu-induced degradation in the endoplasmic reticulum. *J.Virol.* 67:5538 (1993).

99. O.K. Haffar, G.R. Nakamura, and P.W. Berman. The carboxy terminus of human immunodeficiency virus type 1 gp160 limits its proteolytic pro-cessing and transport in transfected cell lines. *J. Virol.* 64:3100 (1990).

100. L. Buonocore, and J.K. Rose. Prevention of HIV-1 glycoprotein transport by soluble CD4 retained in the endoplasmic reticulum. *Nature* 345:625 (1990).

101. A. Adachi, H.E. Gendelman, S. Koenig, et al. Production of acquired immunodeficiency syndrome associated retrovirus in human and non-human cells transfected with an infectious molecular clone. *J. Virol.* 59:284 (1986).

102. P.J. Maddon, D.R. Littman, M. Godfry, et al. The isolation and nucleotide sequence of a cDNA encoding the T cell surface protein T4: a new mem-ber of the immunoglobulin gene gamily. *Cell* 42:93 (1985).

103. H.M. Malim, J. Hauber, L. Shu-Yun, et al. The HIV-1 rev trans-activator acts through a structured target sequence to activate nuclear export of unspliced viral mRNA. *Nature* 338:254 (1989).

104. J. Kimpton, and M. Emerman. Detection of replication-competent and pseudotyped human immunodeficiency virus with a sensitive cell line on the basis of activation of an integrated beta-galactosidase gene. *J. Virol.* 66:2232 (1992).

105. A. Aldovini, and R.A. Young. Mutations of RNA and protein sequences in-volved in human immunodeficiency virus type 1 packaging result in pro-duction of noninfectious virus. *J. Virol.* 64:1920 (1990).

106. J. H. Richardson, L.A. Child, and A.M.L. Lever. Packaging of human immunodeficiency virus type 1 RNA requires cis-acting sequences out-side the 5' leader region. *J. Virol.* 67:3997 (1993).

107. R.A. Morgan, L. Couture, O. Elroy-Stein, et al. Retroviral vectors con-taining putative internal ribosome entry sites: development of a poly-cistronic gene transfer system and applications to human gene therapy. *Nucl. Acids Res.* 20:1293 (1992).

108. A.S. Perelson, D.E. Kirschner, G.W. Nelson, R. DeBoer. The dynamics of HIV infection of CD4+ T cells. *Math. Biosci.* 114:81 (1993).

109. G.W. Nelson, and A.S. Perelson. Modeling defective interfering virus therapy for AIDS. I. Conditions for their survival. (in preparation)

110. M. Eigen. Self-organization of matter and the evolution of biological macromolecules. *Naturwissenschaften* 58:65 (1973).

111. J. Holland, S. Katherine, F. Horodyski, et al. Rapid evolution of RNA genomes. *Science* 215:1577 (1982).

112. K. Saksela, E. Muchmore, M. Girard, P. Fultz, and D. Baltimore. High viral loads in lymph nodes and latent human immunodeficiency virus

(HIV) in peripheral blood cells of HIV-1-infected chimpanzees. *J. Virol.* 67:7423 (1993).

113. H.W. Kestler III, D.J. Ringler, K. Mori, et al. Importance of the nef gene for maintenance of high virus loads and for development of AIDS. *Cell* 65:651 (1991).

FOCUS ON AIDS AND THE NERVOUS SYSTEM: CHALLENGES DURING THE DECADE OF THE BRAIN

TREATMENT OF NEUROLOGICAL COMPLICATIONS IN AIDS: THE AIDS CLINICAL TRIALS GROUP IN THE 1990s

David B. Clifford

Department of Neurology
Washington University School of Medicine
Box 8111, 660 South Euclid Avenue
St. Louis, Missouri 63110

INTRODUCTION

An epidemic of a new infectious disease challenges mankind to respond at multiple levels. Working in medicine in the 1990s leads us to confront the complex challenge of human immunodeficiency virus. By *in vitro* and animal experimental models, we must explore the biology of this infection. Our scientific training recognizes that the most precise way to advance our knowledge is to gain control over as much of the experiment as possible. This can be accomplished in laboratory experiments and is an essential task. By such investigation, more has been learned about HIV than any other virus discovered. Expanding knowledge about the molecular and pathophysiolgic aspects of virology provide increasing hope for new ways to stem this epidemic. However, the name of our opponent in this battle is the <u>human</u> immunodeficiency virus, and it certain that in the end, the only test that will truly matter is whether the knowledge we rough out in simpler systems also can be applied to help infected patients.

Here the challenge of our adversary manifests its great complexity. Not only is there a new and cunning virus incessantly destroying its hosts, but in addition, the host is challenged by multiple simultaneous insults from other often innocuous agents, and by mediators of the defensive battle. The terrain for this conflict varies, prepared in different ways by genetic heritage and prior medical conditions. In the final analysis, each case is unique, making collective judgments about the pathophysiology and results of therapy far more tentative than under controlled experimental conditions.

While the challenge of HIV represents as overly complicated a clinical milieu for research as one can imagine, in truth it is only somewhat more challenging than the usual clinical situation. Controlled clinical trials have become the most convincing means of addressing the critical scientific treatment issues in patients. Recognizing that the "bottom line" in AIDS research is the applicability and success of treatment in patients, the National Institute of Allergy and Infectious Diseases (NIAID) of the National Institutes of Health organized the AIDS Clinical Trial Group (ACTG) to put into place the "biotechnology" necessary to provide answers about the utility of many approaches to HIV therapy.

Technical Advances in AIDS Research in the Human Nervous System
Edited by E.O. Major and J.A. Levy, Plenum Press, New York, 1995

THE AIDS CLINICAL TRIALS GROUP

The current ACTG system consists of 59 units, including pediatric and adult AIDS Clinical Trial Units (ACTUs). With the funding of the ACTUs, trial units complete with local leadership, clinical research personnel including investigators and study nurses, research pharmacies, logistical support for immunology, pharmacology and virology, and data management and statistical design has been assembled. Supporting these units as a part of the ACTG system are two other organizations: (a) the Division of AIDS (DAIDS) Programs; and (b) data and operations support contracts including the Statistics and Data Analysis Center (SDAC) of the Harvard School of Public Health.

These components (ACTUs, DAIDS, SDAC) comprise the ACTG system and cooperatively perform a wide range of scientific planning and coordinating functions related to the conduct of clinical trials. Included among those functions are: assessment of treatment research needs; establishment of scientific priorities among these needs; development of new research protocols addressing these priorities; implementation and analyses of these studies; and the establishment of quality control programs to ensure that accurate data are collected.

The scientific investigators at the ACTUs, through scientific committees and the Executive Committee, with assistance from other agencies, develop a scientific agenda, set priorities for clinical trials, and initiate development of protocols. ACTU investigators initiate most of the ideas for clinical trials.

The group maintains a focus on human immunodeficiency virus (HIV) and its complications, seeking to perform treatment studies rather than attempting to be an epidemiologic study group. All ACTUs perform primary antiviral studies and studies of common opportunistic infections. Implementation of the ACTU structure has resulted in substantial productivity, particularly in the area of anti-retroviral therapeutics and opportunistic infections in HIV. The ACTG probably represents the largest coordinated clinical trial group in the world. It functions as a magnet to HIV patients seeking new therapies. This system follows a substantial population of subjects who could participate in HIV-related neurologic trials. At present, more than 20,000 subjects have participated in over 200 ACTU-supported studies since its inception in 1986.

NEUROLOGY IN THE AIDS CLINICAL TRIAL GROUP

Neurologic HIV involvement is such a prevalent and critical part of the disability experienced by HIV-infected individuals that it must be a crucial target for clinical trials. The distinct possibility of a therapy that is effective against HIV, but fails to control the infection in the brain, leaving its hosts neurologically disabled, would be a tragic failure. Consequently, the ACTG has recognized that continued evaluation of the impact of therapies on neuroAIDS, along with efforts to target specific neurologic complications of the immune deficient state, are significant priorities for clinical research in HIV.

Our efforts to actualize the potential of the ACTG system for neurologic clinical trials has met serious challenges. Among these have been formulation of appropriate ideas for our clinical studies, identifying a cadre of committed investigators, and developing the necessary systems and support. An effective trial system will encourage the synergistic interaction of dedicated people and persuasive ideas to generate discovery and progress.

Our greatest challenge is to develop better ideas about how to approach neurologic AIDS complications. At the onset of the epidemic, there was substantial uncertainty, if not doubt, that the HIV virus had important effects on the brain. Victims of the virus were critically ill and dying, and the change in personality, affect and behavior observed must surely be the consequence of the crushing psychologic impact of the disease along with the systemic impact of the illness. While these interpretations of changes in neurologic performance and behavior remain aspects of the challenge of neuroAIDS, it became apparent several years into the epidemic, that HIV not only entered the brain at an early stage of infection, but resulted in several characteristic changes in thinking and behavior, correlating with distinctive neuropathologic changes. Drs. Richard Price, John Sidtis, Brad Navia[1,2] and their colleagues described the clinical and neuropathologic characteristics of this HIV-related brain disease which they named AIDS dementia complex (ADC). This entity became the prime target of neuroAIDS attention over the ensuing years. I shall refer to this clinical syndrome of central nervous (CNS) system involvement due to HIV as AIDS dementia complex, recognizing the variety of other names that have been applied to it by various investigators, each with its special advantages. However, both because of the frequency of the syndrome, and the severe degradation in the quality of life for patients when it occurs, it has been an important entity for clinical investigation.

AIDS DEMENTIA COMPLEX (ADC)

The ACTG neurology group directed its attention to evaluating the usefulness of the new anti-retroviral drugs for the dementia complex. With a new disease entity, it was important to find appropriate techniques to study it clinically. While changes in brain imaging, cerebrospinal fluid (CSF) findings, or electrophysiologic data might be highly useful, none of these approaches has been practical for quantitative evaluation of ADC in trials. However, the licensing study for zidovudine included a component of neuropsychologic testing under the direction of Dr. Fred Schmidt,[3] which revealed significant improvements in performance of treated AIDS patients receiving zidovudine for the first time. Drs. Price and Sidtis led an effort within the ACTG to develop neuropsychometric testing to follow the course of HIV in the brain. Certainly as dementia develops, these tests provide a reliable indicator of worsening disease. However, a challenge for future investigations is refining our ability to quantitate the impact of HIV in more specific and sensitive ways.

The hope that we are dealing with a potentially treatable and reversible dementia fueled enthusiasm for further studies of ADC. The ACTG organized a double-blind, placebo-controlled study of zidovudine for ADC (protocol 005). After only 40 subjects had been studied, the protocol was terminated because evidence that zidovudine was beneficial to AIDS patients suggested it was not ethical to withhold the drug for the placebo arm of the study. Even with the small numbers enrolled it this study, it was possible to confirm that, at least for a time, zidovudine results in gains in neuropsychologic performance in subjects suffering with ADC.[4] The difficulties experienced in completing this anti-retroviral study within the ACTG foreshadowed the subsequent difficulties in testing anti-retroviral therapy for dementia. With the introduction of didanosine (ddI) and zalcitabine (DDC), demands to rapidly deploy the drugs to the community, particularly those most severely affected, resulted in serious problems implementing trials. Generally, by the time neurologic trials were designed, the drug was so widely used that ADC patients would have tried the drugs before they could be invited to participate in a study. As a result, the ACTG neurology group has not accomplished subsequent directed studies deploying anti-retrovirals for ADC. With anticipated growing options for therapy in the future, information about the relative efficacy of various approaches for neurologic disease will be increasingly needed, and the ACTG will be asked to address that issue. In addition, because the blood-brain barrier is an unique challenge for neurologic therapeutics, the neurology group still must face the challenge of discovering appropriate dosing recommendations for neurologic complications.

An alternate approach to designing controlled trials of antivirals in patients with ADC is based on evaluating the impact of the drugs on neurologic performance prior to dementia. Since HIV enters the brain early in the infection, it is possible that it has less overt effects on the brain which could be monitored in studies of patients without dementia. While the importance of subtle, earlier changes in neuropsychologic performance may be argued, as individuals move from the clinically asymptomatic state to AIDS, there is a concomitant decline in neuropsychometric performance that can be monitored in clinical trials.[5,6] At the present time, the ACTG neurology group is performing "nested" neuropsychometric studies on comparative antiviral protocols to probe the questions about a relative difference in development of neuropsychologic deficits or dementia. We believe that this approach is a cost-efficient way to obtain important information about the neurologic efficacy of both single agents and combination therapy. It adds modest evaluations to already necessary clinical management of the anti-retroviral studies. Our challenge is to continue development of reliable easily tolerated, and economic quantitative measures of neurologic performance.

Implicit in the ideas that have shaped the work of the neurology group in the ACTG up to the present, is that our most important strategy is to obstruct the HIV virus in the brain.[7] While highly effective and specific antiviral therapy might indeed obviate the need for alternate approaches, this does not appear imminent. We are increasingly aware of the serious limitations of our current antiviral therapy, and realize that simple virus replication in the brain is an incomplete and flawed reflection of the impact of viral infection on the nervous system. One of the most important ideas driving future development of clinical trials is that unique pathophysiologic mechanisms may mediate the impact of HIV infection on the brain. Treatments addressing these pathophysiologic elements provide important opportunities to improve the function and outcome of our patients. For example, the importance of calcium-mediated neurotoxicity, of the excitotoxic mechanisms in developing neurologic injury, of the potential role of neurotoxic cytokines, the activity of arachidonic acid metabolites, and the role of nitric oxide in mediating neurologic injury in HIV infection all provide potential targets for therapeutic intervention.[8-11] The ACTG in the 1990s will be asked to determine the importance of some of these hypotheses by testing them in HIV patients suffering from neurologic disease.

The first such trial is in the final stages of treatment. Based on the work of Dr. Stuart Lipton, who demonstrated that in retinal ganglion and hippocampal cells, low levels of the HIV viral envelope glycoprotein, gp120, result in a calcium-mediated neurotoxicity which may be inhibited *in vitro* by calcium channel antagonists drugs, the ACTG has performed a Phase 1-2 study of nimodipine, a centrally active calcium channel antagonist. This study compares addition of one or two doses of nimodipine or placebo to anti-retroviral therapy in patients with ADC. Others are currently performing early studies of pentoxifylline based on its antagonism for tumor necrosis factor. These studies illustrate the eagerness with which the clinical community awaits therapeutic opportunities, and the sincere desire of patients and investigators to test hypotheses in the real world of clinical medicine.

The challenge of the coming years will be to make the wisest determination of potential studies to be undertaken. Because these protocols remain labor-intensive, and appropriate study participants are limited, drugs with the best chance of success must be chosen for study. Critical review of hypotheses and careful selection of agents for evaluation will be a pivotal challenge to the group over the coming years.

EXPANDING NEUROAIDS MISSION

While the initial focus of the neurologic effort within the ACTG has been on ADC, there is growing recognition of important additional topics requiring clinical trial evaluation. A partial list of commonly identified neurologic complications in HIV includes peripheral neuropathies, myopathy, myelopathy, toxoplasma encephalitis, cryptococcal meningitis, cytomegalovirus complications including neuropathy, radiculomyelopathy and encephalitis, JC virus infection presenting as progressive multifocal leukoencephalopathy, primary CNS lymphoma, and neurosyphilis. The coming months require choices deciding which areas require the attention of the neurologic group, and what will be the most fruitful studies. We must include the frequency and severity of the complications, the promise of therapeutic modalities, and the unique ability of this group to successfully perform studies in our decisions regarding which studies to undertake and how to design them. Other ACTG study groups have addressed some of the common and severe problems encountered, including treatment protocols for toxoplasma encephalitis, cryptococcal meningitis and neurosyphilis. Relative early success in these areas has made them less immediate targets for continued intensive investigation by the neurologic community.

PERIPHERAL NEUROPATHY IN AIDS

In contrast to ADC, peripheral neuropathy in HIV has been a sadly neglected area of study. It is well recognized that a distal sensory neuropathy develops in many HIV patients.[12,13] Its analysis is confounded by the frequent use of peripheral neurotoxic drugs such as ddI and DDC. Yet, after a decade of research on HIV, there have been no controlled treatment studies for neuropathy, and the impact of antiviral therapy on neuropathic disease is not well established. Only anecdotal experience is available to direct current treatment practice for this extended, disabling, and common aspect of HIV. Thus, the neurologic group believes that this entity is an important additional area for study. Currently in development is a study to compare amitriptyline, a tricyclic antidepressant compound useful in some other neuropathic pain syndromes, with mexilitene, an antiarrhythmic local anesthetic congener for painful neuropathy in AIDS. The study provides an important opportunity for the group to probe the issue of painful neuropathy in AIDS. It is hoped that this will be a foothold for study efforts that may address the degenerative or toxic process that underlines peripheral nerve damage in HIV. An area of particularly exciting progress in neuroscience deals with the role of neurotropic factors in health and disease. It seems possible that nerve growth factor, now becoming available through genetic engineering, may have a place in combatting neuropathic degeneration. The ACTG neurology group believes that the problem of HIV-associated neuropathy may be an important opportunity to test this approach and to enlarge the domain of therapeutics.

PROGRESSIVE MULTIFOCAL LEUKOENCEPHALOPATHY

Just as the space program provided a stimulus to many areas of progress in science and technology, the AIDS epidemic has generated both the mandate and the opportunity to study diseases that were previously virtually unapproachable. One example of such a situation is JC virus infection, the agent of progressive multifocal leukoencephalopathy (PML). While this condition was well recognized prior to the AIDS epidemic, the cases were so sporadic and infrequent, that it was virtually impossible to mount a controlled treatment study of it.[14] Consequently, after being recognized for 35 years, no therapeutic approach can be honestly recommended as beneficial in this rapidly fatal viral brain infection. PML is found in about 5% of AIDS patients at autopsy, and thus has become a commonly diagnosed problem, providing a new opportunity to design clinical studies of its treatment. After reviewing the anecdotal treatment experience, and informed by *in vitro* studies of viral drug susceptibility performed in Dr. Eugene Major's laboratory at the NINDS/NIH, the ACTG is seizing this opportunity to advance our knowledge about treatment of PML. Both anecdotal experience and *in vitro* studies support the idea that cytosine arabinoside is active against the JC virus. What cannot be judged is the balance of efficacy and toxicity of such a drug in the setting of AIDS. The clinical trial group is mounting the first controlled study of PML, attempting to define the impact of cytosine arabinoside therapy on this infection. It is recognized that an immunosuppressive approach may be harmful, even it it has a spectrum of therapeutic benefit, so the study is planned with a control arm utilizing only aggressive anti-retroviral therapy. Because the best mode of administration for cytosine arabinoside is unknown, there will be arms comparing intrathecal with systemic administration of this agent. The study is seen as an important first step in understanding how to combat this devastating disease. Clearly, less toxic and more efficacious drugs need to be developed. However, the opportunity we have to systematically study this disease should in the end benefit both HIV patients and other immunosuppressed groups subject to this infection.

PRIMARY CENTRAL NERVOUS SYSTEM LYMPHOMA

Primary CNS lymphoma is another rapidly fatal complication encountered in as many as 10% of AIDS patients. The ACTG oncology and neurology groups have developed alliances with National Cancer Institute-supported clinical study groups to perform a clinical trial utilizing chemotherapy followed by radiation for this disease. Here again we encounter the challenge of administering an immunosuppressive treatment to a host already suffering with a damaged immune system. However, systematic study of this problem promises to yield important information about the most efficacious means of dealing with this dilemma.

As can be seen, in the past several years the goals of research for the ACTG neurology group have broadened to include several major neurologic problems. It is very clear that the first studies must be considered stepping stones to more ingenious approaches to these tragic problems. We anticipate that expansion of our understanding of the biology of HIV infection in the nervous system will help us generate more rational and customized tools for the battle against HIV and its complications.

DEVELOPMENT OF THE NEUROLOGIC AIDS RESEARCH CONSORTIUM

As I have indicated, sufficiently promising ideas for therapy are the essential elements limiting our progress. However, we have much work that we can be doing at the present, yet have encountered substantial obstacles. These have revolved around the need to develop a sufficient cadre of interested and dedicated investigators, and to create a research network which is capable of linking them into a productive unit. HIV research and the ACTG derived early leadership from infectious disease specialists and oncologists. Funding for HIV research was concentrated in groups dominated by these medical specialities and interest and support for investigators in neurology has developed more slowly. Several important program project grants from National Institute of Neurological Diseases and Stroke (NINDS) provided support for a nucleus of investigators interested in the impact of HIV in the brain during the first decade of the epidemic. However, the cadre of committed scientists in the neurologic community did not expand very rapidly, and this constriction in development of interested and committed researchers has, in my opinion, generated some of the limitations we have both in concepts and the practical ability of the group to study relatively infrequent complications which demand a sizable multicenter group.

A promising development which addresses these issues is the recently formed collaboration between NIAID and NINDS. These agencies have actively supported and encouraged the development of the "Neurologic AIDS Research Consortium", which consists of a core of 16 centers with investigators committed to coordinated participation in neurologic HIV clinical studies. Through this mechanism, modest funding will flow to a much larger number of medical centers, providing incentive to address the neuroAIDS problems in each of the centers. A substantial number of young investigators will have some support and encouragement both in confronting the problems in neuroAIDS, and in participating in coordinated trials to address the conditions that can be studied in this population. Even before the funding for this group has been released, it is creating interest for additional participation from other university centers, and promises to provide a much needed stimulus. Balanced growth of support for this fledgling subspecialty neurologic field will require that these investigators be able to supplement their support by undertaking other collaborative projects as well as more basic projects. Given adequate support, the 1990s promise to be the decade in which the capability of investigation of HIV neurologic disease matures. As every sensitive person who has lived to this point in the epidemic will understand, the coming progress cannot be too soon. The task is too great, and the need too pressing. However, the wealth of ideas generated by research such as has been discussed here, along with developing support for translation of these concepts into clinical trials via coordinated efforts through several divisions of the NIH gives reason for optimism that much progress will be made during the coming years.

Acknowledgments

This work was supported in part by grant AI-25903 (NIAID) and P01-NS32228 (NINDS).

REFERENCES

1. B.A. Navia, B.D. Jordan and R.W. Price. The AIDS dementia complex. I. Clinical features. *Ann. Neurol.* 19:517 (1986).
2. B.A. Navia, E-S. Cho, C.K. Petito, et al. The AIDS dementia complex. II. Neuropathology. *Ann. Neurol.* 19:525 (1986).
3. F.A. Schmidt, J.W. Bigley, R. McKinnis, et al. Neuropsychological outcome of zidovudine (AZT) treatment of patients with AIDS and AIDS-related complex. *N.Engl. J. Med.* 319:1573 (1988).
4. J.J. Sidtis, C. Gatsonis, R.W. Price, et al. Zidovudine treatment of the AIDS dementia complex: Results of a placebo-controlled trial. *Ann. Neurol.* 33:343 (1993).
5. S.Tross, R.W. Price, B. Navia, et al. Neuropsychological characterization of the AIDS dementia complex: a preliminary report. *AIDS* 2:811 (1988).
6. N. Dunbar, M. Perdices, A. Grunseit, and D.A. Cooper. Changes in neuro-psychological performance of AIDS-related complex patients who progress to AIDS. *AIDS* 6:691 (1992).
7. D.C. Spencer, and R.W. Price. Human immunodeficiency virus and the central nervous system. *Annu. Rev. Microbiol.* 46:655 (1992).
8. E.B. Dreyer, P.K. Kaiser, J.T. Offermann, and S.A. Lipton. HIV-1 coat protein neurotoxicity prevented by calcium channel antagonists. *Science* 248:364 (1990).
9. S.A. Lipton, N.J. Sucher, P.K. Kaiser, and E.B. Dreyer. Synergistic effects of HIV coat protein and NMDA receptor-mediated neurotoxicity. *Neuron* 7:111 (1991).
10. S.L. Wesselingh, C. Power, J.D. Glass, et al. Intracerebral cytokine messenger RNA expression in acquired immunodeficiency syndrome dementia. *Ann. Neurol.* 33:576 (1993).
11. V.L. Dawson, T.M. Dawson, G.R. Uhl, and S.H. Synder. Human immunodeficiency virus type 1 coat protein neurotoxicity mediated by nitric oxide in primary cortical cultures. *Proc. Natl. Acad. Sci. U.S.A.* 90: 3256 (1993).
12. D.R. Cornblath, and J.C. McArthur. Predominantly sensory neuropathy in patients with AIDS and AIDS-related complex. *Neurology* 38:794 (1988).
13. C.D. Hall, C.R. Synder, J.A. Messenheimer, et al. Peripheral neuropathy in a cohort of human immunodeficiency virus-infected patients. *Arch. Neurol.* 48:1273 (1991).
14. E.O. Major, K. Amemiya, C.S. Tornatore, S.A. Houff, and J.R. Berger. Pathogenesis and molecular biology of progressive multifocal leukoencephalopathy: the JC virus-induced demyelinating disease of the human brain. *Clin. Microbiol. Rev.* 5:49 (1992).

TECHNICAL ADVANCES AND THE CHALLENGE OF HIV-RELATED NEUROLOGICAL DISEASES

Richard T. Johnson

The Johns Hopkins University School of Medicine
Department of Neurology
600 North Wolfe Street, Meyer 6-113
Baltimore, Maryland 21287

This chapter will briefly discuss three topics. First, some perspective may be gained from viewing past technical advances related to viral infections of the nervous system. Second, many questions concerning the pathogenesis of human immunodeficiency virus (HIV) infections of the nervous system remain unanswered, and concepts of neuroinvasiveness and neurovirulence confound these questions since they are strangely disconnected with the HIV infections. Third, the magnitude of the problem of AIDS and the human nervous system needs to be reemphasized.

TECHNICAL ADVANCES IN STUDIES OF VIRAL PATHOGENESIS

Prior to the 1920s, conclusions regarding pathogenesis were derived largely from observed clinical signs and pathological studies of the agonal end-stages of diseases. Critical examination of the incubation period began with the studies of Goodpasture and Teague in the 1920s; they sequentially examined tissues of experimental animals throughout the incubation period to determine the cellular progression of infection during the incubation period after varied routes of inoculation.[1,2] Their new insights did not depend, however, on the introduction of new methodology. They used standard histological methods, but in precise and creative ways, they extended established methods beyond previous boundaries.[3] They were also lucky, since their studies involved herpesviruses that left intranuclear inclusions as footprints of the infections.

Quantitation of virus in individual dissected tissues of experimental animals during the incubation period was introduced by Fenner[4] in studies of mice with ectromelia virus infection, but this method failed to identify which cells are infected. Therefore, virulent ectromelia strains that cause death by infection of hepatocytes are not readily distinguished from avirulent strains whose replication is contained within Kupffer cells.[5] Similarly, in other viral infections of experimental animals, virus increases in the brain may reflect an accelerating viremia or growth of virus limited to meningeal, ependymal, or endothelial cells.

Precise identification of infected cells became possible with the introduction of immunocytochemical methods. Fluorescent antibody staining was developed by Coons and his colleagues,[6] but the methodology seemed inadequate in studies of nervous system tissues. Their studies of mumps virus in monkeys showed precipitates that made sections of cerebral cortex not interpretable,[7] and their studies of canine distemper virus in dogs showed fluorescence of nuclei

Technical Advances in AIDS Research in the Human Nervous System
Edited by E.O. Major and J.A. Levy, Plenum Press, New York, 1995

363

in the brain that could not be abolished by absorption of antibody with brain powders.[8] Ultimately, this perceived limitation in studies of neural tissues was overcome with better optics, better antibodies, and counterstains to quench auto-fluorescence. Enzyme immunocytochemistry, immune electron microscopy, *in situ* hybridization and *in situ* polymerase chain reaction (PCR) methodologies have followed; each has posed problems in adaptation to studies of neural tissues resulting in some false positive reports, but these technical problems are also being overcome.

THE PATHOGENESIS OF HIV-ASSOCIATED NEUROLOGICAL DISEASES

A number of questions related to the pathogenesis of HIV-associated neurological diseases remain unanswered, and are as follow:

- How does virus invade the nervous system?
- Are there specific neurotropic and/or neurovirulent strains of virus?
- Is viral burden related to neurological disease and its progression?
- Are only cells of macrophage lineage infected in the nervous system?
- What mediates disease: viral proteins, cytokines, or neurotoxins?
- Do different syndromes have different mechanisms of pathogenesis?
- What is the role of opportunistic infections?
- When and how do antiviral agents modify the course of these diseases?

These questions are compounded by the ambiguous neurotropism and neurovirulence of HIV. Several terms need definition:

Neurotropism:	ability to infect neural cells
Neuronotropism:	ability to infect neurons (as distinct from other nervous system cells)
Neuroinvasiveness:	ability to enter the nervous system
Neurovirulence:	ability to cause neurologic disease

Some neurotropic viruses frequently invade the nervous system yet seldom cause serious disease; for example, mumps frequently invades the nervous system as shown by cerebrospinal fluid changes in most patients with uncomplicated mumps virus infections, yet serious meningitis and encephalitis are rare. Thus, this virus is highly neuroinvasive but shows very limited neurovirulence. In contrast, herpes simplex virus, type 1, is ubiquitous but only rarely infects the nervous system; when this herpesvirus does cause clinical encephalitis, the outcome is fatal in about 70% of untreated patients. This virus shows limited neuroinvasiveness but intense neurovirulence.[9] HIV poses an unique neurotropism. In early infection, there is evidence of high neuroinvasiveness but low neurovirulence; yet with the onset of AIDS there is great neurovirulence and neuronal loss despite the lack of neuronotropism. Whether host or virus changes lead to this shift is unknown. Does host immunodeficiency or evolution of neurovirulent strains of virus affect this change? Does increased virus load or simply longevity of infection lead to the encephalopathy, myelopathy and neuropathies that complicate AIDS?

MAGNITUDE OF THE PROBLEM OF HUMAN NERVOUS SYSTEM DISEASE

Recently a member of the third estate asked what our AIDS laboratories at Johns Hopkins planned to do now that AIDS was a declining problem. This false conception that AIDS is declining may come from several sources: first, the Centers for Disease Control have decreased the estimate of HIV-infected Americans from 1.5 million to 1 million, but this does not represent a loss of infection by one-half million people but by a reassessment of data; the <u>rate</u> of increase in

AIDS cases in the United States has slowed, but the number infected has continued to increase, particularly among intravenous drug users, their sex partners, and their progeny.

Worldwide, over 13 million persons are now infected. In Africa, the burden is overwhelming, with one-half the hospital beds in some areas being occupied with AIDS patients, and with more than one million AIDS orphans. In South and Southeast Asia, seroconversion is being seen at an unprecedented rate, and in the future, AIDS cases in Asia will outnumber those in Africa.[10] Of the 13 million now infected, 8-10 million now have CNS infections with HIV and over the next decade, 20-30% will develop dementia, a similar percentage will develop myelopathy, and 30-50% will develop painful peripheral neuropathies. By the turn of the century, between 20 and 30 million individuals will be infected, and the neurological complications of HIV infections will rank among the world's most common neurological diseases. On a national scale, with an estimated one million infected, an annual incidence of 40,000 cases of HIV dementia alone are anticipated in the United States, approximately five times the annual incidence of multiple sclerosis. HIV will soon become the leading cause of cognitive impairment in young adults.[11]

REFERENCES

1. E.W. Goodpasture. Experimental production of herpetic lesions in organs and tissues of the rabbit. *J. Med. Res.* 44:121 (1925).
2. E.W. Goodpasture, and O. Teague. Transmission of the virus of herpes febrilis among nerves in experimentally infected rabbits. *J. Med. Res.* 44:139 (1925).
3. R.T. Johnson. Herpetic infection, with especial reference to involvement of the nervous system: an appraisal. *Medicine* 72:133 (1993).
4. F. Fenner. Mouse-pox (infectious ectromelia of mice): a review. *J. Immunol.* 63:341 (1949).
5. C.A. Mims. Aspects of the pathogenesis of virus diseases. *Bacteriol. Rev.* 28:30 (1964).
6. A.H. Coons, H.J. Creech, R.N. Joens, and E. Berliner. The demonstration of pneumococcal antigens in tissues by the use of fluorescent antibody. *J. Immunol.* 45:159 (1942).
7. T-H. Chu, F.S. Cheever, A.H. Coons, and J.B. Daniels. Distribution of mumps virus in experimentally infected monkeys. *Proc.Roy. Soc. Exp. Biol. Med.* 76:571 (1951).
8. D.L. Coffin, A.H. Coons, and V.J. Cabasso. A histological study of infectious canine hepatitis by means of fluorescent antibody. *J. Exp. Med.* 98:13 (1953).
9. R.T. Johnson. "Viral Infections of the Nervous System," Raven Press, New York (1982).
10. M.H. Merson. Slowing the spread of HIV: agenda for the 1990s. *Science* 260:1266 (1993).
11. M.J.G. Harrison, and J.C. McArthur. "The Neurology of AIDS," Churchill Livingstone, Edinburgh (1994).

CONTRIBUTORS

Omar Bagasra, M.D., Ph.D.
Division of Infectious Diseases
Thomas Jefferson University
1020 Locust Street, 320 JAH
Philadelphia, Pennsylvania 19107

Dale Benos, Ph.D.
Departments of Physiology and Biophysics
University of Alabama at Birmingham
BHSB 706-UAB Station
Birmingham, Alabama 35294

Joseph Berger, M.D.
Department of Neurology
University of Kentucky
Annex 4, Chambers Building
Room 225E
Lexington, Kentucky 40536

Ruth Brack-Werner, Ph.D.
Institute of Molecular Virology
GSF-Forschungszentrum für Umwelt und Gesundheit
D-85758 Obschleißen
Neuherberg, Germany

Francesca Chiodi, Ph.D.
Department of Virology
Karolinska Institute
Lundagatan 2
S-10521 Stockholm, Sweden

Janice Clements, Ph.D.
Johns Hopkins University School of Medicine
Traylor G-60
720 Rutland Avenue
Baltimore, Maryland 21205

David Clifford, M.D.
Washington University School of Medicine
Box 8111 Neurology
660 South Euclid Avenue
St. Louis, Missouri 63110

Valina Dawson, Ph.D.
Department of Neurology
Johns Hopkins University School of Medicine
Baltimore, Maryland 21237

Monique Dubois-Dalcq, M.D.
Unite de Neurovirologie et Regeneration au System Nerveux
Department de Virologie, Batiment Darre
Institut Pasteur
28 Rue Du Dr. Roux
75724 Paris, Cedex 15, France

Leon Epstein, M.D.
Department of Neurology
University of Rochester Medical Center
601 Elmwood Avenue
Rochester, New York 14642

Volker Erfle, Ph.D.
Institute for Molecular Virology
GSF-Forschungszentrum für Umwelt und Gesundheit GMbH
8042 Neuherberg, Germany

Harris Gelbard, M.D., Ph.D.
University of Rochester Medical Center
601 Elmwood Avenue, Box 631
Rochester, New York 14642

Howard Gendelman, M.D.
Departments of Medicine, Pathology, and Microbiology
Chief, Laboratory of Viral Pathogenesis
University of Nebraska Medical Center
600 South 42nd Street
Omaha, Nebraska 68198

Francisco Gonzalez-Scarano, M.D.
Department of Neurology
University of Pennsylvania
Clinical Research Building
422 Curie Boulevard
Philadelphia, Pennsylvania 19104

John Griffin, M.D.
Department of Neurology and Neuroscience
The Johns Hopkins Hospital
Meyer Building, Room 6-109
600 North Wolfe Street
Baltimore, Maryland 21205

Ashley Haase, M.D.
Department of Microbiology
University of Minnesota Medical School
Box 196 UMHC
420 Delaware Street, S.E.
Minneapolis, Minnesota 55455

Melvyn Heyes, Ph.D.
Laboratory of Clinical Sciences
National Institute of Mental Health
National Institutes of Health
Bethesda, Maryland 20892

Kamel Khalili, Ph.D.
Molecular Neurovirology Section
Thomas Jefferson University
233 South Tenth Street
Philadelphia, Pennsylvania 19107

Peter Lantos, M.D., Ph.D., D.Sc., FRCPath
Department of Neuropathology
Institute of Psychiatry
De Crespigny Park, Denmark Hill
London SE5 8AF, United Kingdom

Jay Levy, M.D.
University of California, San Francisco
Cancer Research Institute
Box 0128, Room S-1280
San Francisco, California 94143

Eugene Major, Ph.D.
National Institute of Neurological Disorders and Stroke
National Institutes of Health
Bethesda, Maryland 20892

Ashlee Moses, Ph.D.
Microbiology/Immunology-L220
Oregon Health Sciences University
3181 S.W. Sam Jackson Park Road
Portland, Oregon 97201

Avindra Nath, M.D.
University of Manitoba
523-730 William Avenue
Winnipeg, Manitoba R3E OW3, Canada

Jay Nelson, Ph.D.
Microbiology/Immunology-L220
Oregon Health Sciences University
3181 S.W. Sam Jackson Park Road
Portland, Oregon 97201

Gerard Nuovo, M.D.
Department of Pathology
SUNY at Stony Brook
Stony Brook, New York 11794

John Oprandy, Ph.D.
IGEN, Inc.
1530 East Jefferson Street
Rockville, Maryland 20852

Roger Pomerantz, M.D.
Director, Division of Infection Diseases
Thomas Jefferson University
1020 Locust Street, 320 JAH
Philadelphia, Pennsylvania 19107

Lynn Pulliam, Ph,.D.
University of California, San Francisco
Veterans Affairs Medical Center
4101 Clement Street (113A)
San Francisco, California 94121

Peter Schmid, M.D.
UCLA, Reed Neurology
Veterans Administration Medical Center
Building 212
Wilshire and Sawtelle Boulevards
Los, Angeles, California 90073

Manfred Schubert, Ph.,D.
National Institute of Neurological Disorders and Stroke
National Institutes of Health
Bethesda, Maryland 20892

Susan Wilt, Ph.D.
Unite de Neurovirologie et Regeneration au System Nerveux
Department de Virologie, Batiment Darre
Institut Pasteur
28 Rue Du Dr. Roux
75724 Paris, Cedex 15, France

INDEX

ACTG, *see* AIDS Clinical Trial Group
ADC, *see* AIDS dementia complex
Adhesion molecules, 206, 215
AIDS Clinical Trial Group, 355-360
AIDS dementia complex, 5, 11-13, 107,
      135, 152, 156, 160, 161, 169, 205,
      217, 223-226, 251, 252, 258, 357-
      359, 365
AIDS-related complex, 205
Antivirals, 17, 41, 42, 327-331, 334-337, 345
Arachidonic acid, 57, 58, 62, 65, 74, 75, 80,
      81, 83, 169, 220, 229
ARC, *see* AIDS-related complex
Astrocytes
  and HIV infection, 33-36, 57, 58, 61-64, 69,
      74-80, 84, 85, 89-97, 100, 117-121,
      125, 130, 152, 153, 163, 167, 169,
      190, 207, 209, 217, 223-230, 237,
      238, 245, 269, 275, 276, 317, 319-
      321
Astrocytoma
  cell lines, 62, 63, 125, 126, 190, 200, 321
AZT, 5, 7, 13, 16, 17, 31, 152, 180-183,
      357

Blood-brain barrier, 14, 16, 17, 35, 36, 58, 73,
      84, 117, 118, 178, 205, 206, 209,
      215, 217, 218, 224, 301, 320, 332
Brain
  aggregates culture, 57, 105-115, 130
  and HIV infection, 4-17, 27-36, 48, 58, 61-
      63, 73-76, 79, 80, 83-85, 117, 118,
      120, 121, 125, 130, 135, 139, 143,
      145, 146, 163-169, 177-184, 189-
      202, 205-207, 213-215, 217, 223,
      224, 226, 229, 230, 237-240, 246,
      251, 258, 259, 288, 291, 301, 305,
      312, 313, 317, 319-321, 328, 329,
      356-360, 363, 364
  in fetal cell culture, 89-101, 237
Cell surface markers
  CD4, 8, 17, 42, 45, 90, 95, 100, 119-121, 135,
      137, 153, 178, 179, 184, 190, 201,
      207, 209, 211, 214, 217, 235-246,
      252-255, 257, 267-269, 271-273,
      275, 305, 306, 308-313, 331-337,
      339-343, 345
  CD8, 8, 13, 17, 90, 95, 223, 224, 252,
      253
Cerebrospinal fluid, 4, 8, 13-16, 118, 153,

Cerebrospinal fluid (*cont'd*)
      156, 177, 178, 180-184, 189-
      193, 195-201, 214, 215, 301, 302,
      305, 306, 308-313, 317, 319
CG4 cells, 156-160
Children
  HIV encephalopathy, 13, 61
CMV, *see* Cytomegalovirus
CSF, *see* Cerebrospinal fluid
Cytokines, 13, 17, 20, 32-36, 45-47, 58, 61-63,
      74-76, 80, 81, 84, 85, 97, 100, 128,
      130 135, 136, 143, 206, 215, 216,
      224-227, 229, 230, 317, 320, 321
Cytomegalovirus , 41, 45, 135

Defective interfering particles (DI), 328-332,
      334-337, 340-345
Defective viruses, 327, 328, 330, 331, 344
Demyelination
  and HIV infection, 152, 156
Dopamine receptors, 61, 64, 68-69

ECL, *see* Electrochemiluminescence
Electrochemiluminescence, 281-287,
      292, 294-296
Encephalitis
  and HIV, 27-29, 73-77, 80-83, 135, 229
Encephalopathy
  and HIV, 5-17, 32, 61, 62, 69, 117, 121, 135,
      143, 145, 364
Endothelium, 125, 130, 206, 207, 213, 217
Excitatory amino acids, 65-69

Gag
  gene, 194, 281, 284-287, 296
  protein, 154, 336, 340, 341
GalCer, *see* Galactosylceramide
Galactosylceramide, 214, 237-246
Gene therapy, 329-331, 335, 336
GFAP, *see* Glial fibrillary acidic protein
Glial cells, 33, 35, 36, 64, 65, 74, 76, 77, 80,
      84, 94, 97-99, 109, 117, 130, 135,
      137-146, 152, 153, 156, 190, 193,
      202, 224, 229, 230, 238, 239, 245,
      252, 253, 269
Glial fibrillary acidic protein , 33, 63, 90-92,
      106, 107, 111-113, 125, 207, 209,
      237, 238, 269, 276
Glioma cell lines, 125-130, 135
Gliosis, 223, 224

Glutamate, 61, 63, 69, 163-169, 224-227, 229, 230
gp120
  and astrocytes, 120-121, 245
  GalCer, 240-244, 246
  HBCE cells, 214
  and HIV infectivity, 81, 84, 235, 239
  and neurotoxicity, 17, 58, 32, 33, 35, 62, 69, 109-113, 130, 163, 166-169, 179, 180, 205, 217, 225-227, 229, 230, 251, 277, 317, 358
HBCE, see Human brain capillary endothelium
Human brain capillary endothelium, 206-217
Immunofluorescence
  and astrocytes, 92
Interferons
  interferon-α, 75, 76
  interferon-γ, 13, 85, 94, 215, 224, 226-229, 319-321
Interleukins
  interleukin-1, 30, 32, 35, 76, 81, 84, 85
  interleukin-1β, 13, 34, 58, 61, 62, 65, 75, 76, 80, 81, 84, 97, 100
  interleukin-6, 13, 85, 252
  interleukin-10, 74, 79, 80, 84

JCV, see JC virus
JC virus (JCV), 89, 96, 97, 135, 143, 145, 146, 281, 284, 288-296, 358, 359

Kainate, 165
Kynurenine, 317-322

Lentiviruses, 89, 189, 211, 212, 334
Leucoencephalopathy, 27-29, 32-34
Long-term repeats (LTR)
  and HIV-1, 91, 96-98, 100, 135-143, 144, 146, 184, 190, 192
Lymphocytes
  and HIV infection, 118-121, 128, 235, 238, 252-255, 257, 267-271
  and meningitis, 30
Lymphoma
  and AIDS, 27, 317, 360

Macrophages
  and cytokines, 48
  and HIV encephalitis, 28-30, 32, 34-36
  HIV-1 infection, 57, 58, 61, 62, 69, 73-76, 80, 81, 83-85, 108-110, 113, 114, 118, 121, 125, 127, 135, 152, 163, 169, 177-179, 182, 184, 189, 200-202, 205, 206, 214-217, 223-226, 229, 237-239, 246, 253, 257, 267-269, 271, 273, 276, 277, 317, 319-321, 239-221, 335
Magnetic resonance imaging (MRI), 14, 15
  and nitric oxide, 164-165, 167

Magnetic resonance imaging (cont'd)
  and peripheral neuropathy, 45
Major histocompatibility complex (MHC)
  and cell surface antigens, 45, 90, 94, 224
Microglial cells
  and AIDS dementia, 107
  brain, 45, 117-119, 125, 151
  in brain aggregates, 106
  and cytokines, 34
  and HIV-1 encephalitis, 28
  and HIV-1 infection, 33, 57, 58, 61, 62, 73, 75, 83, 108, 151-161, 163, 202, 215, 217, 236-239, 246, 251, 252, 258, 269, 275, 276, 313, 329
  and macrophages, 34-35, 118, 119, 165, 167, 169, 177, 178, 180, 184, 223-226, 229, 235, 317, 320, 321
Monocytes
  and HIV encephalitis, 73-85
  and HIV-1 infection, 34, 57, 58, 61-63, 108, 109, 130, 143
  neurotoxicity, 64
MRI, see Magnetic resonance imaging
Myelin, 14, 29, 30, 32-35, 41, 42, 46-48, 62, 74, 76, 83, 84, 89, 90, 97, 117, 118, 145, 152, 156, 161, 321

Na+/H+ antiport, 224, 226, 227
NADPH diaphorase, 174
NMDA, see N-methyl D-aspartic acid
Nef, 33, 62, 127, 131, 189-202, 252
Neuroblastoma cells, 63, 68, 105, 120, 125
Neurotoxicity
  and brain aggregates, 107, 113
  and cytokines, 58, 61-69
  and excitatory amino acids, 65-69
  gp120, 109
  and HIV-1 virus, 62-67, 151-161, 225, 226, 229
  and nitric oxide, 163-167, 169
Neurotoxins, 61, 68, 69, 105, 108, 109, 113
Neurotropism
  and HIV, 177-179, 184, 189, 190, 364
NF-kB transcription factor, 58, 91, 97, 98, 100, 136, 138-140, 146, 153, 160
Nitric oxide, 34, 156, 163-167, 169, 229, 251
Nitric oxide synthase, 164-167, 169
N-methyl-D-aspartic acid (NMDA) receptors, 34, 35, 57, 58, 61, 62, 65, 69, 84, 108-110, 113, 163, 165-167, 169, 226, 227, 229, 230, 317

Oligodendrocytes, 32, 36, 75, 84, 89, 90, 92, 97, 106, 107, 117, 118, 130, 131, 135, 151-153, 156, 158-160, 207, 217

PAF, see Platelet-activating factor
PBMC. see Peripheral blood mononuclear cells

PCR, *see* Polymerase chain reaction
Peripheral blood mononuclear cells, 74, 75, 125, 177, 180, 183, 190-194, 200, 253-255, 257, 271, 359
Peripheral nervous system
and HIV infection, 3, 11, 12, 27, 41-48, 359
Platelet-activating factor, 61-63, 65, 69, 74, 75, 80-84
Pleocytosis, 4, 13, 14
PML, *see* Progressive multifocal leuko-encephalopathy
Pol region
and HIV infection, 180, 340
Polymerase chain reaction , 27, 28, 33, 45, 47, 48, 57, 118, 125, 127-129, 139, 152, 180, 181, 191-195, 197, 200, 235, 252-261, 267-278, 281, 284, 288-296, 301-306, 308, 309, 311-313, 328, 364
Progressive multifocal leukoencephalopathy, 28, 89, 145, 288, 291-294, 317, 359
Psychiatric disorders
and HIV encephalopathy, 12, 13

Quinolinic acid, 14, 35, 36, 229, 317, 319-322
Quisqualic acid, 165, 166, 168, 169

Retroviruses, 177, 207, 251, 254, 275, 327-330, 333-335
Reverse transcriptase
and HIV-1, 45, 48, 74, 100, 127, 129, 177, 180-182, 200, 267, 268
Ribozymes, 336-342, 345
Rubpy, 281-283, 285-287, 289, 292, 294, 295

Simian immunodeficiency virus, 205, 206, 319, 344
SIV, *see* Simian immunodeficiency virus

Skeletal muscle
and HIV infection, 27, 42, 267, 268, 273-275
Syncytia
in HIV-1 infection, 127, 128, 151, 154, 155, 179, 209, 211, 342

TAR, *see* Transactivating responsive element
Tat protein, 135-139, 142-146
T cells, 125, 130, 135, 139, 140, 206, 207, 214, 215, 224
TGF-β, *see* Transforming growth factor-beta
TNF-α, *see* Tumor necrosis factor-alpha
Transactivating responsive element, 137-139, 142, 143, 145, 146
Transforming growth factor-beta
74, 79, 80, 84, 143, 152
Tumor necrosis factor-alpha
and HIV-1 infection, 13, 17, 29, 30, 32, 34, 35, 45, 48, 58, 61-69, 75-77, 80-84,
Tumor necrosis factor-alpha (*cont'd*)
91, 97, 98, 100, 109, 151-161, 251, 273, 275

U87-MG cells, 137-142, 144
U251-MG cells, 74
U373 cells, 237, 239, 252
U937 cells, 84, 200, 201
Uterine cervix
and HIV infection, 267, 268, 271, 277

Variable region 3 (V3), 177, 179-183, 214, 217, 241-243
Vasculitis, 30
Vesicular stomatitis virus (VSV), 333, 334, 336
VSV, *see* Vesicular stomatitis virus

Zidovudine, *see* AZT